Immunology and Pathogenesis of Trypanosomiasis

Editor

Ian Tizard

Department of Veterinary Microbiology and Parasitology
Texas A&M University and Texas
Agricultural Experiment Station
College Station, Texas

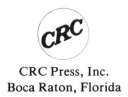

CRC Press, Inc.
Boca Raton, Florida

Library of Congress Cataloging in Publication Data
Main entry under title:

Immunology and pathogenesis of trypanosomiasis.

Bibliography: p.
Includes index.
1. Trypanosomiasis. 2. Trypanosomiasis — Immunological
aspects. I. Tizard, Ian R. [DNLM: 1. Trypanosomiasis —
Immunology. 2. Trypanosomiasis — Etiology. WC 705 I33]
RC186.T82I44   1985   616.9'363   83-26284
ISBN 0-8493-5640-7

Direct all inquiries to CRC Press, Inc., 2000 Corporate Blvd., N.W., Boca Raton, Florida, 33431.

© 1985 by CRC Press, Inc.

International Standard Book Number 0-8493-5640-7
Library of Congress Card Number 83-26284
Printed in the United States

PREFACE

Interest in the Trypanosomiases has increased exponentially over the past 20 years. This renaissance has been fuelled by a new awareness of the significance of the diseases caused by this group of protozoa and by an optimism brought about by the dramatic advances in medical science since 1945.

Recent investigations have centered upon two distinct aspects of the Trypanosomiases. One set of investigators have directed their efforts towards the elucidation of the mechanisms of antigenic variation. As a result we have uncovered a complex and sophisticated set of biochemical and genetic interactions that has provided us with a new insight into the control mechanisms of protein synthesis. Unfortunately, these results have also proved highly discouraging in that they have emphasized the apparently insurmountable difficulties in controlling trypanosomes by means of vaccination. It is becoming increasingly apparent that this route of investigation may not lead to a solution to the trypanosome problem.

The second major route of investigation encompasses the topics discussed in this book, namely the immunopathology and pathophysiology of these diseases. The immunopathological studies have largely centered upon the profound immunosuppression associated with salivarian trypanosome infections in man and domestic animals and on the immunologically mediated lesions associated with disease.

Pathological studies on African trypanosomiasis have evolved from simple morphological descriptions of the lesions observed to a study of the complex pathophysiological changes taking place in infected hosts. Over the past few years this approach has tended to concentrate upon the biological activities of "factors" derived from trypanosomes and there has been a resurgence in the old concept of trypanosome "toxins" although they are clearly much more complex than were once suspected.

The publication of this text is timely since both the immunopathological and the pathophysiological approaches have begun to yield exciting and significant results. This record of the "state of the art" should serve as a benchmark for future investigations into this area and for the development of new, exciting, and innovative therapeutic and preventative approaches to the control of these important diseases.

THE EDITOR

Ian Tizard is Professor and Head of the Department of Veterinary Microbiology and Parasitology, College of Veterinary Medicine, Texas A&M University, College Station, Texas.

Dr. Tizard received his B.V.M.S. degree from the University of Edinburgh in 1965; a B.Sc. in pathology from the same university in 1966 and his Ph.D. from Cambridge University in 1969. He was a post-doctoral fellow in the Department of Veterinary Microbiology and Immunology at the University of Guelph. Canada from 1969 until 1972. After a brief stay in Edinburgh, he joined the faculty at the University of Guelph eventually becoming a Professor in the Department of Veterinary Microbiology and Immunology.

Dr. Tizard's research interests center around the immunology and diagnosis of protozoan diseases, especially Trypanosomiasis and Toxoplasmosis. His research has been supported by the Medical Research Council of Canada, the Natural Science and Engineering Research Council, the Ontario Ministry of Health, the Multiple Sclerosis Society of Canada, and the International Development and Research Center. He has published many research papers and two immunology textbooks and made many presentations at national and international meetings.

Dr. Tizard is a member of the British Society for Immunology, the American Association of Immunologists, the Royal College of Veterinary Surgeons, and is currently president of the American Association of Veterinary Immunologists.

CONTRIBUTORS

Alberto M. Acosta
Department of Pathology
Cornell University Medical College
New York, New York

George W. O. Akol
Research Fellow
Department of Pathology
ILRAD
Nairobi, Kenya

Brigette A. Askonas
Head, Division of Immunology
National Institute for Medical Research
London, England

Greg J. Bancroft
Visiting Worker
Division of Immunology
National Institute for Medical Research
London, England

Peter F. L. Boreham
Senior Parasitologist
Queensland Institute of Medical Research
Queensland, Australia

Markley H. Boyer
Associate Professor
Department of Tropical Public Health
Harvard School of Public Health
Boston, Massachusetts

Christine A. Facer
Lecturer in Hematology
Department of Hematology
The London Hospital Medical College
London, England

James E. Hall
Assistant Professor
Department of Parasitology and
  Laboratory Practice
School of Public Health
University of North Carolina at Chapel
  Hill
Chapel Hill, North Carolina

Rodney Hoff
Assistant Professor
Department of Tropical Public Health
Harvard School of Public Health
Boston, Massachusetts

George C. Jenkins
Professor, Director, and Head
Department of Hematology
The London Hospital Medical College
London, England

Alan Mellors
Professor
Department of Chemistry
University of Guelph
Guelph, Canada

W. Ivan Morrison
Scientist
ILRAD
Nairobi, Kenya

Max Murray
Scientist
ILRAD
Nairobi, Kenya

Klaus H. Nielsen
Associate Professor
Department of Veterinary Pathology
College of Veterinary Medicine
Texas A&M University
College Station, Texas

Charles A. Santos-Buch
Professor of Pathology
Cornell University Medical College
Attending Pathologist
The New York Hospital
Director
Papanicolauo Cytology Laboratory
The New York Hospital
New York, New York

John R. Seed
Professor and Chairman
Department of Parasitology and
  Laboratory Practice
School of Public Health
University of North Carolina at Chapel
  Hill
Chapel Hill, North Carolina

Pierre Viens
Professor
Faculty of Medicine
Department of Microbiology and
  Immunology
University of Montreal
Montreal, Canada

TABLE OF CONTENTS

Chapter 1

PATHOPHYSIOLOGY OF AFRICAN TRYPANOSOMIASIS

John R. Seed and James E. Hall

TABLE OF CONTENTS

I. INTRODUCTION

Animals infected with African trypanosomes have been shown by a number of investigators to differ physiologically from their uninfected counterparts. These differences have included differences in serum amino acid levels of experimental animals,[35] changes in excretion of various urinary catabolites,[19,44,48,49] as well as possible changes in endocrine function.[21,22,61] In addition, there are apparent gross anatomical changes, as well as behavioral changes which would suggest physiological alterations.[43,45] Based upon these studies, it has been suggested that at least a portion of the pathology observed during African trypanosomiasis is due to physiological disturbances.[44,48] However, it is important to note that there are also considerable data available to support the conclusion that pathology is the result of hyper-sensitivity reactions. It has been well documented that immunological antigen-antibody deposits can be found in the kidneys of infected animals.[24] Presumably, these deposits are responsible for the glomerulonephritis which is commonly observed in experimental African trypanosomiasis.[24] They also suggest that similar Arthus-type reactions occur in other organs and are responsible for a variety of clinical symptoms. It has been well documented in experimental animals as well as in man, that the vasoactive agent bradykinin is also increased during a trypanosome infection[5,13] (see Chapter 3). The increase in this agent has been positively correlated with parasite relapses and antigen-antibody reactions.[5,13] The antigen-antibody activated sequence of reactions which leads to the release of kinins has been suggested to be responsible for pathological changes such as increased vascular permeability, edema, and changes in blood coagulation.[5,13-15] Although we do not deny the possible importance of immunopathology, this review will concentrate on the physiological changes observed during African trypanosomiasis and focus on those physiological factors believed to be important in pathogenesis. In addition, although possibly obvious, it should be noted that all pathology suggested to be due to immunological mechanisms has an underlying biochemical or physiological basis. For example, antigen-antibody deposits (with or without complement) in various organs lead to pathology as the result of enzymatic reactions on cellular membranes. It is obvious, therefore, that, ultimately, immunopathology will be described in biochemical and molecular terms. It is our opinion that in the future there should be increased emphasis on the physiological basis of immunological as well as possible direct physiological factors involved in inflammation. A complete understanding of the mechanism should lead to considerable improvement in patient management through dietary supplements or deletions, anti-inflammatory agents, specific enzyme inhibitors, etc. (see Chapter 3).

II. PHYSIOLOGICAL CHANGES: PARASITE INDUCED

A. Macromolecular Products

The idea that trypanosomes produce toxins similar to those produced by bacterial pathogens has been tested by numerous authors.[7,27,41,42] Although an interesting hypothesis, the evidence for such toxins has, until fairly recently, been limited. For an early review of this topic, the reader is referred to Von Brand[61] and Tizard et al.[56] More recently, there are several papers that suggest that the trypanosomes could contain toxic macromolecules. It has been shown that soluble extracts of *Trypanosoma brucei gambiense* are capable of increasing vascular permeability when injected intradermally.[42] It has been suggested that the trypanosomes at relapse release a pyrogenic substance.[47] However, Slotz and van Miert[52] failed to demonstrate a pyrogenic factor in extracts of *T. b. brucei* when soluble extracts were injected into *Escherichia coli* endotoxin-tolerant rabbits. There is also a recent paper by Sanchez et al.[41] reporting that *T. b. brucei* contains a hormone-like substance capable of mobilizing host liver glycogen. Finally, there are several papers which report that trypanosomes contain a mitogenic factor.[11,17,27] These reports are all consistent with the hypothesis that the trypanosomes contain macromolecules that are potentially toxic to the host. More recently, Tizard and associates[11,57] have suggested that the trypanosomes, upon lysis (and relapse), release the enzymes phospholipase A1 and lysophospholipase A1. These workers hypothesized that these enzymes hydrolize phospholipids with the eventual formation of fatty acids that have toxic biological properties.[56,57] Phospholipase Al hydrolyzes phosphatidyl choline which releases free fatty acid plus lysophosphatidylcholine. The lysophosphatidylcholine is further catalyzed by lysophospholipase Al to glyceryl phosphoryl choline with the release of the second fatty acid. Free fatty acids are known to be hypoglycemic, mitogenic, and cytotoxic, which could ultimately produce anemia, disseminated intravascular coagulation, and immunosuppression.

In addition to the possible role of phospholipases in pathogenesis, proteolytic activity has also been demonstrated in trypanosome extracts.[53] Since proteolytic activity can potentially be toxic, it is conceivable that proteases could be involved in the pathology. Similarly, it is possible that other hydrolases could also contribute to the inflammation observed in various tissues. For example, Murray[33] discusses the detection of some proteins from the African trypanosomes with hemolytic activity. It is assumed that these enzymes would be released during the destruction of the trypanosomes at relapse. In addition, the enzymes could also be released (excreted or leaked) from the trypanosome, possibly from the flagellar pocket.[60]

It is apparent that there are a number of macromolecules with biological or enzymic activity that have been demonstrated in extracts of the African trypanosomes. It has been suggested that these macromolecules have either direct toxic activity, or indirectly produce pathology through the release of enzymic by-products. Although these activities have been demonstrated in trypanosome extracts, and, in the case of phospholipase, increases in serum levels observed, there is still no definitive evidence that they are responsible either alone or in combination for pathogenesis. For example, to our knowledge, pathology has not been inhibited by either specific enzyme inhibitors or by the use of specific neutralizing antiserum; nor, in most cases, have changes in activity in body tissues been correlated with specific pathological changes, or with parasitemia levels. Therefore, further work is obviously required before one can state that one or more of these trypanosome factors are involved in the induction of pathology.

B. Small Molecular Weight Products

It has been demonstrated that the members of the family Trypanosomatidae, including the African trypanosomes, are capable of metabolizing the aromatic amino acids to a series of potentially toxic compounds. Tryptophan is catabolized to indole-pyruvate, indole-lactate, indole-acetate, and indole-ethanol (tryptophol). Tyrosine is metabolized to p-hydroxyphenylpyruvate and p-hydroxyphenyllactate and phenylalanine is catabolized to phenylpyruvate. Several of these compounds have been shown to have toxic properties when injected in pharmacological doses. For example, indole-ethanol has been found to induce a sleep-like state,[46] to alter body temperature,[46] and even to be immunosuppressive.[41] It has been suggested that many of these properties are presumably due to the effects of indole-ethanol on the host cell membrane.[50] Indole-ethanol has been shown to alter membrane properties leading to osmotic fragility and lysis.[50] It is also known to rapidly cross the blood-brain barrier[7] and to alter brain metabolism.[8] Finally, it has been shown that these compounds are produced in vivo (reviewed by Tizard et al.[56]) and dramatic increases in most of them have been observed in the urine of infected animals. The only trypanosome catabolite not found in the urine is indole-ethanol, however, this would be expected since indole-ethanol has been shown to be very rapidly metabolized by the host to indole acetic acid which is excreted in elevated concentrations. More recent work has demonstrated that the major aromatic by-products excreted into the urine of infected animals are phenylpyruvate, hydroxyphenylpyruvate, and indole pyruvate.[19] In chronically infected *Microtus montanus*, the concentration of phenylpruvate and hydroxyphenylpyruvate approaches that observed in human phenyl-ketonuria (PKU).[63] Recent studies showed that in infected animals there was no conversion of radiolabeled phenylalanine to tyrosine, and, therefore, a majority, if not all, of the radioactivity was excreted as phenylpyruvate.[49] This suggested that as in PKU the host enzyme phenylalanine hydroxylase should be decreased in activity. This prediction has been shown to be correct, and in chronically infected *Microtus* the activity is decreased by 70% by 21 days.[48] In addition, the increased excretion of phenylpyruvate (and hydroxyphenyl-pyruvate) is also consistent with the elevated tyrosine transaminase activity found in the sera of infected animals.[54] The source of this activity is not known; however, there is suggestive evidence based on cofactor requirements that it is at least partially parasitic in origin. Finally, it has been demonstrated by Newport and associates[35] that both tryptophan and tyrosine are dramatically decreased in the sera of infected animals, whereas phenylalanine levels remain normal or even increased. It has, therefore, been shown that African trypa-nosomiasis has many of the metabolic properties of PKU. In PKU, many of the symptoms observed are suggested to be due to either the altered ratio between phenylalanine and the other aromatic amino acids leading to an inhibition of the cellular transport system, or to direct toxic effects of phenylpyruvate.[25] Phenylpyruvate, again in pharmacological doses, has been shown to have a number of inhibitory effects, including inhibition of mitochondrial function,[40] gluconeogenesis,[25] and proteolytic activity.[25] It is, therefore, conceivable that both phenylpyruvate and hydroxphenylpyruvate are at least partially responsible for the pathology observed. It is hypothesized in Figure 1 that the phenylpyruvate produced during African trypanosomiasis specifically inhibits the enzyme pyruvate translocase[18] and pyruvate carboxylase.[40] The suggested alterations in mitochondrial activity by phenylpyruvate are consistent with the increased pyruvate and α-ketoglutarate observed in the body fluids or the urine of infected animals.[48] Several investigators[11a,14,26] have noted that in livers of chronically infected animals, when examined by electron microscopy, there are abnormal mitochondria. In addition, it is further hypothesized that phenylpyruvate also blocks the enzyme fructose 1-6 diphosphatase. This suggestion is based on the observation that this enzyme is inhibited during African trypanosomiasis,[12] as well as the fact that phenylpyruvate inhibits the gluconeogenic process.

Finally, it should be noted that large increases in both pyruvate and α-ketoglutarate have been observed in animals chronically infected with the African trypanosomes.[14,48] It has been observed that during the metabolism of glucose by *T. b. gambiense,* a dimer of pyruvate is formed.[11b] This dimer (4-hydroxy-4-methyl α-ketoglutarate) has been shown to also be inhibitory to the tricarboxylic acid cycle in mitochondria from rat heart, and, therefore, could directly contribute to the pathology observed.[28,29]

In addition to the direct toxic activity of a number of the catabolites synthesized by the African trypanosomes, the dramatic decreases observed in serum tryptophan and tyrosine could also be detrimental to the host, leading to a specific nutritional deficiency in these essential amino acids. Newport et al.[37] have noted in an abstract that norepinephrine and dopamine are decreased in the hearts of infected animals, and that the catecholamines are reduced in the brains of these animals. In addition, Jose and associates[23] have shown that selective amino acid deficiencies such as tryptophan can lead to significant immunosuppres-sion. Therefore, the decreases in essential nutrients observed in experimental African try-panosomiasis can be detrimental to the host.

III. PHYSIOLOGICAL CHANGES: HOST CHANGES

In the past section, we have attempted to outline a number of biological substances of both large and small molecular weights produced by the parasite that are capable of harming

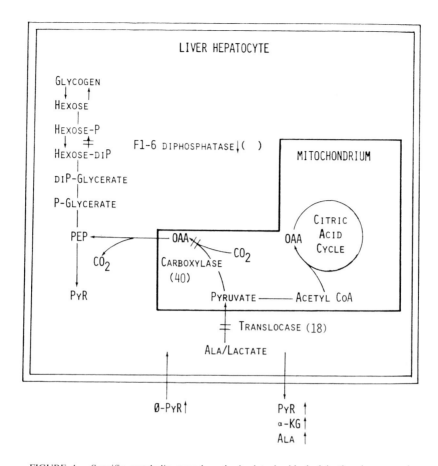

FIGURE 1. Specific metabolic steps hypothesized to be blocked in the gluconeogenic pathway, and in the mitochondria by phenylpyruvate (ϕ-PyR) in hepatocytes of *T. b. gambiense*-infected animals The double-lined box denotes the cell membrane of hepatocytes, and the inner single-lined box represents the mitochondria. Brief summaries of the glycolytic, gluconeogenic, and Kreb's cycle are shown. The lines denote interconnecting pathways, and the short double lines represent predicted enzymic blocks produced by ϕ-PyR. The numbers in parentheses are specific references. It is shown that ϕ-PyR enters the hepatocyte inhibiting three specific metabolic steps which result in increased levels of PyR, α-KG, and ala. The symbols denote the following: ($\downarrow$) decreased levels; ($\uparrow$) increased levels; (PyR) pyruvate; (ϕ-PyR) phenylpyruvate; (ala) alanine; (α-KG) α-ketoglutarate.

the host. In addition, we have briefly described several physiological changes observed during a chronic infection.

In this section we will further investigate the physiological changes observed in the infected host. We will begin by discussing changes in carbohydrate metabolism. In chronically infected animals, it has been demonstrated that there is a very large decrease in the glycogen content from infected livers.[4] There are also greatly elevated levels of pyruvate reported in the blood and urine of infected rabbits as well as increased pyruvate and α-ketoglutarate in the urine of chronically infected *Microtus*.[14,48] These changes are consistent with the presumed drain on host carbohydrate stores to meet the energy demands of the trypanosomes. As previously noted, they are also consistent with the ultrastructural changes found in the livers of infected animals. It has been observed that the livers of guinea pigs chronically infected with *T. b. gambiense* have altered mitochondria ultrastructure, absence of glycogen particles, and large increases in lipid deposits.[26] In addition to the parasite's demand for carbohydrates, these changes also suggest that there are basic changes in the host physiology, for example, decreases in gluconeogenesis and changes in mitochondrial functions. In both examples, changes in various host enzyme systems have been detected during a chronic infection of *Microtus*. Decreases in liver glucose-6-phosphatase and cytochrome oxidase activity have been demonstrated.[26,51] In addition, Diehl and Risby[10] have noticed increases in the lipid concentration of the serum from infected rabbits. Both the liver ultrastructure and the increase in serum lipids would suggest altered lipid metabolism. These profound changes in lipid and carbohydrate metabolism plus presumably mitochondrial function would suggest that the overall energy balance (P/O) ratios are altered, and that the host is in an energy deficit. The excretion of large amounts of energy-rich compounds such as pyruvate and α-ketoglutarate plus the elevated alanine level is consistent with the above hypothesis.[48] Finally, the muscle wasting observed in humans and other chronically infected animals may be an attempt by the host to improve this energy-poor state through the protein catabolism of muscle tissue.

In addition to the changes observed in glycogen, lipid, and protein metabolism in an African trypanosome infection, there are strong indications of endocrine dysfunction. See von Brand[61] for a discussion of earlier work. It is, of course, possible that the metabolic changes which we discussed are also the result of changes in endocrine function. Unfortunately, there is very little direct evidence for endocrine changes in man or experimental animals. The levels of very few, if any, hormones have been monitored; however, the extensive edema (puffy face) observed, changes in body temperature, and the adrenal enlargement observed in infected animals are all consistent with this idea.[45] Finally, the microscopic (pathological) changes which have been observed in the pituitary gland of experimental dogs would suggest changes in pituitary functions.[30] Unquestionably, further work is needed in order to assess the role of endocrine dysfunction in pathogenesis. In addition, in order to present evidence to suggest a role for hormonal imbalance in pathogenesis, work has been summarized from a number of different animal species and is presented in Table 1. To date, there has been no systematic investigation of this problem in a single species.

IV. CONCLUSIONS

As noted in the introduction to this chapter, it is not the intent to deny the importance of immunological factors being involved in pathogenesis. Instead, it was intended to present a balanced approach to this problem. In our opinion, a final explanation of the mechanism(s) of pathogenesis in African trypanosomiasis will be complex, involving both the immunological and physiological factors. It is hypothesized that the deposition of antigen-antibody deposits in the organs of infected animals, as well as soluble antigen-antibody complexes in body fluids, is important and leads to activation of Hageman factor and a cascade of enzymic reactions resulting ultimately in the release of important biological factors such as bradykinin, plasmin, and thrombin. In our opinion, the role of the inflammatory processes in pathogenesis is an area of research that should receive increased attention in the future. Second, there is no doubt that the African trypanosomes themselves produce or contain a number of potentially toxic materials. The release of proteases and phospholipases during relapse could result in pathology.[53,57,60] The catabolites of the aromatic amino acids have properties which mimic many of the clinical symptoms observed in chronically infected animals, such as changes in body temperature. The fact that high concentrations of these compounds are excreted into the urines of infected animals, and that the trypanosomes synthesize the compounds in vivo, would also suggest that their role in pathogenesis should be further examined. Finally, the demonstration that several amino acids are decreased in concentration in infected animals, as well as the fact that changes in the levels of important hormones derived from them have also been recorded, would suggest that the role of amino acid deficiencies in the disease process should be explored.

Table 1
THE TYPES OF PHYSIOLOGICAL CHANGES CURRENTLY OBSERVED IN EXPERIMENTAL ANIMALS CHRONICALLY INFECTED WITH THE AFRICAN TRYPANOSOMES

Physiological parameters		Host	Ref.
Inorganic compounds			
K, Na, Cl, Ca, P	≅	Mouse (acute)	31
K, Na, Cl ↑, Ca ↓, PO_4		Rabbit	14
Fe	△	Cattle	33
Organic compounds: small molecular weight compounds			
CO_2		Mouse ≅, rabbit ↑	14, 31
Creatinine	↑	Mouse, *Microtus*, rabbit	14, 31, 44
Urea		Mouse, ≅ , rabbit ↑, goat ↑	14, 31, 59
Cholesterol	↑	Rabbit	14
Pyruvate	↑	*Microtus*, rabbit	14, 48
α-Ketoglutarate: urine	↑	*Microtus*	48
Bilirubin	≅	Mouse	14
Catecholamines	↓	*Microtus*	37
Amino acids	△	*Microtus*, sheep	20, 35, 36
Glucose		Mouse ↓, rabbit ≅	14, 31
Fatty acids	↑	Rabbit	10
Organic compounds: large molecular weight compounds			
Glycogen: liver	↓	*Microtus*, guinea pig	4, 26
Lipids	↑	Guinea pig, rabbit	14, 26
Protein: synthesis	↓	*Microtus*	49
Protein: total body	↓	Cattle	48
Protein: serum albumin		Mouse ↑, rabbit ↓, cattle ↓	14, 31, 60
Immunoglobulins	↑	Rabbit, cattle	14, 39, 55
Complement	↓	Cattle	39
Protein: urine	↑	*Microtus*, rabbit, goat	14, 44, 59
Organic compounds: specific enzyme activities			
Glucose-6-phosphatase		*Microtus* △, guinea pig ↓	4, 26
Fructose 1-6 diphosphatase	↓	*Microtus*	12
Alkaline phosphatase		Mouse (acute) ≅, rabbit ↓	14, 31
Tyrosine aminotransferase	↑	*Microtus*	54
Glutamic-pyruvic aminotransferase	↑	Mouse	31
Glutamic-oxalocetic aminotransferase	↑	Mouse	31
Aspartate aminotransferase	↑	Rabbit	14
Phenylalanine hydroxylase	↓	*Microtus*	48
Mixed function oxidases	↓	*Microtus*	51
Cytochrome, P-450	↓	*Microtus*	51
Creatinine phosphokinase	↓	Rabbit	14

Note: This list of physiological changes is not intended to be all-inclusive. Instead, it represents examples of the types of physiological parameters which have been measured as well as the variety of hosts examined. The limited number of references reporting physiological changes in human African trypanosomiasis have also been omitted. The reader must refer to the individual papers for details. For example, in some cases, early increases in specific parameters were followed by later, more profound decreases. In this example, only the decrease would be reported in this table. Similarly, in the case where changes were observed in the serum, but not in the tissue fluids, only the changes are recorded. The following symbols were used: (△) indicates that changes were observed; (↑) indicates that an increase was reported; (↓) indicates that a decrease was noted; and, finally, (≅) indicates that no significant change was found.

It should be obvious that physiological changes do occur in infected animals and that systematic investigations into the extent of these changes must be continued. It is believed that such studies will also yield information on the mechanisms of pathogenesis. A summary

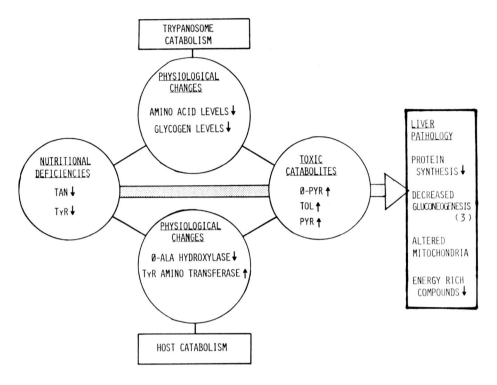

FIGURE 2.   A summary of the major physiological changes occurring during African trypanosomiasis. The small rectangular boxes denote host or parasite catabolism, the circles represent physiological changes associated with host and/or parasite catabolism, and the large thick-lined box shows the resulting liver pathology. The interconnecting lines are intended to represent some of the interactions between the various systems. The arrows within the circles or box denote the direction of these interactions. For example, the increased host tyrosine aminotransferase and parasite amino acid metabolism would lower tyrosine levels, and, thereby, reduce protein synthesis. The symbols denote the following: (↓) decreased levels; (↑) increased levels; (φ-ala) phenylalanine; (φ-PyR) phenylpyruvate; (TyR) tyrosine; (TaN) tryptophan; (TOL) indole ethanol; and (PyR) pyruvate and its dimer.

of the major physiological changes which are predicted to occur in African trypanosomiases is shown in Figure 2. This includes the formation of toxic catabolites and the depletion of essential nutrients. These two factors would alter host metabolism and lead to changes in the major metabolic pathways, such as decreased protein synthesis, gluconeogenesis, and energy production. A more comprehensive figure outlining the predicted physiological factors involved in pathogenesis of chronic African trypanosomiasis has been previously described.[44] The hypothesized specific metabolic lesions which are believed to occur in this disease are, however, shown in Figure 1. The pathology resulting from these physiological changes can be added to that caused by the release of toxic macromolecules during trypanosome death as well as from immunological mechanisms.

It should also be noted that there are numerous precedents described in the literature with other host-parasite systems that suggest physiological mechanisms are involved in pathogenesis. For example, bacterial endotoxins produced profound changes in tryptophan catabolism.[9] Toxic factors have been described in malaria, and tryptophan catabolites produced by *Schistosoma mansoni* have been hypothesized to be responsible for the induction of bladder cancer.[6] Many more examples could be given to document this point, however, it is to be hoped that these few will be sufficient to convince the reader of the potential importance of physiological factors in pathogenesis.

ACKNOWLEDGMENTS

The authors would like to acknowledge the generous financial assistance from the National Institute of Allergy and Infectious Diseases (1-RO1-AIlu185-9) and the UNDP/World Bank/ WHO special program for Research and Training on Tropical Diseases for the support of work conducted in the authors' laboratory, described in this chapter.

REFERENCES

1. **Ackerman, S. B. and Seed, J. R.,** The effects of tryptophol on immune responses and its implications towards trypanosome-induced immunosuppression, *Experientia,* 32, 645, 1976.
2. **Albright, J. W. and Albright, J. R.,** Inhibition of murine humoral immune responses by substances derived from trypanosomes, *J. Immunol.,* 125, 300, 1981.
3. **Arinze, I. J. and Patel, M. S.,** Inhibition by phenylpyruvate of gluconeogenesis in the isolated perfused rat liver, *Biochemistry,* 12, 4473, 1973.
4. **Ashman, P. U. and Seed, J. R.,** Biochemical studies in the vole, *Microtus montanus.* II. The effects of a *Trypanosoma brucei gambiense* infection in the diurnal variation of hepatic glucose-6-phosphatase and liver glycogen, *Comp. Biochem. Physiol.,* 45B, 379, 1973.
5. **Boreham, P. F. L.,** Pharmacologically active substances in *T. brucei* infections, in *Pathogenicity of Trypanosomes,* Losos, G. and Chouinard, A., Eds., International Development Research Centre, Ottawa, Can., 1979.
6. **Cheever, A. N.,** Schistosomiasis and neoplasia, *J. Natl. Cancer Inst.,* 61, 13, 1978.
7. **Cornford, E. M., Bocash, W. D., Brown, L. D., Crane, P. P., MacInnis, A. J., and Oldendorf, W. H.,** Rapid distribution of tryptophol (3-indole-ethanol) to brain and other tissues, *J. Clin. Invest.,* 63, 1241, 1979.
8. **Cornford, E. M., Crane, P. P., Brown, L. D., Bocash, W. D., Myerges, A. M., and Oldendorf, W. H.,** Reduction in brain glucose utilization rate after tryptophol (3-indole ethanol) treatment, *J. Neurochem.,* 36, 1758, 1981.
9. **Curzon, G. and Knott, P. J.,** Environmental toxicological and related aspects of tryptophan metabolism with particular reference to the central nervous system, *CRC Crit. Rev. Toxicol.,* 5, 145, 1977.
10. **Diehl, E. J. and Risby, E. L.,** Serum changes in rabbits experimentally infected with *Trypanosoma gambiense, Am. J. Trop. Med. Hyg.,* 23, 1019, 1974.
11. **Esuruoso, G. O.,** The demonstration *in vitro* of the mitogenic effects of trypanosomal antigen on the spleen cells of normal, athymic and cyclophosphamide-treated mice, *Clin. Exp. Immunol.,* 23, 314, 1976.
11a. **Frommel, T. D., et al.,** unpublished.
11b. **Flynn, I. W., Hall, J. E., Mackenzie, N. E., and Scott, A. I.,** personal communication.
12. **Gonzales, L., Boutte, K. D., Williams, V. R., and Ashman, P. U.,** The effects of a *Trypanosoma brucei gambiense* on two hepatic enzymes in *Microtus montanus, Proc. 2nd Annu. Xavier-MBS Biomed. Symp.,* 2, 47, 1974.
13. **Goodwin, L. G.,** The pathology of African trypanosomiasis, *Trans. R. Soc. Trop. Hyg.,* 64, 797, 1970.
14. **Goodwin, L. G. and Guy, M. W.,** Tissue fluid in rabbits infected with *Trypanosoma (Trypanozoon) brucei, Parasitology,* 66, 499, 1973.
15. **Goodwin, L. G., Guy, M. W., and Brooker, B. E.,** Connective tissue changes in rabbits infected with *Trypanosoma (Trypanozoon) brucei, Parasitology,* 67, 115, 1973.
16. **Greenwood, B. M. and Whittle, H. C.,** Coagulation studies in gambian trypanosomiasis, *Am. J. Trop. Med. Hyg.,* 25, 390, 1976.
17. **Greenwood, B. M. and Oduloju, A. J.,** Mitogenic activity of an extract of *Trypanosoma gambiense, Trans. R. Soc. Trop. Med. Hyg.,* 72, 408, 1978.
18. **Halestrap, A. P., Brand, M. D., and Denton, R. D.,** Inhibition of mitochondrial pyruvate transport by phenylpyruvate and α-ketoisocaproate, *Biochim. Biophys. Acta,* 367, 102, 1974.
19. **Hall, J. E. and Seed, J. R.,** Aromatic ketoaciduria in a mammalian model of chronic African trypanosomiasis, in *The Host Invader Interplay,* Van Den Bossche, H., Ed., Elsevier/North-Holland, Amsterdam, 1980, 503.
20. **Isoun T. T., Isoun, M. J., and Anosa, V. D.,** Free plasma amino acid profiles of normal and *Trypanosoma vivax* infected sheep, *Tropenmed. Parasitol.,* 92, 330, 1978.

21. **Jenkins, A. R. and Robertson, D. H. H.,** Hepatic dysfunction in human trypanosomiasis. I. Abnormalities of excretion function, seroflocculation phenomena and other tests of hepatic function with observations on the alterations of these tests during treatment and convalescence, *Trans. R. Soc. Trop. Med. Hyg.,* 53, 511, 1959.

22. **Jenkins, A. A. and Robertson, D. H. H.,** Hepatic dysfunction in human trypanosomiasis. II. Serum proteins in *Trypanosoma rhodesiense* infections, and observations on the alterations found after treatment and during convalescence, *Trans. R. Soc. Trop. Med. Hyg.,* 53, 524, 1959.

23. **Jose, D. G. and Good, R. A.,** Quantitative effects of nutritional essential amino acid deficiency upon immune responses to tumors in mice, *J. Exp. Med.,* 137, 1, 1973.

24. **Lambert, P. H. and Houba, V.,** Immune complexes in parasitic diseases in *Progress in Immunology II,* Vol. 5, Brent, L. and Holbroow, J., Eds., North-Holland, Amsterdam, 1974.

25. **Lane, J. E. and Neuhoff, V.,** Phenylketonuria: clinical and experimental considerations revealed by the use of animal models, *Naturwissenschaften,* 67, 227, 1980.

26. **Lumsden, R. D., Marciacq, Y., and Seed, J. R.,** *Trypanosoma gambiense:* cytopathologic changes in guinea pig hepatocytes, *Exp. Parasitol.,* 32, 369, 1972.

27. **Mansfield, J. M., Craig, S. A., and Stelzer, G. T.,** Lymphocyte function in experimental African trypanosomiasis: mitogenic effects of Trypanosome extracts, *in vitro, Infect. Immun.,* 14, 976, 1976.

28. **Montgomery, C. M. and Webb, J. L.,** Metabolic studies on heart mitochondria. II. The inhibitory action of parapyruvate on the tricarboxylic acid cycle, *J. Biol. Chem.,* 221, 359, 1956.

29. **Montgomery, C. M., Fairhurst, A. S., and Webb, J. L.,** Metabolic studies on heart mitochondria. III. The action of parapyruvate on α-ketoglutaric oxidase, *J. Biol. Chem.,* 221, 369, 1956.

30. **Morrison, W. I., Murray, M., Sayer, P. D., and Preston, J. M.,** The pathogenesis of experimentally induced *Trypanosoma brucei* infection in the dog, *Am. J. Pathol.,* 102, 168, 1981.

31. **Moon, A. P., Williams, J. S., and Witherspoon, C.,** Serum biochemical changes in mice infected with *Trypanosoma rhodesiense* and *Trypanosoma duttoni, Exp. Parasitol.,* 22, 112, 1968.

32. **Moulton, J. E. and Coleman, J. L.,** A soluble immunosuppressor substance in spleen in deer mice infected with *Trypanosoma brucei, Am. J. Vet. Res.,* 40, 1131, 1978.

33. **Murray, M.,** Anemia of bovine African trypanosomiasis: an overview, in *Pathogenicity of Trypanosomes,* Losos, G. and Chouinard, A., Eds., International Development Research Centre, Ottawa, Can., 1979.

34. **Musoke, A. J. and Barbet, A. F.,** Activation of complement by variant-specific surface antigen of *Trypanosoma brucei, Nature (London),* 270, 438, 1977.

35. **Newport, G. R., Page, C. R., III, Ashman, P. U., Stibbs, H. H., and Seed, J. R.,** Alteration of free serum amino acids in voles infected with *Trypanosoma brucei gambiense, J. Parasitol.,* 63, 15, 1977.

36. **Newport, G. R. and Page, C. R., III,** Free amino acids in brain, liver, skeletal muscle tissue of voles infected with *Trypanosoma brucei gambiense, J. Parasitol,* 63, 1060, 1977.

37. **Newport, G. R., Sferruzza, A., and Page, C. R., III,** Catecholamine and indoleamine levels in tissue of infected field voles, *Abstr. 54th Annu. Meet. Am. Soc. Parasitol.,* 1979, 53.

38. **Newton, B. A.,** The metabolism of African trypanosomes in relation to pathogenic mechanisms, in *Pathogenicity of Trypanosomes,* Losos, G. and Chouinard, A., Eds., International Development Research Centre, Ottawa, Can., 1979.

39. **Nielsen, K., Sheppard, J., Holmes, W., and Tizard, I.,** Experimental bovine trypanosomiasis. Changes in serum immunoglobulins, complement and complement components in infected animals, *Immunology,* 35, 817, 1978.

40. **Patel, T. B., Booth, R. F. G., and Clark, J. B.,** Inhibition of acetoacetate oxidation by brain mitochondria from the suckling rat by phenylpyruvate and ketoisocaproate, *J. Neurochem.,* 29, 1151, 1977.

41. **Sanchez, G., Lockwood, J., and Chavez, R.,** Liver glycogen mobilization by *Trypanosoma brucei* sonicates, *Comp. Biochem. Physiol.,* 70B, 447, 1981.

42. **Seed, J. R.,** *Trypanosoma gambiense* and *T. lewisi:* increased vascular permeability and skin lesions in rabbits, *Exp. Parasitol.,* 26, 214, 1969.

43. **Seed, J. R. and Khalili, N.,** The changes in locomotor rhythms of *Microtus montanus* infected with *Trypanosoma gambiense, J. Interdiscipl. Cycle Res.,* 2, 91, 1971.

44. **Seed, J. R.,** The possible role of aromatic amino acid catabolites in the pathogenicity of *Trypanosoma brucei gambiense,* in *The Host Invader Interplay,* Van Den Bossche, H., Ed., Elsevier/North-Holland, Amsterdam, 1980, 273.

45. **Seed, J. R. and Hall, J. E.,** A review on the use of *Microtus montanus* as an applicable experimental model for the study of African trypanosomiasis, *Ann. Soc. Belge. Med. Trop.,* 60, 341, 1980.

46. **Seed, J. R. and Sechelski, J.,** Tryptophol levels in mice infected with pharmacological doses of tryptophol, and the effect of pyrazole and ethanol on these levels, *Life Sci.,* 21, 1603, 1977.

47. **Seed, J. R. and Varney, J. R.,** *Trypanosoma brucei gambiense:* changes in body temperature rhythms of infected New Zealand albino rabbits, *Exp. Parasitol.,* 40, 238, 1976.

48. **Seed, J. R., Hall, J. E., and Price, C. C.,** A physiological mechanism to explain pathogenesis in African trypanosomiasis, in *From Parasitic Infection to Parasitic Disease,* Gigase, P. L., Ed., S. Karger, Basel, 1982.

49. **Seed, J. R., Hall, J. E., and Sechelski, J.,** Phenylalanine metabolism in *Microtus montanus* chronically infected with *Trypanosoma brucei gambiense, Comp. Biochem. Physiol.,* 71B, 209, 1982.

50. **Seed, J. R., Seed, T. M., and Sechelski, J.,** The biological effects of tryptophol (indole-3-ethanol) hemolytic, biochemical and behavior modifying activity, *Comp. Biochem. Physiol.,* 60, 175, 1978.

51. **Shertzer, H. G., Hall, J. E., and Seed, J. R.,** Hepatic microsomal alterations during chronic trypanosomiasis in the field vole *Microtus montanus, Mol. Biochem. Parasitol.,* 6, 25, 1982.

52. **Slotz, J. M. M., van Miert, A. S. J. P. A. M., Akkerman, J. W. N., and de Gee, A. L. W.,** *Trypanosoma brucei* and *Trypanosoma vivax:* antigen-antibody complexes as a cause of platelet serotonin release *in vitro* and *in vivo, Exp. Parasitol.,* 43, 211, 1977.

53. **Steiger, R. F., Opperdoes, F. R., and Bontemps, J.,** Subcellular fractionation of *Trypanosoma brucei* bloodstream forms with special reference to hydrolases, *Eur. J. Biochem.,* 105, 163, 1980.

54. **Stibbs, H. H. and Seed, J. R.,** Elevated serum and hepatic tyrosine aminotransferase in voles chronically infected with *Trypanosoma brucei gambiense, Exp. Parasitol.,* 29, 1, 1976.

55. **Tabel, H.,** Serum protein changes in bovine trypanosomiasis: a review, in *Pathogenicity of Trypanosomes,* Losos, G. and Chouinard, A., Eds., International Development Research Centre, Ottawa, Can., 1979.

56. **Tizard, I., Nielsen, K. H., Seed, J. R., and Hall, J. E.,** Biologically active products from African trypanosomes, *Microbiol. Rev.,* 42, 661, 1978.

57. **Tizard, I. R., Nielsen, K. H., Mellors, A., and Assoku, R. V. G.,** Biologically active lipids generated by autolysis of *T. congolense,* in *Pathogenicity of Trypanosomes,* Losos, G. and Chouinard, A., Eds., International Development Research Centre, Ottawa, Can., 1979.

58. **Valli, V. E. O., Forsberg, C. M., and Mills, J. N.,** Pathology of *T. congolense* in calves, in *Pathogenicity of Trypanosomes,* Losos, G. and Chouinard, A., Eds., International Development Research Centre, Ottawa, Can., 1979.

59. **Van den Ingh, T. S. G. A. M., Zwart, D., Schotman, A. J. H., van Miert, A. S. J. P. A. M., and Veenendaal, G. H.,** The pathology and pathogenesis of *Trypanosoma vivax* infection in the goat, *Res. Vet. Sci.,* 21, 264, 1976.

60. **Vickerman, K. and Tetley, L.,** Biology and ultrastructure of trypanosomes in relation to pathogenesis, in *Pathogenicity of Trypanosomes,* Losos, G. and Chouinard, A., Eds., International Development Research Centre, Ottawa, Can., 1979.

61. **von Brand, T.,** *Biocemistry of Parasites,* Academic Press, New York, 1966.

62. **Yokigoshi, H. and Yoshida, A.,** Effects of supplementation and depletion of a single essential amino acid on hepatic polyribosome profile in rats, *J. Nutr.,* 110, 375, 1980.

63. **Zelnicek, E. and Slama, J.,** Phenylpyruvate and O-hydroxyphenylacetate in phenylketonuric urine, *Clin. Chem. Acta,* 35, 496, 1971.

64. **Zwart, D. and Veenendaal, G. H.,** Pharmacologically, active substances in *T. vivax* infections, in *Pathogenicity of Trypanosomes,* Losos, G. and Chouinard, A., Eds., International Development Research Centre, Ottawa, Can., 1979.

Chapter 2

HEMATOLOGY OF AFRICAN TRYPANOSOMIASIS

George C. Jenkins and Christine A. Facer

TABLE OF CONTENTS

I. INTRODUCTION

Over the years, many workers have made observations on the ways in which African trypanosomiasis affects the hemopoietic tissue. It is now apparent that although there are a number of fundamental effects, some such effects are more prominent in the pathogenesis of the disease caused by one species of organism compared with another and that different species affect different mammalian hosts with varying emphasis on the possible hematological consequences.

II. ANEMIA

Anemia is a significant feature of the disease in mammals. The severity of the anemia depends not only on the species of the organism, but also on the isolate of the species as well as the species of host and the acuteness or chronicity of the infection.

The significance of anemia on the overall morbidity of African trypanosomiasis, both in man and livestock, is often difficult to assess since many other causes of severe anemia (nutritional and parasitic) are concurrently present in endemic areas. However, a recent hematologic study on Nigerian cattle indicated that trypanosomiasis produced the most severe anemia of all blood protozoan and gastrointestinal helminth infections encountered among the animals.[1] Mamo and Holmes,[2] in their Ethiopian field studies of Zebu cattle infected with *Trypanosoma congolense,* pronounced anemia to be the primary cause of death. Severe anemia in a previously healthy student (presumably well nourished) has been recorded following infection with *T. rhodesiense.*[3] Similarly, experimental infections of rabbits with *T. brucei* produced a severe anemia with a drop in the hemoglobin level to 6.0 g/dℓ, that is, to half the initial volume.[4]

It is becoming increasingly obvious that the etiology of the anemia in trypanosomiasis is multifactorial with hemolysis, hemodilution, and disordered and/or noncompensatory erythropoiesis all playing a part and the contribution of each varying throughout the infection (Table 1).

A. Hemolysis

There is now considerable evidence that hemolysis is the major component of the anemia in African trypanosomiasis as indicated by a number of different studies. Indications for intravascular hemolysis, such as increased serum bilirubin and decreased haptoglobin levels, are not consistent features, and it would appear that extravascular hemolysis is a much more important contributor. Thus, the histological evidence for intravascular hemolysis, viz. presence of erythrophagocytosis in the spleen, liver, and lymph nodes, together with hemosiderin deposition, have been described in animal trypanosomiasis.[5-9] The spleen was shown to be the major site of red cell sequestration and destruction in animals with mild anemia, while the liver was the major site in severely anemic animals.[10,11] Confirmatory evidence for increased peripheral red cell destruction comes from erythrokinetic data. In all animals studied to date, a shortened half-life of DF^{32}P or ^{51}Cr-labeled red cells, an accelerated urinary excretion of ^{51}Cr from the labeled cells, and the retention of ^{59}Fe in the body have been demonstrated and are indicative of anemia of hemolytic origin.[2,4,6,10-13] A decreased ^{51}Cr-labeled red cell survival is also a feature of Rhodesiense sleeping sickness.[14]

Detailed hematological investigations using rabbits infected with *T. brucei,*[4,15] showed a progressive fall in hemoglobin and red cell counts commensurate with a decreased ^{51}Cr survival of autologous red cells. No difference was found between syringe passaged and fly-transmitted infections.

Splenectomy delayed the onset of the anemia and lessened its severity although there was only a slight decrease in the half-life (T50) of labeled cells in splenectomized, infected

Table 1
**CAUSES OF ANEMIA IN ACUTE AND CHRONIC
AFRICAN TRYPANOSOMIASIS**

Increased red cell destruction
    Extravascular and intravascular hemolysis
        Immune (trypanosome Ag/Ab complexes; antierythrocyte antibodies?)
        Hemolysins
        Nonspecific RE activation
        Direct traumatic effect of trypanosomes
        Microangiopathy associated with DIC

Splenic phagocytosis and splenic pooling

Increased plasma volume

Noncompensatory and/or decreased erythropoiesis
    Anemia of chronic disorders

animals. Interestingly, intact infected animals splenectomized at mid-infection showed a marked increase in T50 shortly after the operation (Figure 1). These experiments demonstrate the importance of the spleen in the extra-vascular hemolysis of trypanosomiasis. Reticulocyte counts were raised as evidenced by high levels of red cell pyruvate kinase, reflecting the emerging young cell community in response to the hemolytic stimulus.

There is increasing interest in the possibility that different stocks (zymodemes) of one species of trypanosome can give rise to varying pathogenicity in a given host. This is particularly true of American trypanosomiasis in man caused by different zymodemes of *T. cruzi*.[16] This possibility has been investigated among the African trypanosomes using anemia as an indicator of the degree of pathogenicity.[17] Rabbits were infected with one of the three stocks of *T. congolense* — either GAMB 19, TSW 99/77, or a laboratory-maintained stock S104. The newly isolated stocks, GAMB 19 and TSW 99/77, produced a chronic infection lasting >150 days, whereas survival was between 39 and 100 days with S104. The pattern of parasitemia produced (given the same inoculum) was quite different and this was reflected in the degree of anemia. TSW 99/77 characteristically produced a very high parasitemia 15 to 20 days after infection, whereas the same level was attained in GAMB 19 and S104 only towards the end of infection. There was a corresponding decrease in hemoglobin and red cell survival was normal during the first week of infection in the GAMB 19 infection and only slightly reduced in the TSW 99/77 infection. However, during the second week, whereas the red cell survival in the former became only slightly reduced it was markedly reduced in the latter correlating well with the parasitemia. This study, therefore, shows that different stocks of African trypanosomes can produce quite a different pathological response as occurs with *T. cruzi* in man. More work is needed to apply results of laboratory infections like this to the field situation.

Various mechanisms for the hemolysis in trypanosomiasis have been demonstrated as shown in Table 1.

1. Immune
There is cumulative evidence for immune sensitization of the red cells in trypanosome infections and this has been supported by the observation that corticosteroids attenuate the anemia and that as the host becomes immunosuppressed the waves of anemia cease. In 1973 Herbert and Inglis[20] demonstrated that in infected mice, trypanosome antigen(s) can attach to the red cell membrane, thereby rendering them susceptible to phagocytosis by the reticuloendothelial system (RES). Confirming this was the observation that sonicated *T. brucei*

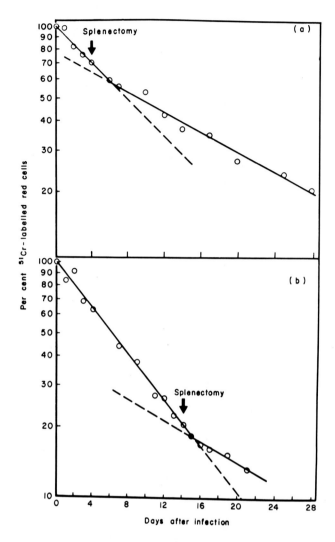

FIGURE 1.   ^{51}Cr-labeled red cell survival curves in two rabbits infected with *T. brucei* S42. Effect of splenectomy after infection: (a) splenectomy at 4 days; (b) at 14 days.

antigen(s) readily adsorbs onto the surface of rabbit red cells in vitro. The antigen-coated cells could then be lysed following the addition of antitrypanosome antibody plus complement.[21,22] Furthermore, when rabbits, immunized with sonicated *T. brucei* antigen and adjuvant, were given challenge intravenous doses of homologous trypanosome antigen, a marked decrease in hemoglobin and hematocrit followed. This did not occur in control nonimmunized animals.[22]

A positive direct Coombs antiglobulin test (DAT) recorded in both animal and human trypanosomiasis provides evidence for immune sensitization in vivo.[3,14,19,23-26] It was more difficult to demonstrate antibody on the surface of red cells of rabbits infected with *T. brucei* necessitating a "build-up" antiglobulin test which showed consistent red cell sensitization 3 to 5 days after infection.[27] Erythrocyte sensitization has been examined in detail in calves infected with *T. vivax*. Animals became anemic after the first parasitemic peak (7 to 10 days after infection) and this coincided with the demonstration of erythrocyte-bound IgG and IgM with or without C'.[26] Sensitized red cells were removed promptly from the circulation since the DAT became negative 2 to 4 days later. Immunoglobulin eluted from sensitized erythrocytes had specificity for *T. vivax* antigen. The exact mechanism of erythrocyte sensitization is unknown, but the results are consistent with a type II or type III cytotoxic reaction involving trypanosome antigen-antibody complexes.[28] Immune complexes are elevated in trypanosomiasis and it has recently been suggested that red cells function in the removal of soluble immune complexes from the peripheral circulation.[29-31] Trypanosome antigen has also been demonstrated on the red cells of sheep infected with *T. congolense*.[32] The DAT has been reported as either positive or negative in infected calves possibly as a result of the different stocks of parasites and breed of cattle used.[33,34]

Autoantibodies to erythrocyte antigens have not yet been positively implicated in the pathogenesis of the anemia. Elevated cold-reacting IgM anti-I antibodies are produced in *T. brucei*-infected rabbits and similar cold-reacting hemagglutinins have been described in other experimental infections, although their specificity has not been defined.[35,36] An antibody reacting to trypsinized red cells also occurs although, again, its specificity is unknown.[35,37] The presence of this antibody suggests that a ''cryptic'' red cell antigen may be exposed during infection. Trypanosomes contain proteases such as cathepsin-D released on autolysis, and *T. brucei* homogenates contain significant amounts of trypsin-like activity.[35,38] It is possible, therefore, that considerable amounts of trypanosome-derived proteolytic activity is released during periods of trypanolysis, and this may expose the ''cryptic'' red cell antigen. Evidence for this possibility in vivo follows the observation that the net negative charge on the red cells of infected rats was reduced during high parasitemia coincident with increased plasma sialic acid content and developing anemia.[39]

2. Hemolysins

Considerable attention has been focused on the possibility that trypanosomes produce a hemolytic factor causing direct lysis of the circulating red cells. Huan and colleagues[40] described a slow-acting hemolysin in suspensions of *T. brucei*, *T. congolense*, *T. gambiense*, and *T. vivax*. The lytic factor is of low molecular weight (about 10,000 daltons) and protein in nature.

The pathogenic trypanosomes also generate phospholipase-A activity.[41,42] The action of this enzyme on endogenous phospholipid results in the generation in vivo of large quantities of hemolytic free fatty acids (FFA) with linoleic acid primary responsible for the hemolytic properties. However, the effect of FFA on hemolysis in vivo is considered unlikely since serum albumin binds to FFA, so blocking its hemolytic effect.[43]

3. Nonspecific Reticuloendothelial Activation

The RES shows intense proliferation during trypanosomiasis as evidenced from an increased rate of clearance of intravenously injected particles.[44] In many other infections where there is increased RES activity with associated splenomegaly and hepatomegaly, phagocytic cells are known to consume normal red cells in a nonspecific manner. Certainly, erythrophagocytosis is a marked feature in trypanosomiasis, but whether the phagocytosed red cells are ''normal'' has not been assessed.

4. Direct Traumatic Effect on the Red Cells

In 1965 Holwill[45] demonstrated that *T. brucei* visibly distorted the red cells of mice. Using a cine-microphotographic technique with Nomarski light interference, filmed sequences have shown a process of pinching out red cells by adherent trypanosomes in wet preparations of infected mouse blood.[46] It is most likely that this process affects the subsequent integrity of the cell, though how significant it is in vivo remains in doubt and, presumably, only occurs when parasitemia is at a high level.

B. Role of the Spleen

1. Nonspecific Effect of Splenic Enlargement

Splenomegaly is a feature of infections with African trypanosomes, and the spleens of rabbits infected with *T. brucei* can reach ten times the normal size.[47] As in the case of other conditions of splenic enlargement such as tropical splenomegaly syndrome, even normal red cells in their extended travel through the lengthened vascular network are exposed for a more protracted time to the macrophages lining the channels and, therefore, a greater number are removed from the circulation. Several workers have shown that the slow mixing and stagnation of red cells in the large extra-sinusoidal compartments of infiltrated spleens have an injurious effect on red cells with increased osmotic fragility and a decrease in the red cells with increased osmotic fragility and a decrease in the red cell K^+/Na^+ ratio.[48,49] Anosa[50] demonstrated that low cholesterol and glucose levels in the splenic environment may be harmful to red cells.

2. Specific Red Cell Destruction in the Spleen

As referred to previously, if red cells are coated with immune complexes or sensitized in some way as demonstrated by positive direct antiglobulin tests, they are likely to be removed, at least in some measure, by the splenic reticuloendothelial tissue as in other immunohematological conditions. Chronological studies of the histology of the spleen in the course of *T. brucei* infections in rabbits showed an increase in lymphoid tissue between 6 and 12 days following infection. Histiocytes increased in nearly all animals with time and almost all showed erythrophagocytosis and hemosiderin deposition.[9]

3. Red Cell "Pooling"

Enlarged spleens pool red cells. That is to say, the red cells are trapped or sequestered within their substances with only a slow exchange rate with the general circulation. This process may be responsible for depriving the body circulation of a large volume of red cells at any one time. However, the contribution of sequestration to the anemia in infected rabbits was found to be relatively small.[15]

C. Increased Blood and Plasma Volume

This is an almost constant sequel to splenic enlargement. It appears to be nonspecific and is found in enlarged spleens of patients in temperate climates as often as in, for example, chronic malaria and tropical splenomegaly syndrome. It was originally suggested by Naylor[51] that in trypanosome-infected cattle the plasma volume may increase disproportionately, thereby enhancing the anemia by a hemodilution effect. Similarly, in experimental infections in laboratory animals an expanded blood and plasma volume was encountered as infection progressed.[12,19]

Further attempts to study the contribution of plasma volume changes to the anemia of bovine trypanosomiasis have resulted in conflicting reports. This has largely been due to the various radioactive labels used in the studies. Mamo and Holmes,[2] using ^{59}Fe-labeled transferrin, showed that *T. congolense*-infected cattle had an increase in plasma volume per unit of body weight which was accompanied by a lowering of the hematocrit, although the effect appeared to be secondary to the red cell loss in causing the anemia. Hemodilution resulting from increased plasma and blood volume was also found in *T. vivax*-infected ruminants employing a combination of ^{131}I-labeled albumin and ^{51}Cr-labeled red cells.[52] However, the detailed studies of Dargie et al.[53] showed that because of its rapid transfer from the plasma, ^{59}Fe does not equilibrate with the total plasma space and seriously overestimates the plasma volume in anemic animals. Concurrent ^{125}I-labeled albumin studies showed that the true plasma volumes of infected cattle were, in fact, significantly higher and the circulating red cell volumes significantly lower than the corresponding control values. The total blood volume was not altered by infection.

D. The Anemia of Chronic Disorders

There is evidence that factors other than hemolysis contribute to anemia in the infected host, particularly in the later stages of infection. In both intact and splenectomized animals there is marked bone marrow erythroid hyperplasia in accordance with the demands of peripheral red cell destruction (see Section VI). Holmes[54] demonstrated an increased rate of removal of ^{59}Fe and incorporation into red cells with an increase plasma iron turnover in cattle 12 to 16 weeks after infection with *T. congolense*. The conclusion was that there was no evidence of marrow depression. However, the hyperplasia of the red cell precursors seems to fluctuate during the evolution of the disease, and with the gradual development of noncompensatory erythropoiesis the hemolytic episodes cause a rapidly increasing anemia. In experimental infections in rabbits there was a fall off of reticulocyte response in the late stages of infection, and the development of anemia at this time was not reflected in decreased red cell survival and probably related to marrow failure.[55] Dargie,[53] in his studies in cattle, suggested that in the early stages the degree of anemia depended upon the rate of red cell destruction which, in turn, depended on the level of parasitemia. Later, as the parasitemia declines, hemoglobin levels and PCV values stabilize at a higher level, although some red cell destruction continues due to the active mononuclear phagocytic system; however, in the intermediate stages this is compensated by an increased marrow erythroid hyperplasia. Finally, the anemia of chronic disorders becomes evident.[56] There is then a lack of incorporation of iron into the developing red cell precursors, a decrease in red cell production by the bone marrow, and an intrinsic modest reduction in red cell survival. The principle defect at this stage lies in the bone marrow where there is a large excess of storage iron not used for hemoglobin synthesis.

III. LEUKOCYTE CHANGES

Edwards et al.[57] did not observe any consistent changes in the leukocyte values of sheep and goats infected with *T. vivax*. However, Saror[8] described an initial leukopenia over the first 3 weeks of infection in cattle with values subsequently rising above the preinfection levels. Anosa and Isoun[11] subsequently confirmed these findings in sheep and goats infected with *T. vivax* and demonstrated that leukopenia lasted for several weeks of the clinically critical "crisis" phase followed by a leukocytosis in the animals that survived. The leukopenia was due to a combination of lymphopenia and neutropenia. Naylor[51] studied hematological changes in cattle infected with *T. congolense* and showed that eosinophils, lymphocytes, and neutrophils were all depressed early on in the infection. Monocyte levels showed little change, basophils tended to disappear, but plasma cells increased in number. The leukopenia was followed by leukocytosis about 14 weeks after infection. Similar studies by Valli and Mills[58] demonstrated that lymphocytosis was responsible for the rise in leukocytes in the chronic phase and that infected calves had a marked reduction in granulocyte mobilization for the first 14 weeks of infection with a reduced ability to mount an inflammatory response. Moretti et al.[59] remarked upon the lymphocytosis which included a high percentage of cells containing granulations which stained positive with periodic acid-Schiff reagent.

IV. ABNORMAL HEMOSTASIS

Bleeding manifestations are often associated with trypanosome infections although these are rarely sufficiently severe as to be life threatening. Minor hemorrhage and multiple petechiae are frequently observed in human sleeping sickness although severe gastrointestinal hemorrhage, associated with a low platelet count, was the cause of death in one patient with Rhodesiense sleeping sickness.[3,60,61] Likewise, focal hemorrhages in various organs have been described in experimental infections in laboratory animals and livestock (for review see Section IV.D), and prolonged bleeding times are frequently observed during infection.[62]

Four major hemostatic factors appear to be involved in the pathology of trypanosomiasis: vascular injury, coagulopathy with increased fibrinolysis, and thrombocytopenia.

A. Vascular Injury

Vasculopathy, readily recognized and manifested by petechiae and leakage of fluid and protein into extravascular spaces, is particularly noticeable in infections with the *T. brucei* subgroup trypanosomes as a result of their predilection for connective tissue.[63] In experimental *T. brucei* infections of rabbits, for example, endothelial cells become swollen and endothelial gaps appear.[63,64] Collections of platelets and circulating leukocytes cause occlusions and the blood vessels finally disintegrate.[63] It has been suggested that the cause of these vascular changes are brought about by the release of pharmacologically active substances. Vascular injury, however, has not been described as a feature of the human disease.

B. Coagulopathy

Over the past 10 years the role of abnormalities in coagulation and fibrinolysis in the pathogenesis of African trypanosomiasis has become apparent as a result of comprehensive analysis of this compartment in both experimental and natural infections. The identification of the causes of coagulopathy and abnormal hemostasis is necessary since it may indicate useful methods for therapy in the acute infection. The general consensus among hematologists is that mild to moderate consumption coagulopathy with disseminated intravascular coagulation (DIC) occurs in the acute disease only. Thus, the overall view combining histological and laboratory test data indicates that widespread intravascular coagulation with associated primary fibrino(geno)lysis and secondary fibrinolysis is an important mediator in the pathology of the acute phase of the disease. However, consideration of the importance of coagulation in the pathology may reflect differences in the relative dynamics of coagulation between different host species.[65] For example, clotting is very rapid in the domestic pig and this may explain why widespread intravascular coagulation is the dominant feature in the pathogenesis of *T. simaie* infection in pigs.[66-68]

1. Disseminated Intravascular Coagulation (DIC)

The contribution of DIC (also known as consumption coagulopathy or defibrination syndrome) to the pathophysiology of trypanosomiasis has attracted considerable attention in recent years. Thus, the thrombosis, hemorrhage, tissue necrosis, and microangiopathic anemia found in the acute disease has been attributed to this condition. DIC is a dynamic pathological process triggered by activation of the clotting cascade and can be manifest as a wide clinical spectrum.[69] For example, if the intravascular coagulation process is dominant and secondary fibrino(geno)lysis minimal, DIC may be expressed primarily as diffuse thrombosis. Alternatively, if the secondary fibrinolysis which occurs with DIC is dominant and the drive toward procoagulant activity minimal, then hemorrhage will result. In trypanosomiasis a wide spectrum of findings demonstrating combinations of these two clinical manifestations of DIC has been described using both histological and laboratory tests of hemostasis.

a. Histological Evidence for DIC

Various investigations into the histopathology of natural and experimental trypanosomiasis record the presence of microthrombi in various organs. Of frequent occurrence are microthrombi within capillary loops of the glomerulus and vessels within the brain, liver, lungs, heart, and plexus pampiniformis of the testes.[50,52,68,70-77] In most cases the thrombi were mixed, composed of platelets, fibrin, trypanosomes, and some monocytoid cells.

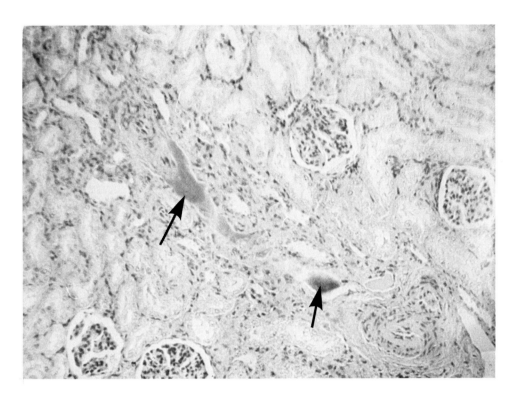

FIGURE 2. Fibrin microthrombus (arrowed) occluding a renal tubule vessel from a calf infected with *T. vivax*. (MSB stain; magnification × 100.)

It is notable that all observations of microthrombus formation report a high parasitemia in infected animals. For example, the basic histological lesion in mice with an acute *T. vivax* infection lasting 8 days was shown to be generalized fibrin thrombus formation in the heart, lung, spleen, and brain, the development of which correlated with increasing parasitemia.[78] Infections with *T. vivax* in other host species produces a similar pathology. Thus, in infected goats intravascular coagulation is a predominant feature of the disease.[72,77,79] Both acute and chronic forms of the disease occur in *T. vivax* infections in goats. The main difference between the two forms seems to be the presence of thrombus formation in the acute disease directly related to the high parasitemia. The thrombosis results in ischemia which could explain the hemorrhages and necrotic changes found in several organs in infected animals. Similarly, in calves with experimental *T. vivax* infections widespread microthrombus formation (Figure 2) occurred.[80,81]

b. Laboratory Diagnosis of DIC in Trypanosomiasis

Supporting evidence for intravascular coagulopathy in trypanosomiasis also comes from the results of sequential clotting screening tests made during infection which indicate defects in the extrinsic and intrinsic coagulation pathways. The criteria for the diagnosis of DIC are not well defined and there is considerable variability in laboratory findings. These depend first on the severity of the condition and second on other complicating factors involving the disease (hepatic dysfunction will also reduce factor V and antithrombin III levels). As a result, DIC may be decompensated, compensated, or overcompensated. However, it is generally agreed that a combination of the laboratory findings listed in Table 2 are diagnostic of DIC. The observations of these features in acute trypanosomiasis are also listed in Table 2.

Table 2
LABORATORY FINDINGS DIAGNOSTIC OF DIC AND PRESENT IN ACUTE TRYPANOSOMIASIS

Laboratory diagnosis of DIC	Observation in acute trypanosomiasis
The APTT and PT are prolonged in acute DIC	APTT prolonged; PT normal or occasionally prolonged
Fibrinogen usually low, may be raised in infection as an acute phase reactant	Usually raised
Platelet count is low and platelet survival reduced	Yes
Thrombin time is prolonged	Yes
High levels of FDPs in serum, occasionally in urine; may result from primary fibrinolysis	Frequently raised
Factor V and factor VIII-C activity reduced (former reduced in hepatic dysfunction)	Yes
Decreased plasminogen	Yes
Presence of fibrinopeptide-A in serum	N/M[a]
Presence of circulating fibrin monomer	Yes
Presence of a double-D-dimer degradation product	N/M[a]
Decreased T50 fibrinogen survival	Yes

[a] N/M = not measured.

It was a chance observation that the activated partial thromboplastin time test (APTT) was grossly abnormal in a psychiatric patient whose disease was subsequently shown to be due to infection with *T. gambiense*.[82] On treatment the APTT returned to normal. The APTT is a screening test for the intrinsic pathway of coagulation and, therefore, measures the adequacy of factors VIII-C, IX, XI, and XII as well as factors V and X which are common to both the intrinsic and extrinsic pathways. Unfortunately, the prothrombin time (PT), a measure of the extrinsic system (factor VII) as well as factors common to both systems (factors X, V, prothrombin, and fibrinogen) was not performed. Prolongation of clotting times beyond those of normal "control" plasma in the test system will indicate a deficiency either as a result of inadequate production (as in liver disease) or excessive utilization of clotting factors. It is unlikely that impairment of liver function is responsible for the coagulation abnormalities since microscopic examination of livers from trypanosome-infected animals has revealed no evidence of cirrhosis and only minimal hepatic abnormalities.[83]

Using various combinations of these laboratory tests, three independent observations of naturally acquired *T. rhodesiense* infections of man implicate DIC as a feature of the disease. One case report on a Caucasian with acute trypanosomiasis lists abnormal coagulation tests on admission with prolonged APTT and PT times, elevated serum fibrin/fibrinogen degradation products (FDPs; see under Fibrinolysis section), decreased plasma fibrinogen, and marked thrombocytopenia.[3] In another study, elevated FDPs and fibrinogen were found in 13 patients with Rhodesiense sleeping sickness.[84] Similarly, three out of four patients with Rhodesiense trypanosomiasis studied by Robins-Browne et al.[61] demonstrated evidence of DIC. In these patients there was a fall in fibrinogen, marked elevation of serum FDP, and decreased factor V and VIII levels, all indicative of consumption coagulopathy. This was confirmed by a shortened ^{125}I-fibrinogen half-life in two of these cases. The third patient had a normal fibrinogen half-life which was attributed to the institution of heparin therapy 1 day prior to the injection of labeled fibrinogen. Following administration of trypanosomal therapy (suramin) all coagulation system abnormalities, except the platelet count which remained low, returned to normal. There was one exception where the coagulation abnormalities actually followed administration of suramin. In this patient DIC may have been precipitated by the lysis of trypanosomes, release of large amounts of soluble antigen, and the subsequent formation of immune complexes.

Intravascular coagulation appears to be a more frequent accompaniment of Rhodesiense than Gambiense sleeping sickness. This may be related to the more marked parasitemia and more acute nature of the Rhodesian form of the disease. Thus, patients with advanced *T. gambiense* infection did not show a significant rise in serum FDPs.[85] Unfortunately, additional coagulation tests were not documented in this study to support the absence of intravascular coagulation.

Since elevated serum FDPs can also arise from primary fibrinolysis (see next section), the laboratory diagnosis of DIC should be supported by evidence that thrombin has cleaved the fibrinogen molecule. This reaction is demonstrated by the presence of fibrin monomer-fibrinogen complexes in plasma using either the protamine sulfate or ethanol paracoagulation tests. Rabbits infected with *T. brucei* gave positive protamine sulfate tests for fibrin monomer indicating that a proportion of the elevated FDPs were as a result of DIC.[84] Similarly, positive tests for fibrin monomer have been obtained in other experimental infections.[62,74,86,87]

Coagulation screening tests in experimental infections in laboratory animals provide a similar picture to the case reports on the human disease. Infected animals have prolonged APTT times and fibrinogen and serum FDPs are elevated.[62,84,88,89] Electron microscopy frequently demonstrates widespread fibrin formation in damaged capillaries, thereby confirming DIC.[64]

Similarly, clotting studies in experimental infections in cattle have also permitted a reliable estimate of the involvement of coagulopathy in the disease caused by *T. congolense*. Acutely infected calves, with high parasitemias, had a consistent prolongation of the APTT although this was not apparent in chronic infections with *T. congolense* TREU 112 despite hypofibrinogenemia and shortened fibrinogen half-life.[87,88]

In horses, goats, and sheep experimentally infected with *T. brucei* or *T. congolense*, the APTT was found to be regularly and abnormally prolonged (100 to 300 times) in all animals during infection, although the one-stage PT was normal.[90] In animals which achieved spontaneous cure, the first indication of recovery was the reversion of the APTT to normal. In the absence of data relating to parasitemia in this study, no comment can be made in its relationship to the coagulation abnormalities. An interesting observation was that factor VIII-C, but not factor IX, was significantly elevated suggesting that the defect in the APTT may be a result of coagulation inhibitors rather than factor deficiency. The differentiation between the two in trypanosomiasis is an area which requires further investigation.

The triggering events for DIC in trypanosomiasis are undefined although the contenders are many. The existence of DIC during the acute disease, itself related to a high parasitemia, suggests that trypanosomes or their products act directly or indirectly as initiating factors. In addition, the vast amount of connective and vascular tissue damage that occurs in experimental infections[91] would result in the local release of activator substances into the blood. Other factors might activate the extrinsic coagulation pathway including endothelial injury and antigen-antibody complexes. A hemolytic anemia is a feature of acute trypanosomiasis (see Section II) and a common cause of DIC is intravascular hemolysis. In this situation the release of red cell ADP may initiate the platelet release reaction with generation of platelet factor 3 activity and subsequent activation of coagulation. Additionally, the release of red cell membrane phospholipoprotein during hemolysis may independently initiate the clotting sequence and, perhaps, also, a platelet release reaction.[69]

C. Fibrinolysis

It is the function of the fibrinolytic system to digest intracapillary fibrin deposition following the restoration of hemostasis, a process known as secondary fibrinolysis. Primary fibrinolysis, or fibrinogenolysis, does not occur under normal conditions and usually follows acute episodes of secondary fibrinolysis. The appearance of increased levels of the breakdown products of plasmin digestion of fibrin and fibrinogen (FDPs) in the serum as either "early"

FDP fragments (X and Y) or "late" FDP fragments (D and E) are good indicators of the degree of fibrinolysis.

As mentioned in the previous section, increased serum FDPs have frequently been demonstrated during trypanosome infections. However, detection of FDPs in serum does not differentiate between primary or secondary fibrinolysis. The breakdown of fibrin is a more complex affair and involves the formation of unique fragments including fibrin monomer.[92] The detection of circulating fibrin monomer in trypanosomiasis (as discussed in Section IV.B.1) is evidence for intravascular coagulation followed by secondary fibrinolysis.

Activation of plasminogen to plasmin is the major pathway for the observed increased fibrinolysis in experimental *T. brucei* infections. Thus, the administration of two inhibitors of plasminogen and plasmin, EACA (ε-aminocaproic acid) and Trasylol®, to infected rabbits caused a fall in serum FDPs.[84,89] Both endogenous and exogenous activation of fibrinolysis is likely. First, endogenous activation may occur following the release of known activators (plasma kinase, tissue kinase, and other proteolytic enzymes) which results from tissue damage, particularly, damage to the endothelium which is rich in tissue activator. As previously discussed, widespread vasculopathy is a classical feature of certain experimental trypanosome infections.

Trypanosomes per se have been found to cause exogenous activation of fibrinolysis in an in vitro system.[84] Following the addition of a soluble fraction from a *T. brucei* homogenate to a plasminogen-rich fibrinogen solution, complete fibrinogenolysis occurred over a 24-hr period. EACA only partially inhibited the reaction, suggesting that a trypanosome-derived protease capable of hydrolyzing fibrinogen was present. This was confirmed when Trasylol®, a potent inhibitor of a wide range of proteolytic enzymes, was added. A very marked reduction in fibrinogen proteolysis was apparent (Figure 3). Electrophoretic characteristics of the digests indicated two protein components with the electrophoretic mobility common to those of fragments D and E (Figure 4). Obviously, these in vitro results must be interpreted with caution when extrapolating them to the in vivo situation since antiplasmins in the serum may negate their effect.

Antigen-antibody complexes (either trypanosomal or trypanosome unrelated) are also likely candidates for initiating exogenous activation of plasminogen. Increased serum levels of immune complexes are a feature of trypanosomiasis.[29]

The complex series of events leading to the formation of microthrombi and pathological fibrinolysis are shown diagrammatically in Figure 5. The demonstration of increased serum FDPs is not only important for the diagnosis of DIC and increased fibrinolysis but has important physiopathological implications. For example, the "early" fragments X and Y are powerful inhibitors of blood coagulation having antithrombin effects and promoting ADP-induced platelet aggregation.[93,94] Other effects involve the "late" FDP and relate to potentiation of biogenic amines and peptides, increased vascular permeability, and distinct immunosuppressive activity.[95-97] The latter effect may be a contributory factor to the immunosuppression characteristic of trypanosomiasis.

D. Platelets

A platelet defect, either in number or function, will result in abnormal hemostasis. Thus, in man, if platelet numbers fall below 50×10^9 then petechial hemorrhage, purpura, and abnormal bleeding may occur. In many natural and experimental trypanosome infections, thrombocytopenia and in vivo platelet clumping are characteristic features. For example, decreased platelets have been reported in naturally acquired trypanosomiasis of both the Rhodesian and Gambian types.[3,60,61,85] The cause of the mild thrombocytopenia seen in Gambiense sleeping sickness has been attributed to enhanced activity of the reticuloendothelial system, whereas the severe thrombocytopenia characteristic of *T. rhodesiense* infections probably results from DIC. The cause of death in one patient with Rhodesiense sleeping

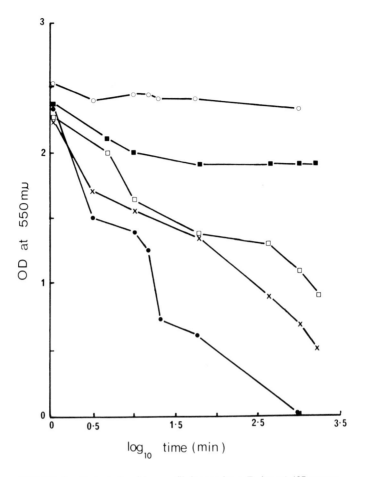

FIGURE 3. Proteolysis of human fibrinogen by a *T. brucei* 427 extract. Fibrinogen concentrations plotted as optical density (OD) at 550 μm. ○—○, Incubation control: buffer + fibrinogen (fbg); ●—●, tryp. extract + fbg; □—□, tryp. extract + fbg + EACA (8 mg/mℓ); ■—■, tryp. extract + fbg + Trasylol® (200 KIU/mℓ); x—x, tryp. extract + fbg + additional thrombin (500 U/mℓ) during clotting process.

sickness was severe gastrointestinal hemorrhage almost certainly precipitated by his extremely low platelet count.[61] Other reports of thrombocytopenia in patients with *T. rhodesiense* infection described minor hemorrhage or the formation of multiple petechiae.[3,60]

Experimental *T. rhodesiense* infections in rhesus monkeys and rats produced a pronounced thrombocytopenia.[62,83,98] Likewise, a decreased platelet count is described as a clinical feature in *T. brucei* infections in rabbits.[99,100] Dogs experimentally infected with *T. congolense* had severe thrombocytopenia which was associated with focal hemorrhages in the brain and "thin, watery blood which failed to clot."[101]

Thrombocytopenia complicating trypanosomiasis is best documented in ruminants. Cattle infected with *T. congolense* had very low platelet levels which were most severe during periods of high parasitemia.[74,86,87,102-104] Petechial hemorrhages were frequently observed in the sclera, nostrils, and visceral organs of acutely infected animals. Curative therapy with antitrypanosomal drugs usually induced a rapid transient rebound thrombocytosis and reestablishment of normal circulatory concentrations of platelets. This picture is also consistent with that of *T. vivax* infections in cattle.[100,103] The severity of the thrombocytopenia was reflected in the development of extramedullary thrombopoiesis in the liver of calves dying

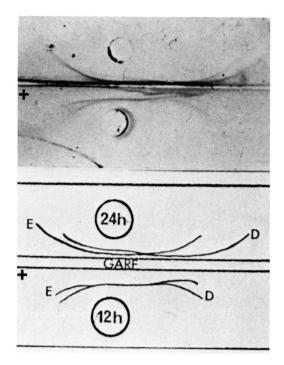

FIGURE 4.   Electrophoresis of fibrinogen following proteolysis with a *T. brucei* homogenate. Upper well: 24-hr digest;
lower well: 12-hr digest; trough: goat antirabbit fibrinogen
(GARF).

with acute trypanosomiasis (Figure 6). An inverse relationship between numbers of trypanosomes and platelets in the peripheral blood is a characteristic feature of chronically infected
animals which had intermittent parasitemia.[74-76]

The etiology of the thrombocytopenia is less well documented. Thrombocytopenia may
result from a failure of platelet production as part of general bone marrow failure, selective
megakaryocyte depression, or ineffective thrombopoiesis, increased platelet destruction, or
the dilutional effect of increased plasma volume. It is becoming apparent that the cause of
the thrombocytopenia in trypanosomiasis is multifactorial and evidence is accumulating
which suggests one or more of the above known cases may operate in the disease (Table
3).

1. Increased Platelet Destruction

Accelerated destruction and consumption of normal or immunologically damaged platelets
by the reticuloendothelial system involves changes in platelet kinetics. Thrombokinetic
studies in trypanosomiasis indicate that both platelet pooling in the enlarged spleen and
excessive removal of platelets from the circulation occurs in the disease. Thus, recovery of
^{51}Cr-labeled platelets after injection (which varies inversely with the size of the splenic
platelet pool) was greatly reduced in patients with Rhodesiense sleeping sickness.[61] Values
for platelet recovery were as low as those reported in patients with congestive splenomegaly.[105] Thus, platelet pooling in the spleen is a major contributor to the thrombocytopenia
of human trypanosomiasis. However, in thrombocytopenic states due only to excessive
pooling of platelets in the spleen, platelet life span is usually normal or near normal.[105] This
was not the case in the patients with sleeping sickness. Platelet life span was significantly
shortened to between 7 and 60% of normal.

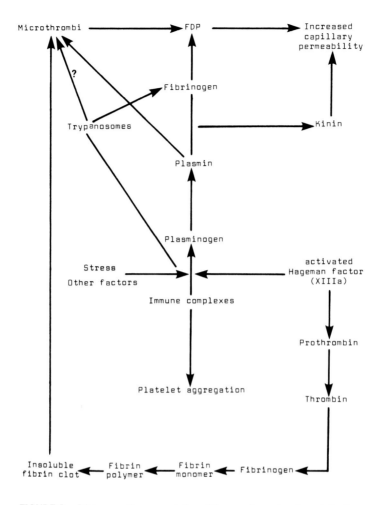

FIGURE 5. Diagrammatic representation of the complex series of events leading to the formation of microthrombi and pathological fibrinolysis in acute trypanosomiasis.

Likewise, in parallel with depressed platelet levels in cattle with *T. congolense*, the half-life of ^{51}Cr-labeled platelets was found to be reduced by 50%.[104] It is of interest that although no determination was made of the contribution of splenic pooling in this study, thrombocytopenia was still observed in splenectomized *T. congolense*-infected cattle.[106] Conflicting evidence for platelet destruction in infected calves was reported earlier although the normal platelet life span was assessed by incorporation of ^{35}S-methionine.[87] Care must be taken in interpreting survival data using ^{35}S-methionine since the period during which this compound remains available for labeling megakaryocytes or platelets is long compared with the mean platelet survival.[107] Thus, a decreased platelet life span may be assessed as normal.

In a recent extensive study into the pathogenesis of thrombocytopenia in experimental trypanosomiasis, platelet kinetics have been carefully investigated using the radioisotope [111]Indium (^{111}In) complexed to 8-hydroxyquinoline (oxine).[100] The availability of this isotope is relatively new and has recently been recognized as the best and most accurate technique for determining platelet life span since there is minimal release, elution, and reutilization of the ^{111}In label.[108] Calf platelets were labeled with ^{111}In and the pre- and postinfection (with *T. vivax*) survival data fitted to a multiple hit model. Estimations of the life span using this technique support earlier findings of significant peripheral destruction of platelets (Table

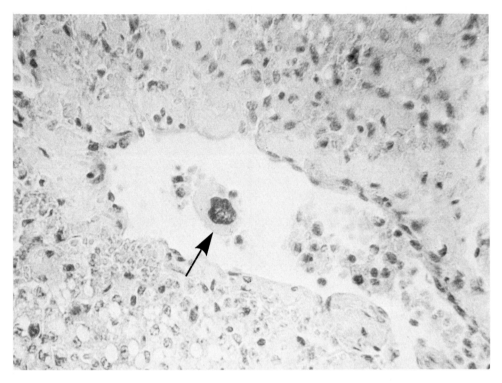

FIGURE 6.   Extramedullary erythropoiesis in the liver of a calf infected with *T. vivax*. Arrow indicates the megakaryocyte. (Magnification × 250.)

Table 3
CAUSES OF THROMBOCYTOPENIA IN TRYPANOSOMIASIS

Increased destruction of platelets
    Disseminated intravascular coagulation
    Antiplatelet antibodies (?)
    Type II-mediated hypersensitivity
    Type III immune complex-mediated hypersensitivity
    Direct damage (activation) by trypanosomes
    Nonspecific as a result of hyperplasia and increased RE activity

Failure of platelet production
    Ineffective thrombopoiesis

Abnormal distribution of platelets
    Splenomegaly

Dilution loss
    Increased plasma volume

4). The same platelet labeling technique was also applied to study thrombokinetics in rabbits infected with *T. brucei*. Platelet life span was reduced again by approximately 50% and the timing coincided with a high parasitemia. A useful feature of ^{111}In is that it enables in vivo accumulations of labeled platelets to be visualized using a gamma camera, thereby indicating the sites of platelet destruction. The scintigraphic distribution of platelets showed that significant destruction of platelets occurred in the spleen of infected animals.

The cause of the shortened platelet life span in both human and animal trypanosomiasis is unknown, but various mechanisms have been proposed as listed in Table 3. Consumption

Table 4
PLATELET LIFE SPAN IN CALVES
INFECTED WITH *T. VIVAX* 64/23 AND
RABBITS WITH *T. BRUCEI* S42

	Infected			
	Preinfection	Week 1	Week 4	After Berenil (days)
Calf No.[a]				
1	3.02	1.08	N/D	[b]
2	2.92	1.92	N/D	4.38 (4)
3	3.49	2.61	N/D	4.16 (22)
Rabbit No.[a]				
1	2.01	1.64	[b]	N/D
2	2.40	N/D	0.96	N/D
3	2.39	1.98	1.24	N/D

Note: Life span was assessed using a multiple hit model; N/D = not done.

[a] Differences between preinfection infected, and post-Berenil values significant $p < 0.05$.

[b] Animal died.

of platelets in DIC is probably most important in the acute disease when other features of DIC are present as discussed previously. It is also possible that autoantibodies to specific antigens on platelets may be produced, but this has not been confirmed in the one study to date.[61]

The reduced red cell life span described in patients with trypanosomiasis and experimental bovine trypanosomiasis has been attributed to immune hemolysis resulting from either a type II (absorption of trypanosomal antigens onto red cells) or type III (immune complex) cytotoxic hypersensitivity as specified by Coombs and Gell.[26,28,109] The decreased platelet life span could similarly be mediated by complement fixing immune complexes. In fact, immune complexes are known to cause platelet aggregation in vitro and have become a recognizable cause of thrombocytopenia in disease states.[110-112] The high levels of antigen-antibody complexes found in trypanosomiasis may be mediators of platelet destruction by binding to platelets via the platelet Fc or C3b receptor. This mechanism of immune damage is considered very likely since severe thrombocytopenia occurs during or just after a parasitemic peak.[103] Confirmatory evidence for this suggestion comes from studies on goats and cattle infected with *T. vivax*.[75,93] There was a good correlation in the disease between numbers of *T. vivax* in the peripheral blood, platelet aggregation, and blood serotonin release. Mixtures of *T. vivax* with plasma containing *T. vivax* antibodies induced the release of ^{14}C-serotonin from prelabeled goat platelets in vitro.[113] Furthermore, in vivo studies showed that immunization of endotoxin-tolerant rabbits with a lyophilized preparation of *T. brucei* caused a rise in body temperature accompanied by a decrease in blood serotonin level related to the formation of trypanosome antigen-antibody immune complexes during this immunization procedure. These results indicate that the formation of circulating antigen-antibody complexes plays an important role in the pathogenesis of the febrile response, thrombocytopenia, and the decrease in whole blood serotonin levels during the acute phase of trypanosomiasis.

The suggestion that trypanosomes per se be mediators of the thrombocytopenia also arose from the correlation of low platelet numbers with an increasing parasitemia. It has been claimed that living *T. rhodesiense* or a supernatant from lysed trypanosome induced rat platelet aggregation in vitro, although the involvement of immune complexes in these studies cannot be excluded.[98] Subsequent studies using *T. gambiense* with human and rat platelets *T. vivax* and *T. brucei* with goat platelets, and *T. brucei* with rabbit platelets have been unable to reproduce these observations.[85,100,113] Whether the ability to induce platelet aggregation reflects a specific biological characteristic of *T. rhodesiense* requires further study.

2. Failure of Platelet Production

One study has indicated ineffective thrombopoiesis as the cause of thrombocytopenia in bovine trypanosomiasis.[87] Ineffective platelet production from normal or increased numbers of megakaryocytes is normally a feature of megaloblastic anemias in man. The suggestion that this may be the mechanism of decreased platelets in *T. congolense* infections in calves arose from the finding of a normal platelet life span (using ^{35}S-methionine as a label — see earlier discussion) and five times as many megakaryocytes per area of marrow which were also larger than normal.[87] However, this latter observation might be expected since mega-karyocytosis is stimulated by thrombocytopenia as a result of an increase in thrombopoietin levels and this is accompanied by macrocytosis.[114] The increased number of megakaryocytes per unit area of marrow does indicate, however, that the stem cell input was increased and, therefore, was not the limiting factor in the reduction of circulating platelets. One abnormal histological feature noted was an increase in megakaryocyte nuclear size without increased cytoplasmic diameter, which the authors considered suggestive of dysthrombopoiesis or inadequate maturation of megakaryocytes. However, the rapid recovery of peripheral platelet number, usually wthin 24 hr following trypanosomal chemotherapy (which has frequently been recorded), does not support a defect in thrombopoiesis which might be expected to take longer than this to recover. Obviously, more work investigating bone marrow platelet turnover is needed.

3. Splenic Pooling

The rebound thrombocytosis following chemotherapy and the concurrent return of normal platelet function (see below) is an interesting observation with at least two explanations. First, there may be rapid maturation of the large numbers of bone marrow megakaryocytes and release of platelets into the circulation. This possibility could be determined by making a histological examination of the bone marrow following chemotherapy. The second consideration is the splenic pooling effect. Normally, platelets in the general circulation exchange freely with a "reservoir", a "pool" of platelets in the splenic circulation which accounts for about one third of the platelet numbers. In splenomegaly, the fraction of the exchangeable pool increases and may represent the bulk, e.g., 90% of the marrow output. Splenic pooling in the enlarged spleen was found to be the main cause of the thrombocytopenia in Rhodesiense sleeping sickness.[61] Following treatment these platelets may be suddenly released into the circulation. It would be of interest to see if rebound thrombocytosis occurred in splenectomized infected animals following antitrypanosomal chemotherapy.

E. Platelet Function

This is an area in the hematology of trypanosomiasis which has only recently received attention. A moderate thrombocytopenia may have equally important pathophysiological effects as severe thrombocytopenia if those platelets are already activated and are not functioning adequately. One technique used for assessing congenital and acquired abnormalities of platelet function is the measurement of platelet aggregation monitored in an aggregometer. Studies in our laboratory indicate a rapid development of abnormal platelet function in bovine. (*T. vivax*) trypanosomiasis.[100] When compared to platelets taken from normal non-infected calves, "infected" platelets showed minimal aggregation responses to both collagen and ADP by the seventh day of infection (Figure 7). Two weeks after infection platelets taken from infected animals showed no response to any of the aggregating agents. Following treatment with Berenil, all trypanosomes disappeared from the blood within 24 hr and platelet aggregation responses returned to normal. The cause of the complete loss of platelet function is not known. The presence of inhibitors or activators of platelet function must be considered. Trypanosomes may be producing substances directly inhibiting aggregation. C-reactive protein (CRP), an acute phase-reactant protein found in the serum in increasing levels in trypanosome infections, has been shown to inhibit many platelet reactivities such as inhibition of aggregation induced by collagen, ADP, immunoglobulin, thrombin, and adrenalin.[115,116] Another consideration is that trypanosomes or trypanosome antigen-antibody complexes may activate platelets, thereby, releasing their active agents so that they can no longer reaggregate. This possibility is supported by electronmicrographs showing that peripheral platelets taken from infected animals are activated (Figure 8) and peripheral blood films showing large platelet clumps (unpublished observations).

Platelet aggregation or clumping in vivo is frequently observed in trypanosomiasis. The aggregation in vivo was accompanied by a thrombocytopenia and reduced blood serotonin levels in goats and cattle infected with *T. vivax*.[73,74] An attempt was made to inhibit platelet aggregation in infected animals using the nonsteroidal anti-inflammatory agent flurbiprofen.[76] Intraplatelet levels of cyclic AMP and platelet prostaglandin synthesis are central factors involved in platelet aggregation in vitro.[117] Flurbiprofen is a potent inhibitor of prostaglandin synthesis and blocks the fomation of both PGI_2 and TXA_2 (thromboxane A_2). It is, therefore, capable of inhibiting platelet aggregation induced by ADP, collagen, and adrenalin and also blocks serotonin release from human platelets.[118,119] But administration of this drug to infected goats did not block either platelet aggregation or serotonin release. However, the failure to block prostaglandin synthesis in this study may be related to the fact that a prostaglandin-mediated pathway for aggregation may not operate in goat platelets since malondialdehyde (MDA), one product of the cyclo-oxygenase system of platelets, is not produced in this species.

Antibodies to thymocytes and β_2-microglobulin have also been shown to cause activation of human platelets.[120] Autoantibodies to thymocytes have been described in murine trypanosomiasis and, thus, are possible contenders for platelet activation in the disease.[121]

Defects in platelet storage pool and release in trypanosomiasis need to be examined using labeled adenine nucleotides and serotonin. Whatever the cause of the platelet dysfunction it is certain that the pathological result will be abnormal hemostasis and bleeding as described earlier.

V. HEMORHEOLOGY

Alterations in the viscosity of blood play an important role in governing microcirculatory function. The hyperviscosity syndrome (HVS), as described by Fahey et al.,[122] is commonly linked with those diseases involving abnormal plasma protein synthesis such as IgA or IgG myeloma and both primary and secondary macroglobulinemia.[123] In addition, peripheral vascular disease typified by an increase in plasma macromolecules, such as fibrinogen and lipoproteins, is associated with blood hyperviscosity.[124] Decreased cell deformability may also cause a rise in whole blood viscosity.[123]

Many of the above determinants of blood viscosity are raised during natural and experimental infections with pathogenic trypanosomes. Thus, a characteristic feature of the humoral immune response with African trypanosomes is the marked IgM production with an

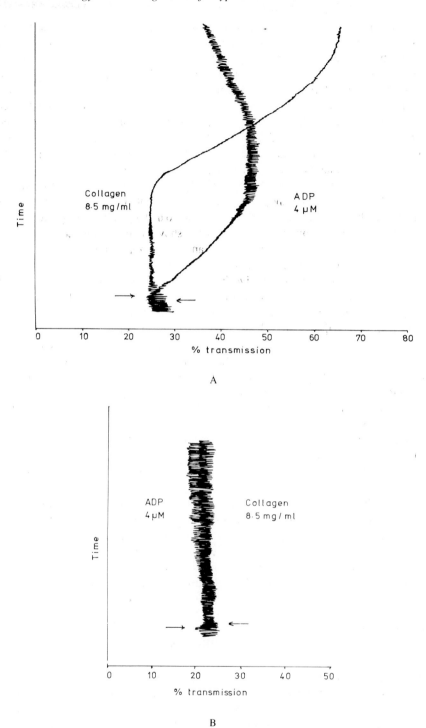

FIGURE 7. (A)   Aggregation response of normal calf platelets to collagen and ADP; (B) platelets taken from a calf 2 weeks after infection with *T. vivax* fails to aggregate when exposed to ADP or collagen.

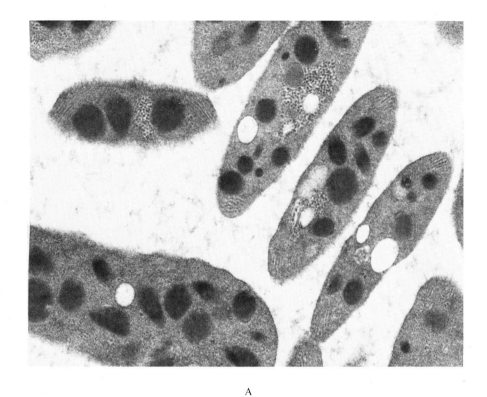

A

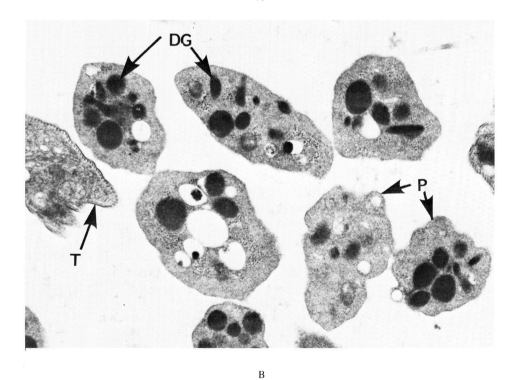

B

FIGURE 8. Electronmicrographs of platelets taken from a normal calf (A) and from a calf 2 weeks after infection with *T. vivax* (B). "Infected" platelets show features typical of activated platelets, namely, shape change (become more rounded), increased pseudopodia (P), and a decrease in the number of dense granules (DG). A trypanosome (T) is also seen in this section. (Magnification (A) × 42,000; (B) × 12,000.)

accompanying but lesser increase in IgG. The diagnosis of macroglobulinemia is based upon the demonstration of serum IgM (19S IgM) in excess of five times the normal level.[122] In trypanosomiasis numerous reports indicate an increase in IgM 8 to 16 times the normal level.[125] Complicating the macroglobulinemia is an increase in other large molecular weight proteins such as fibrinogen and lipoproteins.[84,126] Although a considerable amount of effort has gone into detailing concentrations, specificity, and causes of the high serum IgM, little attention has been given to the hematological consequences of such a vast amount of macroglobulin in the circulation. The blood proteins influence important biophysical characteristics of circulating blood such as suspension stability, osmotic pressure, and viscosity, and changes in these properties, in turn, affect the rate of blood flow, caliber of the small vessels, and permeability through vessel walls.

A study in experimental *T. brucei* infections in rabbits has indicated that the changes in peripheral blood proteins during the disease have a profound effect on blood viscosity. A rise in whole blood viscosity occurred within the first week of infection, and after 3 weeks this had reached a peak with a 33% increase above normal.[84,127] Plasma and serum viscosity reflected the same pattern of increase with the exception that the percentage increase was considerably higher (60% above normal). The relatively smaller increase in whole blood viscosity was attributed to the concurrent anemia, since the hematocrit is an important determinant of whole blood viscosity. The etiology of the elevated blood viscosity was investigated and found to be related to a combination of the high fibrinogen and globulin levels.[127] Attempts were made to differentiate the contribution of these two to the increased viscosity. First, in vitro defibrination of infected plasma resulted in a slight fall in the viscosity, indicating that although fibrinogen was an important determinant of the viscosity, it was not a major one. This was confirmed in vivo by the administration of the drug Clofibrate (ethyl-p-chlorophenoxyisobutyrate or Atromid-S®) to infected rabbits. This drug has gained widespread attention as an effective agent for lowering both a raised fibrinogen level and blood lipids.[128,129] Clofibrate, administered to rabbits prior to and during infection with trypanosomes, prevented the rise in fibrinogen and lipid levels and, at the same time, reduced blood viscosity, although the viscosity still remained significantly above normal.[130]

It is, therefore, certain that the increased serum IgM is the major determinant of hyperviscosity in trypanosomiasis. Supportive evidence for this suggestion comes from the observation of maximal levels of IgM 3 weeks after infection coinciding with the peak of whole blood, serum, and plasma viscosity.[131]

The contribution of blood hyperviscosity to the pathology of trypanosomiasis must be considered. The primary effect will be a decrease in blood flow. There is now direct evidence linking hemorheological abnormalities to the development of thrombosis where an increase in whole blood viscosity, by slowing blood flow velocity, may play a primary etiological role.[132] A 10 to 30% increase in blood viscosity results in a 20 to 60% decrease in blood flow.[124] Following the onset of reduced or stagnant blood flow, adverse effects of tissue perfusion and oxygenation would be expected. A vicious circle of events may be set up between ischemia and decreased red cell deformability (caused by anoxia) which, in turn, produces microcirculatory stagnation and the development of macrothrombi. Such events probably contribute to the significant vascular degeneration observed in trypanosomiasis.[63,64]

The clinical features described during experimental rabbit trypanosomiasis which could be attributed to hyperviscosity have also been described in human and bovine trypanosomiasis. Many other symptoms seen in patients with macroglobulinemia, such as headache, dizziness, dysequilibria, and motor weakness, are typical of human trypanosomiasis. Further work needs to be carried out on the importance of blood viscosity in sleeping sickness, since, if the rheological picture is similar to that described above, then various treatments such as plasmapheresis might be indicated to help alleviate the symptoms.

Table 5
SUMMARY OF THE BONE MARROW HEMOPOIETIC RESPONSE IN TRYPANOSOMIASIS

	Early infection	Late infection normally following the first parasitemic peak
Erythropoiesis	Increased which compensates for red cell loss	Increased but ineffective and does not compensate. The cause probably results from a failure of Fe incorporation into hemoglobin as a result of Fe trapping in the RE system
Myelopoiesis	Increased which is compensatory	Decreased with maturation arrest resulting in leukopenia. Two causes: (1) increased erythropoiesis possible at the expense of myelopoiesis; (2) inhibition factor(s) in the serum (antitrypanosome antibodies and/or lymphokines)
Megakaryopoiesis	Increased	Increased but possibility of maturation arrest

VI. THE BONE MARROW IN TRYPANOSOMIASIS

A limited number of detailed observations have been made on the bone marrow in animal trypanosomiasis and none in the human disease. However, it is clear from the reports available that the bone marrow becomes markedly hyperplastic during the course of infection in both experimental infections of laboratory animals and ruminants.[8,71,73,74,77,103,133] The following discussion relates to changes during trypanosomiasis in the three lines of hemopoiesis, viz. erythropoiesis, myelopoiesis, and megakaryopoiesis. A summary of these events is shown in Table 5.

A. Erythropoiesis

An active erythropoietic response by the bone marrow might be expected in response to the ongoing hemolytic anemia (see section on Anemia). Thus, the data available indicate that shortly after infection, when the animal shows a high parasitemia and concomitant accelerated red cell destruction, an increased bone marrow erythropoiesis results. However, as the infection progresses, this does not adequately compensate for the red cell loss and the host becomes severely anemic. Even so, it must be remembered that even in the normal marrow, erythropoiesis is not entirely efficient since about 10 to 15% of erythropoiesis is ineffective, i.e., the developing erythroblasts die within the marrow.[134] This ineffective erythropoiesis is substantially increased in a number of chronic anemias, for example, megaloblastic anemias.

Various tests can be performed to assess both total erythropoiesis (the myeloid to erythroid [M:E] ratio and plasma iron turnover) and effective erythropoiesis (^{59}Fe incorporation into red cells). Both have been applied to the study of erythropoiesis during trypanosomiasis. In a recent detailed study of the hemopoietic response in *T. brucei* infections in rabbits, sequential bone marrows taken throughout infection showed a progressive increased cellularity which was apparent 1 week after infection.[9] The fatty marrow, comprising approximately 50% of the total marrow in normal noninfected animals, was gradually replaced by hemopoietic marrow until by 3 weeks postinfection, few fat spaces were visible and the marrow was packed with cells. The M:E ratio, that is, the proportion of granulocyte precursors to red cell precursors in the bone marrow (normally 2:1 to 12:1), was calculated. Within 1 week of infection the M:E ratio increased indicating selective myelopoiesis predominantly as a result of increased mononuclear cells (Figure 9). However, as the infection progressed there was a rapid reversal in the M:E ratio indicating a selective increase in total

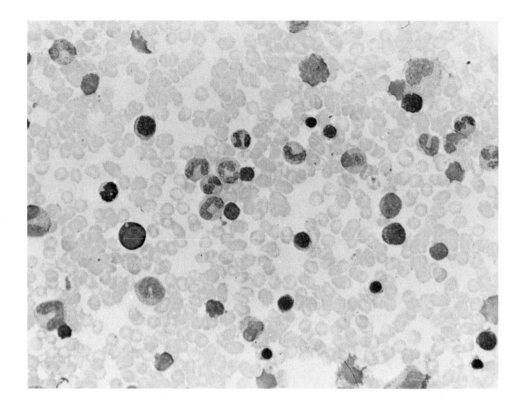

A

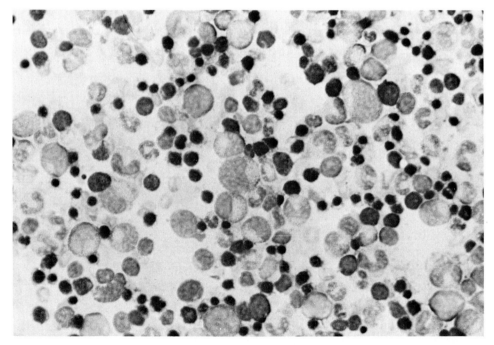

B

FIGURE 9.   Bone marrow taken from the femoral shaft of a normal rabbit (A) and from a rabbit 24 days after infection with *T. brucei* S42 (B). The "infected" marrow shows considerable erythropoiesis and marked myelopoiesis.

erythropoiesis during this period, presumably in response to the ongoing peripheral hemolysis. This marked erythropoietic activity has also been noted in trypanosomiasis in goats, monkeys, and cattle.[8,71,74,77,83]

Interesting observations have come from the extensive studies on the pathology of bovine trypanosomiasis caused by *T. vivax* and *T. congolense*.[103] The first peak of parasitemia was closely associated with the development of pancytopenia, i.e., anemia, leukopenia, and thrombocytopenia. This was accompanied by a reduced M:E ratio and macrocytosis which was more marked in the *T. congolense* group indicating a more vigorous marrow erythroid response in these animals. Nevertheless, the erythron could not be returned to normal levels which implies more marked ongoing red cell destruction in the *T. congolense* infection. Furthermore, the initial leukopenia common to both infected groups became very severe in the *T. congolense* group, whereas animals in the *T. vivax* group were apparently able to increase hemopoiesis sufficiently to maintain normal leukocyte concentrations. The persistently depressed leukocyte count in the *T. congolense* group may have resulted from increasing demands on the bone marrow for erythropoiesis leaving only a small population of stem cells available for granulopoiesis. This suggestion is supported by the greater reduction in the M:E ratio in the *T. congolense* group. Alternatively, the findings might be explained by inhibition of granulopoiesis (see later).

The kinetics of erythropoiesis have been extensively studied in the bovine with experimental *T. congolense* infections.[2,12,135] However, between them the studies disagreed on the relative importance of hemodilution and dyshemopoiesis in long-standing infections. In view of these differences of opinion further erythrokinetic studies were carried out on *T. congolense*-infected N'Dama and Zebu cattle.[13,53] Judging from the rates of plasma iron turnover and red cell iron utilization early in infection, erythropoiesis was enhanced and there was no evidence of overt dyshemopoiesis. Later in the disease, in most cases red cell synthesis was less than expected from the degree of anemia, suggesting impairment of bone marrow function. Measurement of red cell iron utilization indicated this was the case and that it resulted from defective iron reutilization from degraded red cells arising from reticuloendothelial blockade. The extent of total erythropoiesis, as measured by the rate of removal of transferrin-bound iron from the plasma, was increased two to three times the normal rate suggesting a two- to threefold expansion of erythropoiesis. The effectiveness of this response was determined by calculating radioactive iron incorporation into circulating red cells. The percentage incorporation was reduced indicating diminished or ineffective erythropoiesis. Thus, these ferrokinetic studies suggest defective iron metabolism with iron retention and trapping in the mononuclear phagocytic system, as the cause of ineffective erythropoiesis. In such a situation the bone marrow becomes effectively starved of iron, a situation kinetically analogous to the anemias of chronic disorders in man.[56] The possibility of depressed erythropoietin levels in trypanosome infections, as recently shown to occur in malaria, has not been considered and should be investigated in light of the above observations.[136]

That red cell synthesis was less than expected in infected cattle in relation to the number of red cells being removed may relate to the reduced erythropoietic capacity in the bovine when compared to other species. It is known, for example, that cattle are slow in mobilizing their stem cell pool and any limitation in proliferative potential would be most critical when there is simultaneous stress on the myeloid and erythroid systems as in trypanosomiasis.[137] In a series of experiments, Lawson et al.[138] have used in vitro bone marrow techniques to determine whether the pancytopenia of bovine trypanosomiasis is due to a reduction in stem cell numbers or depressed differentiation. No reduction in the number of erythroid colonies (CFU-E) produced was found and the degree of maturation was decreased in only 2 out of 12 animals. Search for erythroid inhibitors in the sera of cattle infected with *T. congolense* or *T. vivax* proved negative and, surprisingly, sonicated *T. brucei*, *T. congolense*, and *T. theileri* actually stimulated bovine CFU-E colonies in vitro, sometimes resulting in a 20-fold increase in colony formation.[139,140]

B. Myelopoiesis

Leukopenia and a shift to the left in the differential count is a characteristic feature of African trypanosomiasis. There is no concensus of opinion on the pathogenesis of the leukopenia but it is believed to result from a combination of increased peripheral utilization, leukophagocytosis, and increased bone marrow erythropoiesis at the expense of leukopoiesis.[5,10,51]

However, more recent evidence indicates that there is significant inhibition of myelopoiesis in the bone marrow. When bone marrow taken from *T. congolense*-infected calves was grown in vitro in the presence of colony stimulating factor, there was a marked decrease in the number of myeloid colonies (CFC-C) produced compared to normal marrows.[139] Furthermore, serum collected from infected cattle inhibited the bovine granulocyte/macrophage colony formation in vitro with maximum inhibition caused by serum collected 2 to 3 weeks postinfection. The degree of inhibition was related to the degree of parasitemia. An attempt to characterize the inhibitory factor or factors in serum showed that a globulin with a molecular weight of between 100,000 and 200,000 daltons could inhibit CFU-C colony formation.[140] It was suggested that in bovine trypanosomiasis, the granulocyte/macrophage progenitor cells might adsorb trypanosomal antigen and, subsequently, be injured by anti-trypanosomal antibody. An alternative explanation is that a lymphokine, produced by lymphocytes present in the marrow cultures, was causing inhibition of myeloid colony formation. T cells have been shown to play an important role in the regulation of hemopoiesis. For example, purified T lymphocytes derived from the marrow or peripheral blood of patients with severe aplastic anemia inhibit colony growth in vitro and the CFC-C suppressive effect is restricted to T cells with receptors for the Fc of IgG (T_G cells). The supernatant of T_G cells from normal individuals fails to have suppressor activity unless mitogen stimulated. Trypanosomal products can act as mitogens.[142] However, the contribution of mitogen stimulation of T_G cells in the suppression of myeloid colony formation in trypanosomiasis is unlikely since neither *T. brucei, T. congolense,* or *T. theileri,* when added directly to cultures, had any effect on depressing CFC-C formation.[140]

C. Megakaryopoiesis

A normal or increased bone marrow megakaryocyte population is the usual observation in trypanosomiasis.[8,77,83,87,103] However, maturation arrest of megakaryocytes may be a feature of certain infections as deduced from an increase in nuclear size without increased cytoplasmic diameter.[87]

D. Extramedullary Hemopoiesis

Compensatory extramedullary hemopoiesis, whereby the liver and spleen resume their fetal hemopoietic role, has frequently been observed in experimental infections. Thus, the stimulus for increased erythropoiesis and megakaryopoiesis to compensate for the increased red cell and platelet destruction, respectively, has been observed in trypanosomiasis in cattle (Figure 6), in goats, and in rabbits.[8,9,73,74,77,80]

VII. BLOOD TRANSFUSION

There are few reported incidents of transfusion-induced African trypanosomiasis. One report describes a Zambian child contracting a *T. rhodesiense* infection following a blood transfusion.[143] The donors were traced and found to be asymptomatic carriers of the disease. It has now been confirmed that a small proportion of persons harboring *T. rhodesiense* may be clinically asymptomatic for a considerable period after acquiring the infection. Obviously, better screening facilities for potential donors are required.

Congenital trypanosomiasis, due to transplacental infection by both *T. rhodesiense* and *T. gambiense,* has been described.[144,145]

It would appear that there is no link between the susceptibility to trypanosomiasis and the host blood group status. Thus, ABO blood group status in man showed no association with susceptibility to infection with *T. rhodesiense*.[146] Likewise, the level of parasitemia in experimental *T. congolense* infections was not influenced by bovine J blood group antigens.[147]

REFERENCES

1. **Obi, T. U. and Anosa, V. O.,** Haematological studies on domestic animals in Nigeria. IV. Clinico-haematological features of bovine trypanosomiasis, theileriosis, anaplasmosis, eperythrozoonosis and helminthiasis, *Zentralbl. Veterinaermed., Reihe B.,* 27, 789, 1980.
2. **Mamo, E. and Holmes, P. H.,** The erythrokinetics of Zebu cattle chronically infected with *Trypanosoma congolense, Res. Vet. Sci.,* 18, 105, 1975.
3. **Barrett-Connor, E., Ugoretz, R. J., and Braude, A. I.,** Disseminated intravascular coagulation in trypanosomiasis, *Arch. Int. Med.,* 131, 574, 1973.
4. **Jenkins, G. C., McCrorie, P., Forsberg, C. M., and Brown, J. L.,** Studies on the anaemia in rabbits infected with *Trypanosoma brucei.* I. Evidence for haemolysis, *J. Comp. Pathol.,* 90, 107, 1980.
5. **Mackenzie, P. K. I. and Cruickshank, J. G.,** Phagocytosis of erythrocytes and leucocytes in sheep infected with *Trypanosoma congolense, Res. Vet. Sci.,* 15, 256, 1973.
6. **Jennings, F. W., Murray, P. K., Murray, M., and Urquhart, G. M.,** Anaemia in trypanosomiasis: studies in rats and mice infected with *Trypanosoma brucei, Res. Vet. Sci.,* 16, 70, 1974.
7. **Murray, M. and Morrison, W. I.,** Pathogenesis and pathology of African trypanosomiasis, in FAO Appendix VIII, Report on the Expert Committee on Research in Trypanosomiasis, Food and Agriculture Organization, Rome, 1979, 70.
8. **Saror, D. I.,** Observations on the course and pathology of *Trypanosoma vivax* in Red Sokoto goats, *Res. Vet. Sci.,* 28, 36, 1980.
9. **Colvin, B. E., McCrorie, P., Facer, C. A., Revell, P., and Jenkins, G. C.,** in preparation.
10. **Valli, V. E. O., Forsberg, C. M., and Robinson, G. A.,** The pathogenesis of *Trypanosoma congolense* in calves. II. Anaemia and erythroid response, *Vet. Pathol.,* 16, 96, 1979.
11. **Anosa, V. O. and Isoun, T. T.,** Haematological studies on *Trypanosoma vivax* infection of goats and intact and splenectomised sheep, *J. Comp. Pathol.,* 90, 155, 1980.
12. **Holmes, P. H. and Jennings, F. W.,** The effect of treatment on the anaemia of African trypanosomiasis, in *The Pathophysiology of Parasitic Infections,* Soulsby, E. J. L., Ed., Academic Press, New York, 1976, 119.
13. **Dargie, J. D.,** *Pathophysiology of Trypanosomiasis in the Bovine,* International Atomic Energy Agency Rep. 240/28, Vienna, 1980, 121.
14. **Woodruff, A. W., Ziegler, J. L., Hathaway, A., and Gwata, T.,** Anaemia in African trypanosomiasis and 'big spleen' disease in Uganda, *Trans. R. Soc. Trop. Med. Hyg.,* 67, 329, 1973.
15. **McCrorie, P., Jenkins, G. C., Brown, J. L., and Ramsey, C. E.,** Studies on the anaemia in rabbits infected with *Trypanosoma brucei brucei.* II. Haematoloical studies on the role of the spleen, *J. Comp. Pathol.,* 90, 123, 1980.
16. **Miles, M.,** personal communication, 1979.
17. **Jenkins, G. C., Syndercombe - Court, D., Facer, C. A., Smith, P., and Young, C.,** in preparation.
18. **Balber, A. E.,** *Trypanosoma brucei:* attenuation by corticosteroids of the anaemia of infected mice, *Exp. Parasitol.,* 35, 209, 1974.
19. **Amole, B. O., Clarkson, A. B., and Shear, M. L.,** Pathogenesis of anaemia in *Trypanosome brucei*-infected mice, *Infect. Immun.,* 36, 1060, 1982.
20. **Herbert, W. J. and Inglis, M. D.,** Immunisation of mice against *T. brucei* infections by administration of released antigens adsorbed to erythrocytes, *Trans. R. Soc. Trop. Med. Hyg.,* 67, 268, 1973.
21. **Woo, P. T. K. and Kobayashi, A.,** Studies on the anaemia in experimental African trypanosomiasis. I. A preliminary communication on the mechanism of the anaemia, *Ann. Soc. Belge. Med. Trop.,* 55, 37, 1975.
22. **Facer, C. A.,** unpublished observations, 1974.
23. **Zoutendyk, A. and Gear, J.,** Autoantibodies in the pathogenesis of disease. A preliminary study of auto-sensitisation of red cells in various diseases, *S. Afr. Med. J.,* 25, 665, 1951.
24. **Mackenzie, A. R. and Boreham, P. F. L.,** Autoimmunity in trypanosome infections. III. The antiglobulin (Coombs) test, *Acta Trop.,* 4, 360, 1974.

25. **Jarvinen, J. A. and Dalmasso, A. P.,** *Trypanosoma musculi:* immunologic features of the anaemia in infected mice, *Exp. Parasitol.,* 3, 203, 1977.
26. **Facer, C. A., Crosskey, J. M., Clarkson, M. J., and Jenkins, G. C.,** Immune haemolytic anaemia in bovine trypanosomiasis, *J. Comp. Pathol.,* 92, 393, 1982.
27. **Dodd, B. E., Jenkins, G. C., Lincoln, P. J., and McCrorie, P.,** The advantage of a build-up antiglobulin technique for the detection of immunoglobulin on the red cells of rabbits infected with trypanosomes. A preliminary report, *Trans. R. Soc. Trop. Med. Hyg.,* 72, 501, 1978.
28. **Coombs, R. R. A. and Gell, P. G. H.,** *Clinical Aspects of Immunology,* 3rd ed., Gell, P. G.H., Coombs, R. R. A., and Lachmann, P. J., Eds., Blackwell Scientific, Oxford, 1974, chap. 25.
29. **Fruit, J., Santoro, F., Afchain, D., Duvallet, G., and Capron, A.,** Les immunocomplexes circulants dans la trypanosomiase Africaine humaine et experimentale, *Ann. Soc. Belge, Med. Trop.,* 57, 257, 1977.
30. **Lindsley, H. B., Nagle, R. B., Werner, P. A., and Stechschulte, D. J.,** Variable severity of glomerulonephritis in inbred rats infected with *Trypanosoma rhodesiense, Am. J. Trop. Med. Hyg.,* 29, 348, 1980.
31. **Siegal, I., Liu, T. L., and Gleicher, N.,** The red cell immune system, *Lancet,* 2, 556, 1981.
32. **Mackenzie, P. K. I., Boyt, W. P., Nesham, V. W., and Pirie, E.,** The aetiology and significance of the phagocytosis of erythrocytes and leucocytes in sheep infected with *Trypanosoma congolense* (Broden, 1904), *Res. Vet. Sci.,* 24, 4, 1978.
33. **Kobayashi, A., Tizard, I. R., and Woo, P. J. K.,** Studies on the anaemia in experimental African trypanosomiasis. II. The pathogenesis of the anaemia in calves infected with *Trypanosoma congolense, Am. J. Trop. Med. Hyg.,* 25, 401, 1976.
34. **Maxie, H. G., Losos, G. J., and Tabel, H.,** A comparative study of the haematological aspects of the diseases caused by *Trypanosoma vivax* and *T. congolense* in cattle, in *Pathophysiology of Parasitic Infections,* Soulsby, E. J., Ed., Academic Press, London, 1976, 183.
35. **Facer, C. A.,** unpublished observations, 1975.
36. **Rickman, W. J. and Cox, H. W.,** Association of autoantibodies with anaemia, splenomegaly and glomerulonephritis in experimental African trypanosomiasis, *J. Parasitol.,* 65, 65, 1979.
37. **Rickman, W. J., Cox, H. W., and Thoongsuwan, S.,** Interactions of immunoconglutinin and immune complexes and cold autohaemagglutination associated with African trypanosomiasis, *J. Parasitol.,* 67, 159, 1981.
38. **Venkatsen, S., Bird, R. G., and Ormerod, W. E.,** Intracellular enzymes and their localisation in slender and stumpy forms of *Trypanosoma brucei rhodesiense, Int. J. Parasitol.,* 7, 139, 1977.
39. **Lanhan, S.,** personal communication, 1976.
40. **Huan, C. N., Webb, L., Lambert, P. M., and Miescher, P. A.,** Pathogenesis of the anaemia of African trypanosomiasis: characterisation and purification of a haemolytic factor, *Schweiz. Med. Wochenschr.,* 105, 1582, 1975.
41. **Tizard, I. R. and Holmes, W. L.,** The generation of toxic activity from *Trypanosoma congolense, Experientia,* 32, 1533, 1976.
42. **Hambrey, P. N., Tizard, I. R., and Mellors, A.,** Accumulation of phospholipase-A1 in tissue fluid of rabbits infected with *Trypanosoma brucei, Tropenmed. Parasitol.,* 31, 439, 1980.
43. **Tizard, I. R., Mellors, A., and Nielson, K.,** Role of biologically active substances in the pathogenesis and immunology of trypanosomiasis, in *Isotope and Radiation Research on Animal Diseases and Their Vectors,* IAEA-SM-240/15, International Atomic Energy Agency, Vienna, 1980, 149.
44. **Murray, P. K., Jennings, F. W., Murray, M., and Urquhart, G. M.,** The nature of immunosuppression in *Trypanosoma brucei* infections in mice. I. The role of the macrophage, *Immunology,* 27, 815, 1974.
45. **Holwill, M. E. J.,** Deformation of erythrocytes by trypanosomes, *Exp. Cell. Res.,* 37, 306, 1965.
46. **Jenkins, G. C., Brown, J., and Swettenham, K.,** unpublished observations, 1973.
47. **Greenwood, B. M. and Whittle, H. C,** The pathogenesis of sleeping sickness, *Trans. R. Soc. Trop. Med. Hyg.,* 74, 716, 1980.
48. **Prankard, T. A. J.,** The spleen and anaemia, *Br. Med. J.,* 2, 517, 1963.
49. **Richmond, J., Donaldson, G. W. K., Williams, R., Hamilton, P. J. S., and Hutt, M. S. R.,** Haematological effects of the idiopathic splenomegaly seen in Uganda, *Br. J. Haematol.,* 13, 348, 1967.
50. **Anosa, V. O.,** Studies on the Mechanism of Anaemia and the Pathology of Experimental *Trypanosoma vivax* Infection in Sheep and Goats, Ph.D. thesis, University of Ibadan, Nigeria, 1977.
51. **Naylor, D. C.,** The haematology and histology of *Trypanosoma congolense* infection in cattle. II. Haematology (including symptoms), *Trop. Anim. Health Prod.,* 3, 159, 1971.
52. **Isoun, T. T.,** *Animal Protein, Malnutrition and the Science of Disease,* inaugural lecture, University of Ibaden, Ibaden University Press, Nigeria, 1980, 12.
53. **Dargie, J. D., Murray, P. K., Murray, M., Grimshaw, W. R. T., and McIntyre, W. I. M.,** Bovine trypanosomiasis: the red cell kinetics of N'dama and Zebu cattle infected with *Trypanosoma congolense, Parasitology,* 78, 271, 1979.

54. **Holmes, P. H.,** The use of radioisotope tracer techniques in the study of the pathogenesis of trypanosomiasis, in *Nuclear Techniques in Animal Production and Health,* International Atomic Energy Agency, Vienna, 1976, 463.

55. **Jenkins, G. C., Brown, J. L., and Forsberg, C. M.,** unpublished observation, 1973.

56. **Cartwright, G. E. and Lee, R.,** The anemia of chronic disorders, *Br. J. Haematol.,* 21, 147, 1975.

57. **Edwards, E. E., Judd, J. M., and Squire, F. A.,** Observations on trypanosomiasis in domestic animals in West Africa. The daily index of infection and the weekly haematological values in goats and sheep infected with *T. vivax, T. congolense* and *T. brucei, Ann. Trop. Med. Parasitol.,* 50, 223, 1956.

58. **Valli, V. E. O. and Mills, J. N.,** The quantitation of *Trypanosoma congolense* in calves. I. Haematological changes, *Tropenmed. Parasitol.,* 31, 215, 1980.

59. **Moretti, G., Veyret, V., and Broustet, A.,** Interet de la recherche des lymphocytes a granulations P. A. S. positives dans le sang des trypanosomes, *Bull. Soc. Pathol. Exot.,* 60, 420, 1967.

60. **Ottman, P. and Zumwalt, J.,** African trypanosomiasis — California, *Morbid. Mortal.,* 19, 233, 1970.

61. **Robins-Browne, R. M., Schneider, J., and Metz, J.,** Thrombocytopenia in trypanosomiasis, *Am. J. Trop. Med. Hyg.,* 24, 226, 1975.

62. **Rickman, W. J. and Cox, H. W.,** Immunologic reactions associated with anaemia, thrombocytopenia and coagulopathy in experimental African trypanosomiasis, *J. Parasitol.,* 66, 28, 1980.

63. **Goodwin, L. G.,** The pathology of African trypanosomiasis, *Trans. R. Soc. Trop. Med. Hyg.,* 64, 797, 1970.

64. **Edeghere, H. I. U. F.,** Morphological and Ultrastructural Changes in Small Blood Vessels of Rabbits Infected with *T. brucei,* Ph.D. thesis, University of London, 1980.

65. **Didisheim, P., Hattovi, I., and Lewis, J. H.,** Haematologic and coagulation studies in various animal species, *J. Lab. Clin. Med.,* 53, 866, 1959.

66. **Mews, A.,** personal communication, 1978.

67. **Isoun, T. T.,** The pathology of *Trypanosoma simiae* infection in pigs, *Ann. Trop. Med. Parasitol.,* 62, 188, 1968.

68. **Van Dijk, J. E., Zwart, D., and Leeflang, P. A.,** Contribution to the pathology of *Trypanosoma simiae* in pigs, *Zentralbl. Veterinaermed.,* 20, 374, 1973.

69. **Bick, R. L.,** Disseminated intravascular coagulation and related syndromes: aetiology, pathophysiology, diagnosis and management, *Am. J. Haematol.,* 5, 265, 1978.

70. **Isoun, T. T. and Anosa, V. O.,** Lesions in the reproductive organs of sheep and goats experimentally infected with *Trypanosoma vivax, Tropenmed. Parasitol.,* 25, 469, 1974.

71. **Murray, M.,** The pathology of African trypanosomiasis, *Prog. Immun.,* 2(4), 181, 1974.

72. **Van Den Ingh, T. S. G. A. M.,** Pathology and Pathogenesis of *Trypanosoma brucei* Infection in the Rabbit, Ph.D. thesis, University of Utrecht, The Netherlands, 1976.

73. **Van Den Ingh, T. S. G. A. M., Zwart, D., Schotman, A. J. H., Van Miert, A. S. J. P. A. M., and Veneendaal, G. H.,** The pathology and pathogensis of *Trypanosoma vivax* infection in the goat, *Res. Vet. Sci.,* 21, 264, 1976a.

74. **Van Den Ingh, T. S. G. A. M., Zwart, D., Van Miert, A. S. J. P. A. M., and Schotman, A. J. H.,** Clinico-pathological and pathomorphological observations in *Trypanosoma vivax* infection in cattle, *Vet. Parasitol.,* 2, 237, 1976b.

75. **Veenendaal, G. H., Van Miert, A. S. J. P. A. M., Van Den Ingh, T. S. G. A. M., Schotman, A. J. H., and Zwart, D.,** A comparison of the role of kinins and serotonin in endotoxin-induced fever and *Trypanosoma vivax* infections in the goat, *Res. Vet. Sci.,* 21, 271, 1976.

76. **Van Miert, A. S. J. P. A. M., Van Duin, C. Th., Busser, F. J. M., Perie, N., Van Den Ingh, T. S. G. A. M., and Neys-Backers, M. H. H.,** The effect of flurbiprofen, a potent non-steroidal anti-inflammatory agent, upon *Trypanosoma vivax* infection in goats, *J. Vet. Pharm. Ther.,* 1, 69, 1978.

77. **Masake, R. A.,** The pathogenesis of infection with *Trypanosoma vivax* in goats and cattle, *Vet. Rec.,* 107, 551, 1980.

78. **Isoun, T. T.,** The histopathology of experimental disease produced in mice infected with *Trypanosoma vivax, Acta Trop.,* 32, 267, 1975.

79. **Losos, G. L. and Ikede, B. O.,** Review of the pathology of diseases in domestic and laboratory animals caused by *Trypanosoma congolense, T. vivax, T. rhodesiense* and *T. gambiense, Vet. Pathol.,* 9 (Suppl.), 1972.

80. **Facer, C. A.,** unpublished observations, 1976.

81. **Isoun, T. T. and Esuruoso, G. O.,** Pathology of natural infection of *Trypanosoma vivax* in cattle, *Niger. Vet. J.,* 1, 42, 1972.

82. **Langdell, R. D., Wagner, R. H., and Brinkhous, M. M.,** Effect of antihaemophilic factor on one-stage clotting tests; presumptive test for haemophilia and simple one-stage antihaemophilic factor assay procedure, *J. Lab. Clin. Med.,* 42, 637, 1953.

83. **Sadun, E. H., Johnson, A. J., Nagle, R. B., and Duxbury, R. E.,** Experimental infections with African trypanosomes. V. Preliminary parasitological, clinical, haematological, serological and pathological observations in Rhesus monkeys infected with *Trypanosoma rhodesiense, Am. Trop. Med. Hyg.,* 22, 323, 1973.

84. **Facer, C. A.,** Physiopathological Changes in the Blood of Animals Infected with African Trypanosomes, Ph.D. thesis, University of London, 1974.

85. **Greenwood, B. M. and Whittle, H. C.,** Coagulation studies in Gambian trypanosomiasis, *Am. J. Trop. Med. Hyg.,* 25, 390, 1976.

86. **Wellde, B. T., Kovatch, R. M., Chumo, D. A., and Wykoff, D. E.,** *Trypanosoma congolense:* thrombocytopenia in experimentally infected cattle, *Exp. Parasitol.,* 45, 26, 1978.

87. **Forsberg, C. M., Valli, V. E. O., Gentry, P. W., and Donworth, R. M.,** The pathogenesis of *Trypanosome congolense* infection in calves. IV. The kinetics of blood coagulation, *Vet. Pathol.,* 16, 229, 1979.

88. **Boulton, F. E., Jenkins, G. C., and Lloyd, M. J.,** unpublished observations, 1973.

89. **Boreham, P. F. L. and Facer, C. A.,** Fibrinogen and fibrinogen/fibrin degradation products in experimental African trypanosomiasis, *Int. J. Parasitol.,* 4, 143, 1974.

90. **Essien, E. M. and Ikede, B. O.,** Coagulation defect in experimental trypanosomial infection, *Haemostasis,* 5, 341, 1976.

91. **Goodwin, L. G.,** Pathological effects of *Trypanosoma brucei* on the small blood vessels in rabbit ear chambers, *Trans. R. Soc. Trop. Med. Hyg.,* 65, 82, 1971.

92. **Marsh, N.,** *Fibrinolysis,* John Wiley & Sons, Chichester, 1981, 52.

93. **Niewiarowski, S. and Kowalski, E.,** Anti-thrombin formation during proteolysis of fibrinogen, in Transactions of the 6th Congress of the European Society for Haematology, Copenhagen, 1957.

94. **Holt, J. C., Mahmoud, M., and Gaffney, P. J.,** The ability of fibrinogen fragments to support ADP-induced platelet aggregation, *Thromb. Res.,* 16, 427, 1979.

95. **Barnhart, M. I.,** Role of blood coagulation in acute inflammation, *Biochem. Pharmacol.,* Suppl., 205, 1968.

96. **Triantaphyllopoulos, D. C. and Triantophyllopoulos, E.,** Physiological effects of fibrinogen degradation products, *Thromb. Diath. Haemorrh.,* 39 (Suppl.), 175, 1970.

97. **Girman, G., Pees, H., Schwarze, G., and Scheurlen, P. G.,** Immunosuppression by micromolecular fibrinogen degradation products in cancer, *Nature (London),* 259, 399, 1976.

98. **Davis, C. E., Robbins, R. S., Weller, R. D., and Braude, A. I.,** Thrombocytopenia in experimental trypanosomiasis, *J. Clin. Invest.,* 53, 1359, 1974.

99. **Jenkins, G. C., Forsberg, C. M., Brown, J. C., and Parr, C. W.,** Some haematological investigations on experimental *Trypanosoma brucei* infections in rabbits, *Trans. R. Soc. Trop. Med. Hyg.,* 68, 154, 1974.

100. **Syndercombe-Court, D.,** unpublished observations, 1982.

101. **Hildebrandt, P. K., Johnson, A. J., Anderson, J. S., and Sadun, E. H.,** The clinical course and pathology of dogs experimentally infected with *Trypanosoma congolense,* unpublished observations, 1972.

102. **Maxie, M. G., Losos, G. J., and Tabel, H.,** A comparative study of the haematological aspects of the diseases caused by *Trypanosoma vivax* and *T. congolense* in cattle, in *Pathophysiology of Parasitic Infection,* Soulsby, E. J. L., Ed., Academic Press, New York, 1976, 183.

103. **Maxie, M. G., Losos, G. L., and Tabel, H.,** Experimental bovine trypanosomiasis *(Trypanosoma vivax* and *T. congolense).* I. Symptomatology and clinical pathology, *Tropenmed. Parasitol.,* 30, 274, 1979.

104. **Preston, J. M., Kovatch, R. M., and Wellde, B. T.,** *Trypanosoma congolense:* thrombocyte survival in infected steers, *Exp. Parasitol.,* 54, 129, 1982.

105. **Harker, L. A. and Finch, C. A.,** Thrombokinetics in man, *J. Clin. Invest.,* 48, 963, 1969.

106. **Bhogal, M. S. and Wellde, B. T.,** unpublished observations, 1982.

107. International Committee for Standardization in Haematology, Recommended methods for radioisotope platelet survival studies, *Blood,* 50, 1137, 1979.

108. **Heaton, W. A., Davis, H. H., Welch, M. J., Mathias, C. J., Joist, J. H., Sherman, L. A., and Siegal, B. A.,** Indium-111: a new radionuclide label for studying human platelet kinetics, *Br. J. Haematol.,* 42, 613, 1979.

109. **Woodruff, A. W.,** Mechanisms involved in anaemia associated with infection and splenomegaly in the tropics, *Trans. R. Soc. Trop. Med. Hyg.,* 67, 313, 1973.

110. **Miescher, P. and Cooper, N.,** The fixation of soluble antigen-antibody complexes upon thrombocytes, *Vox Sang.,* 5, 138, 1960.

111. **Lurhuma, A. Z., Riccomi, P. L., and Masson, P. L.,** The occurrence of circulating immune complexes and viral antigens in idiopathic thrombocytopenia purpura, *Clin. Exp. Immunol.,* 27, 45, 1977.

112. **Clancy, R., Trent, R., Danis, V., and Davidson, R.,** Autosensitisation and immune complexes in chronic idiopathic thrombocytopenic purpura, *Clin. Exp. Immunol.,* 39, 170, 1980.

113. **Slots, J. M. M., Van Miert, A. S. J. P. A. M., Akkerman, J. W. N., and Gee, A. L. W.,** *Trypanosoma brucei* and *T. vivax:* antigen-antibody complexes as a cause of platelet serotonin release *in vitro* and *in vivo, Exp. Parasitol.,* 43, 211, 1977.

114. **Johnson, S., Ed.,** *The Circulating Platelet,* Academic Press, New York, 1971, 25.

115. **Thomasson, D. L., Mansfield, J. M., Doyle, R. J., and Wallace, J. H.,** C-reactive protein levels in experimental African trypanosomiasis, *J. Parasitol.,* 59, 738, 1973.

116. **Fiedal, B. A. and Gewurz, H.,** Effects of C-reactive protein on platelet function. I. Inhibition of platelet aggregation and release reaction, *J. Immunol.,* 116, 1289, 1976.

117. **Vermylen, J., de Gaetano, G., and Verstraete, M.,** *Recent Advances in Thrombosis,.* Poller, L., Ed., Churchill Livingstone, Edinburgh, 1973, 113.

118. **Nishizawa, E. E., Wynalda, D. J., and Suyda, M. D. E.,** Effect of flurbiprofen on platelet function, *Thromb. Diath. Haemorr.,* Suppl., 415, 1974.

119. **Davies, T., Lederer, D. A., Spencer, A. A., and McNicol, G. P.,** The effect of flurbiprofen (2- (2-fluoro-4-biphenyl) propionic acid) on platelet function and blood coagulation, *Thromb. Res.,* 5, 669, 1974.

120. **Csako, G., Suba, E. A., and Wistar, R.,** Activation of human platelets by antibodies to thymocytes and β_2-microglobulin. III. Effect of cell absorptions on the platelet aggregating and lymphocytotoxic activities of HAIG and SA-beta-2mG, *Clin. Lab. Immunol.,* 7, 199, 1982.

121. **Hudson, K.,** personal communication, 1982.

122. **Fahey, J. L., Barth, U. F., and Solomon, A.,** Serum hyperviscosity syndrome, *JAMA,* 192, 464, 1965.

123. **Stuart, J. and Kenny, M. W.,** Blood rheology, *J. Clin. Pathol.,* 33, 417, 1980.

124. **Dormandy, J. A.,** Clinical significance of blood viscosity, *Ann. R. Coll. Surg. Engl.,* 47, 211, 1970.

125. **Clarkson, M.,** Immunoglobulin M in trypanosomiasis, in *Pathophysiology of Parasitic Infection,* Soulsby, E. J. L., Ed., Academic Press, London, 1976, 171.

126. **Diehl, E. J. and Risby, E. L.,** Serum changes in rabbits experimentally infected with *Trypanosoma gambiense, Am. J. Trop. Med. Hyg.,* 23, 1019, 1974.

127. **Facer, C. A.,** Blood hyperviscosity during *Trypanosoma brucei* infections of rabbits, *J. Comp. Pathol.,* 86, 393, 1976.

128. **Grundy, S. M., Ahrens, E. H., Salen, G., Schreibman, P. H., and Nestel, P. J.,** Mechanisms of action of clofibrate on cholesterol metabolism in patients with hyperlipidemia, *J. Lipid Res.,* 13, 531, 1972.

129. **Dormandy, J. A., Gutteridge, J. M. C., Hoare, E., and Dormandy, T. L.,** The effect of clofibrate on blood viscosity in intermittent claudication, *Br. Med. J.,* 4, 259, 1974.

130. **Facer, C. A.,** unpublished observations, 1981.

131. **Seed, J. R., Cornille, R. L., Risby, E. L., and Gam, A. A.,** The presence of agglutinating antibody in the IgM immunoglobulin fraction of rabbit anti-serum during experimental African trypanosomiasis, *Parasitology,* 59, 283, 1969.

132. **Dormandy, J. A.,** Haemorheological aspects of thrombosis, *Br. J. Haematol.,* 45, 519, 1980.

133. **Nagle, R. B., Dong, S., Guillot, J. M., McDaniel, K. M., and Lindsley, H. B.,** Pathology of experimental African trypanosomiasis in rabbits infected with *Trypanosoma rhodesiense, Am. J. Trop. Med. Hyg.,* 29, 1187, 1980.

134. **Hoffbrand, A. V. and Pettit, J. E.,** *Essential Haematology,* Blackwell Scientific, London, 1980, 24.

135. **Preston, J. M. and Wellde, B. T.,** Studies on African Trypanosomiasis, final report to Department of the Army, Walter Reed Army Institute of Research, DAMD 17-76-9412, Washington, D.C., 1976.

136. **Noyes, W. D., Srichakul, T., Choawanakul, V., Chaisiripumkeeree, W., and Dunn, C. D. R.,** Erythropoietin levels in the anaemia of malaria, presented at Int. Congr. of Haematology and Blood Transfusion, Abstr. No. Tu-247, Budapest, 1982.

137. **Valli, V. E. O., McSherry, B. J., Robinson, G. A., and Willoughby, R. A.,** Leukaphoresis in calves and dogs by extracorporeal circulation of blood through siliconised glass wool, *Res. Vet. Sci.,* 10, 267, 1969.

138. **Lawson, B. M., Valli, V. E. O., Mills, J. N., and Forsberg, C. M.,** The quantitation of *Trypanosoma congolense* in calves. IV. *In vitro* culture of myeloid and erythroid marrow cells, *Tropenmed. Parasitol.,* 31, 425, 1980.

139. **Kaaya, G. P., Valli, V. E. O., Maxie, M. G., and Losos, G. J.,** Inhibition of bovine bone marrow granulocyte/macrophage colony formation *in vitro* by serum collected from cattle infected with *Trypanosoma vivax* or *T. congolense, Tropenmed. Parasitol.,* 30, 230, 1979.

140. **Kaaya, G. P., Tizard, I. R., Maxie, M. G., and Valli, V. E. O.,** Inhibition of leukopoiesis by sera from *Trypanosoma congolense* infected calves, *Tropenmed. Parasitol.,* 31, 232, 1980.

141. **Bacigalupo, A. and Moretta, L.,** T-cell mediated suppression of hemopoiesis, *Immunol. Today,* 2, 47, 1981.

142. **Greenwood, B. M.,** Possible role of a B-cell mitogen in the hypergammaglobulinaemia in malaria and trypanosomiasis, *Lancet,* 1, 435, 1974.

143. **Hira, P. R. and Husein, S. F.,** Some transfusion-induced parasitic infections in Zambia, *Hyg. Epid. Microbiol. Immunol.,* 23, 436, 1979.
144. **Traub, N., Hira, P. R., Chintu, C., and Mhango, C.,** Congenital trypanosomiasis: report of a case due to *Trypanosoma brucei rhodesiense, East. Afr. Med. J.,* 55, 477, 1978.
145. **Burke, J., Bengoni, K., and Diantete, N. L.,** Un cas de trypanosomiase Africaine (*T. cambiense*) congenitale, *Ann. Soc. Belge Med. Trop.,* 54, 1, 1974.
146. **Jenkins, G. C., Parr, C. W., and Welch, S.,** unpublished observations, 1973.
147. **Tabel, H., Losos, G. J., and Maxie, M. G.,** Experimental bovine trypanosomiasis (*Trypanosoma congolense*). Lack of relation of the level of parasitaemia to the J blood group, *Tropenmed. Parasitol.,* 32, 99, 1981.

Chapter 3

AUTOCOIDS: THEIR RELEASE AND POSSIBLE ROLE IN THE PATHOGENESIS OF AFRICAN TRYPANOSOMIASIS

Peter F. L. Boreham

TABLE OF CONTENTS

I. INTRODUCTION

It is now well over 20 years since Goodwin[1] first reported the release of autocoids in experimental trypanosome infections. The term autocoid is applied to a variety of amines, peptides, and lipids which are found in tissues and have pharmacological activity. These substances have also been referred to as local hormones. In hindsight, however, it is possible to see that some of the earlier work predicted that potent autocoids were released during trypanosomiasis and could play a role in its pathogenesis. For example, in 1925 Dukelsky[2] recorded that mice heavily infected with trypanosomes often died a few hours after administration of Bayer® 205 (suramin) but not after treatment with salvarsan (arsphenamine). He postulated that suramin caused an anaphylactic reaction which, by this date, was known to involve the release of histamine.[3] Another early study compared the Jarisch-Herxheimer reactions of syphilis and trypanosomiasis and concluded that host cell destruction and release of histamine resulted from an interaction of the arsenical drug used with the parasite-induced cellular exudate.[4]

The release of pharmacologically active substances in cattle trypanosomiasis was clearly predicted by Fiennes[5] in 1950 when he wrote: ''Factors favourable to the development of anaphylactic states are present in trypanosomiasis and other relapsing conditions. At each crisis, trypanosomes are destroyed in the blood in very large numbers, and the system presumably becomes permeated with dead trypanosome protein . . . The animal may therefore become sensitized to trypanosome protein at each crisis, and at any crisis except the first — but especially at the major one — anaphylactic shock may be induced . . . Death follows collapse, and usually occurs after the temperature-curve has fallen and after trypanosomes have to a large degree been eliminated from the blood. The picture certainly suggests anaphylactic shock.''

Three facts led Goodwin[1] to initiate studies into the release of autocoids in parasitic diseases and, in particular, trypanosomiasis.

1. The paradox that death in trypanosomiasis often occurred when only a few organisms were present, thus suggesting that the parasite alone was not responsible, but that host factors were also involved
2. That severe adverse reactions sometimes occurred following the treatment of trypanosomiasis and other infectious diseases which were not due simply to drug toxicity[4,6-11]
3. The hypothesis put forward by Maegraith and colleagues[12,13] that the shock-like reactions that occur in *Plasmodium knowlesi* infections of monkeys and *Babesia canis* infections of dogs were caused by simple physiologically active substances which were derived either from the host or the parasite

Most authors writing about the pathogenesis of trypanosomiasis have pointed out the complexity of the subject, the fact that many biological systems are involved, and our general lack of knowledge and understanding in this area. Many different approaches to the subject have been taken which are reviewed elsewhere in this book, including cellular and humoral immunological mechanisms, toxic substances produced by parasites, biochemical mechanisms, especially the role of indole amines, hematological mechanisms, and pathological studies on biopsy and autopsy material. The intricacy and multifarious nature of the process has led to many theories being propounded in an attempt to explain its etiology.[14-23] Despite these complexities which have been described as a vicious circle,[15] it is essential to try to unravel the mechanisms involved and especially to attempt to delineate the initiating factor(s). Once the process has been established it will be much easier to suggest ways of reversing or attenuating it, thus providing better methods of prophylaxis or therapy.

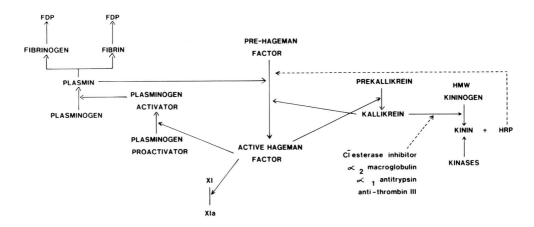

FIGURE 1. Diagram of the main components of the kallikrein-kinin system to show its interrelationships with the blood coagulation, fibrinolytic, and complement cascades. Broken lines indicate inhibitory reactions. FDP, fibrin/fibrinogen degradation products; HRP, histidine-rich peptides; XI and XIa, factor XI and activated factor XI (plasma thromboplastin antecedent) of the clotting system.

This chapter will review the current state of our knowledge of autocoids released in trypanosomiasis in humans, cattle, and experimental laboratory animals, discuss the mechanism of their release, and consider the possible implications to the pathogenesis of the disease. Since some readers may not be familiar with the production, storage, and actions of the autocoids, a brief review is included of those autocoids known to be released in trypanosomiasis. For a more detailed consideration the reader is referred to standard pharmacological textbooks.[24,25] There are several other potentially important autocoids such as the prostaglandins, substance P, renin, angiotensin, and the leukotrienes which await systematic study in trypanosomiasis. Previously published reviews have considered the release of autocoids in protozoal and helminthic infections[10,26] and the kallikrein-kinin system in hemoprotozoan infections.[27,28]

II. THE KALLIKREIN-KININ SYSTEM IN TRYPANOSOMIASIS

A. Pharmacology of the Kallikrein-Kinin System

The kallikrein-kinin system consists of a complex series of reactions involving the formation of polypeptides (kinins) from α_2-globulins in the blood (kininogens) by serine proteases (kallikreins). Kallikreins are present as inactive precursors (prekallikreins) and the whole system is modulated by inhibitors and feedback mechanisms[29,30] (Figure 1). The kallikrein-kinin system is closely linked to the coagulation, fibrinolytic, and complement cascades.[31-33] The key reaction which leads to the activation of all four systems is the activation of Hageman factor (factor XII). This occurs (1) when blood comes into contact with negatively charged surfaces such as glass or kaolin, (2) in various pathological conditions where immune complexes, inflammatory exudates, or other acidic conditions are produced, or (3) by proteolytic cleavage.[30] Formation of activated Hageman factor initiates the intrinsic coagulation pathway, converts plasminogen proactivator to an activator, which in turn, converts plasminogen to plasmin, and activates the first component of complement.

Three major kinins have been described which have similar pharmacological properties, although showing quantitative differences. Bradykinin is a nonapeptide produced by the action of plasma kallikrein on high molecular weight kininogen. Tissue kallikrein releases kallidin (lysyl-bradykinin) from low molecular weight kininogen. A third naturally occurring kinin, methionyl-lysyl-bradykinin, has been found in bovine plasma and human urine. During the activation of complement via the classical pathway, a C2 fragment with kinin-like activity is also produced.[33] These peptides have a number of important biological properties including increasing vascular permeability, causing a reversible hypotension, and contraction of many smooth muscle preparations.[29] The action of kinins on smooth muscle appears to be direct and involves two types of receptors: B1 receptors which cause contraction, such as that seen in the rabbit aorta, and B2 receptors causing relaxation which are present in the rabbit jugular vein and dog carotid artery.[34]

In addition to their enzymatic activity kallikreins have been shown to have direct effects on the cardiovascular system.[29,30] Renal kallikrein has been suggested to have a physiological role in maintaining renal blood pressure directly and by regulating aldosterone secretion.[35] There is also evidence to suggest that there is a link between the kallikrein-kinin system and prostaglandins, that kallikrein has a role as a growth factor, and that it is important in reproductive physiology.[30] When bovine plasma kallikrein releases bradykinin from high molecular weight kininogen two other peptide fragments are produced. One of these has been designated the histidine-rich peptide (HRP) which is a potent inhibitor of prehageman factor activation.[36] Several proteolytic enzymes (kininases) present in blood or located on the surface of endothelial and other cells are able to break down kinins. These kininases include aminopeptidases which cleave the lysyl group from kallidin and two metalloproteins, kininase I and II, which act at the C-terminal end of the molecule.

Kinins (and angiotensins) differ from other autocoids in that they are not synthesized and stored in specialized cells within the body.

B. Kinin Release

In considering the role of autocoids in trypanosomiasis it is important to clearly distinguish between acute infection produced by some trypanosome strains in laboratory animals, such as rats and mice, and the chronic infections of cattle and man which may persist for months or even years. In the former the animal may die with an overwhelming parasitemia in as little as 3 to 5 days, before an effective immune response is mounted. In this case utilization of essential nutrients[37,38] and the production of toxic substances by trypanosomes[20] may be important mechanisms leading to the death of the host. However, in chronic infections, such as that seen in experimental *Trypanosoma brucei* infections of the rabbit, the general condition of the animal gradually deteriorates with lethargy, weakness, anemia, intermittent fever, and edema being the most common signs.[19,21,39] In chronic infections parasitemia is often very scanty.

1. Acute Infections

Kinin release was first demonstrated in mice infected with *T. rhodesiense* and it was shown that activity in plasma, urine, ears, skin, and feet progressively increased during the infection.[1,40] Concentrations three to five times higher than control levels were recorded just prior to death. Similar results were found when kinins were extracted from the urine of rats infected with *T. brucei*[41,42] and plasma taken from guinea pigs with a heavy parasitemia of *T. evansi*.[43] Since it has been shown that kinins are released in a number of acute protozoal infections, including *P. knowlesi* of monkeys,[44] *P. berghei*, *B. rhodaini* of mice,[1] and *B. bovis* of cattle,[45] it appears that such release is a general phenomenon of pathogenic hemoprotozoa. This conclusion is supported by the fact that no increase in kinins were found in the urine of rats infected with the nonpathogenic *T. lewisi*[41] or in avirulent infections of *B. bovis*.

2. Chronic Infections

Most of the studies on chronic infections relate to *T. brucei* subgroup infections of rabbits,[47,48] cattle,[47] and man,[49] although some studies on *T. vivax* infections of goats[50] and

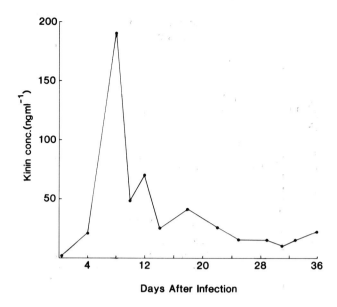

FIGURE 2. Kinin concentration in the blood of rabbits infected with *Trypanosoma brucei* expressed as ng of synthetic bradykinin mℓ^{-1}. (From Boreham, P. F. L., *Br. J. Pharmacol. Chemother.*, 32, 493, 1968. With permission.)

cattle[51] have been undertaken. However, there is no information on *T. congolense* infections. The pattern of kinin release in all these infections is similar and is illustrated for the rabbit in Figure 2. About 10 days postinfection (DPI) a peak of kinin release occurs coinciding with, or immediately subsequent to, the first major parasitemic wave. Subsequent peaks of kinin release occurred at 5- to 10-day intervals but always in lower concentrations than the initial peak. In some cases of man infected with *T. rhodesiense*[49] and cattle and goats infected with *T. vivax*,[50-52] an additional small peak of kinin release was reported, about 4 DPI. Increases in urinary kinin were detected in the rabbit 4 DPI with *T. brucei* and, although the concentrations remained high throughout, the greatest concentrations were found early in the infection.[41]

Studies on cattle infected with *T. brucei* gave the first clue to the mechanism of kinin release.[47] Concentrations of plasma kinins were inversely correlated with kininogen, and at maximum kinin concentration (approximately 35 ng mℓ^{-1} blood) the amount of kininogen in the plasma fell from approximately 6 to 3 μg mℓ^{-1} plasma. After treatment of the cattle with diminazene aceturate (7 mg kg^{-1}) kinin levels returned to control values, while kininogen levels rose rapidly to twice control values (Figure 3). These results indicate, first, that only a small portion of the kinin released from kininogen is detected in the blood. Thus, measurement of kinin as an indication of activation of the kallikrein-kinin system is extremely insensitive, probably due to the rapid breakdown of kinins by kininases. The half-life of bradykinin is known to be less than one complete circulation of the blood.[53] Second, the rapid increase in kininogen after treatment indicated increased synthesis of this protein during the infection.

Figure 3 also shows the pattern of antibody production in cattle. Variant specific antibodies were detected 4 DPI using neutralization and agglutination tests, whereas common antibodies were first detected by precipitation reactions 8 to 10 DPI and by fluorescence tests 9 to 13 DPI. Correlation of maximal kinin release with the appearance of the first antigenic variant suggested that the immune reaction, resulting in the death of most of the organisms, might also lead to the formation of kinins. Studies with a human volunteer which correlated the

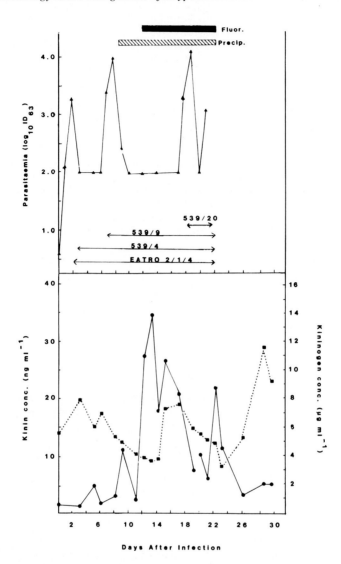

FIGURE 3.   Parasitemia and antibody response (upper section) and kinin and kininogen concentrations in cow number 539 after infection with *Trypanosoma brucei* EATRO 2/1/4. Parasitemia is expressed in mouse $\log_{10}\text{ID}_{63}$ mℓ^{-1} blood. The period when common fluorescent antibodies (solid horizontal bar) and precipitating antibodies (hatched bar) are found is shown, together with the presence of variant specific neutralizing antibodies to the original stabilate and stabilates prepared on day 4 (539/4), day 9 (539/9), and day 20 (539/20) of the infection. Kinin concentrations (●━━━●) are expressed as ng of synthetic bradykinin mℓ^{-1} blood and kininogen concentrations (■━━━■) as μg of synthetic bradykinin released by trypsin mℓ^{-1} plasma. (Adapted from Boreham, P. F. L., *Br. J. Pharmacol Chemother.*, 32, 493, 1968. With permission.)

production of antibodies with kinin production after infection with *T. rhodesiense* gave essentially the same results.[49] In goats infected with *T. vivax* no correlation was found between the rise in kinin levels, fever, and decreased ruminal motility even though injection of 1 to 4 μg kg^{-1} of synthetic bradykinin evoked a strong inhibition of gastric activity.[50,52]

C. Kallikrein Activation

Kinin-forming enzymes (kallikreins) have, to date, been studied in rats acutely infected with *T. brucei*[54] and in rabbits chronically infected with *T. brucei*.[55-58] In acute infections

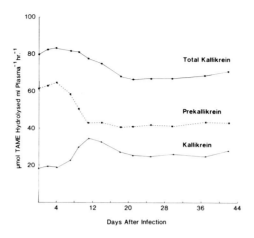

FIGURE 4. Total kallikrein (●━━━●), prekallikrein (■━━━■), and
free kallikrein concentration in rabbits infected with *Trypanosoma brucei*.
Values are expressed as μmol TAME hydrolyzed mℓ plasma^{-1} hr^{-1}. Each
point represents the mean value from six rabbits. (Drawn from data in
Parry, M. G., Kallikrein and Its Activation in Experimental *Trypanosoma
brucei* Infections of Rabbits, Ph.D. thesis, University of London, 1980.
With permission.)

of rats, plasma kallikrein levels fell from 38 ± 5.4 to 9.5 ± 1.0 ng/mℓ$^{-1}$ bradykinin
equivalent on the 5 DPI just prior to death. Concentrations of the precursor fell from 223.7
± 24.9 to 110.8 ± 10.2 ng/mℓ$^{-1}$ bradykinin equivalent. This was interpreted as an indication
of kallikrein activation.[54]

In the rabbit urinary kallikrein concentrations, measured either biologically on anesthetized
rabbit blood pressure or enzymatically using *N*-tosyl-L-arginine methyl ester as a substrate,
rose four- to eightfold after infection. Maximum concentrations were detected in the urine
6 to 7 DPI. Throughout the whole of the infection urinary kallikrein levels were elevated
with a second peak of activity 17 DPI and a third peak 24 DPI. Both the biological and
enzymatic activity of urinary kallikrein were inhibited by aprotonin, a protease inhibitor,
but by not soya bean trypsin inhibitor,[56] which is indicative of glandular and not plasma
kallikrein. An increase in free kallikrein of approximately 100% was seen in rabbit plasma
reaching a peak 10 to 14 DPI. This was associated with a fall of about 30% in prekallikrein
levels.[57,58] Total kallikrein did not differ markedly from control values but free plasma
kallikrein levels remained raised throughout the whole of the infection (Figure 4). Plasma
kallikrein was inhibited by both aprotonin (1000 IU mℓ$^{-1}$) and soya bean trypsin inhibitor
(100 mg mℓ$^{-1}$). Since increased concentrations of urinary kallikrein were detected several
days before plasma kallikrein levels increased, it seems unlikely that the urinary kallikrein
resulted from leakage of plasma kallikrein through the glomerulus. This conclusion is supported by the different responses of urinary and plasma kallikreins to protease inhibitors.

D. Kininases

The only other component of the kallikrein-kinin system to have been measured in trypanosomiasis is plasma kininase in rats acutely infected with *T. brucei*.[54] No difference was
found in the ability of control and infected plasma to break down synthetic bradykinin. No
kinin-forming enzymes were present in washed, separated trypanosomes but a small amount
of kininase was detected within parasites after disruption.

E. Mechanisms of Kallikrein Activation

Trypanosomes themselves are neither able to activate salivary kallikrein nor do they contain
plasma or erythrocyte kininase inhibitors.[54] The experiments on rabbits, cattle, and man

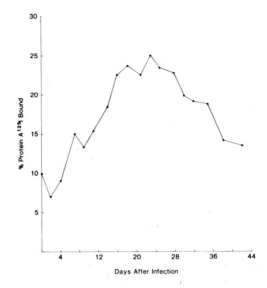

FIGURE 5. Circulating immune complex concentrations in rabbits infected with *Trypanosoma brucei* estimated as amount of ^{125}I protein A bound. (Drawn from data in Parry, M. G., Kallikrein and Its Activation in Experimental *Trypanosoma brucei* Infections of Rabbits, Ph.D. thesis, University of London, 1980. With permission.)

described above suggested an association of kinin release with peaks in parasitemia and suggested that the formation of immune complexes, which reduce the parasitemia, might also be responsible for activation of the kallikrein-kinin system. Antigen-antibody complexes are known to be able to activate Hageman factor.[59] Evidence confirming that complexes of trypanosomes and antibody can cause the release of kinins comes from three sources:

1. Kinins are released in vitro from a kininogen substrate by immune complexes of trypanosomes and antibody but not by either component alone.[60] This ability is lost by heating the immune plasma used to prepare the complexes at 65°C but not at 56°C. This suggests that Hageman factor is involved.
2. Trypanosome antigen added to isolated infected rabbit or guinea pig intestine caused the release of pharmacologically active substances.[10] This did not occur with pieces of intestine taken from noninfected animals.
3. Injection of trypanosome-antibody complexes intravenously into uninfected rabbits will cause a profound hypotension which can be blocked by aprotonin.[61] Similarly, injection of washed trypanosomes into infected animals, but not uninfected rabbits, produced a fall in blood pressure. The fall in blood pressure was biphasic and prolonged. On occasions it was so severe that death resulted. In rabbits infected with *T. brucei* the production of circulating immune complexes corresponds to the activation of kallikrein (Figure 5).[57,58,62]

It is thus apparent that the formation of immune complexes is one cause of activation of the kallikrein-kinin system in trypanosomiasis.

Attempts to inhibit immune complex formation in rabbits by penicillamine (5 or 25 mg kg^{-1} daily), indomethacin (5 mg kg^{-1} daily), or a single dose of cyclophosphamide (750 mg kg^{-1}) were unsuccessful, although dexamethasome (1 mg kg^{-1}) daily did reduce the amount of circulating complexes and the amount of kallikrein released.[58] It is of interest to note that while dexamethasone reduced the amount of kallikrein at the 10-day peak, it also caused an alteration in the parasitemia. Large numbers of trypanosomes were present 4 DPI and this coincided with an increase in plasma kallikrein. Similar early peaks of plasma kallikrein in trypanosome infections have been reported as mentioned above, indicating a second mechanism of release. In *B. bovis* infections it has been conclusively shown that kallikrein is activated by a serine esterase enzyme present in the parasite.[27] Such a system does not occur in trypanosomes,[54] but it is possible that kinin release may result from complement activation by variant specific glycoproteins on the surface of the parasite.[20,63] Alternatively, proteases such as cathepsin D found in the lysosomes of trypanosomes[64] or kinin-generating enzymes found in the lysosomes of polymorphonuclear leukocytes may be involved.[65] The mechanism for the production of urinary kallikrein is also unknown. Urinary kallikrein is synthesized in the kidney, probably in the juxta-glomerular complex.[66] Since the release of urinary kallikrein is regulated by the levels of sodium-retaining steroids, such as aldosterone,[67] it may be that trypanosomes in some way are able to modulate aldosterone levels.

III. HISTAMINE AND TRYPANOSOMIASIS

A. Pharmacology

Histamine is the most widely studied autocoid and it has been shown to be important in inflammatory, allergic, and anaphylactic reactions. It is formed by decarboxylation of histidine, a reaction which is catalyzed by two enzymes, L-histidine decarboxylase and aromatic amino acid decarboxylase. Histamine is widely distributed in almost all organs and body fluids, although there is considerable variation in concentrations between different host species and different tissues.[68] The major source of histamine is the mast cell, where it is stored in large basophilic granules together with ATP and heparin. Release of histamine from mast cells occurs in three main ways: first, it may be displaced by a compound that competes for the binding site; second, it is released when the process of exocytosis is stimulated; and, third, when damage to the mast cell occurs.[25] Many drugs, including the trypanocidal diamidines, are histamine releasers.

The pharmacological properties of histamine are demonstrated by the triple response resulting from its administration by intradermal injection. The response consists of a flush reaction due to arteriole vasodilatation, a flare reaction brought about by stimulation of sensory nerves, leading to an itch and localized pain response, and a wheal reaction caused by localized edema due to an increase in capillary permeability. Histamine also causes a fall in blood pressure, contraction of bronchial smooth muscle in most species, and contraction of many isolated smooth muscle preparations. It will also stimulate hydrogen ion secretion in the gastric mucosa and increase mucosal secretions. Two types of receptors (H1 and H2) are involved.[69] Specific inhibitors for both types of receptors are now available.

B. Release in Trypanosomiasis

Histamine was first reported to be released in trypanosomiasis when an increase was detected in the plasma, urine, ears, skin, and feet of mice with acute infections of *T. brucei*.[40] In all cases increases were detected on the day following infection, reaching maximum values two to three times greater than control levels, 3 to 4 DPI. A subsequent fall occurred prior to death on day 5. Although trypanosomes contain small amounts of histamine,[40] this is unlikely to be the major source, since increases in plasma histamine levels were found before parasites could be detected in the circulation. Yates[70,71] was unable to repeat this work and detected neither changes in the histamine content of blood or tissues, nor could he detect any differences in histidine decarboxylase levels in livers of mice acutely or chronically infected with *T. brucei*. No free histamine was found in the urine of infected rats.

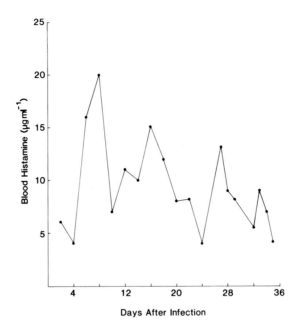

FIGURE 6.   Total blood histamine concentrations in rabbits infected with *Trypanosoma brucei*. Each point represents the mean
of estimations made on five animals. (From Yates, D. B., Involvement of Biogenic Amines, Enzymes and the Cardiovascular System
in the Pathology of Trypanosomiasis in Laboratory Animals, Ph.D.
thesis, University of London, 1978. With permission.)

Figure 6 shows the results of histamine changes in the blood of rabbits infected with *T. brucei*. Blood histamine concentrations increased 6 DPI with *T. brucei* and reached peak levels of nearly 20 μg mℓ$^{-1}$ 8 DPI. Subsequent peaks were seen around days 15 and 23, but the concentrations of histamine in the blood on these occasions were lower than at the first peak.[72] This pattern is very similar to that seen for kinin release (Figure 2) raising the possibility that similar release mechanisms exist. Preparations made from the subcutaneous tissues and ears of mice show that the numbers of mast cells present and their degree of granulation do not differ significantly at any stage of the trypanosome infection.[42] This suggests that histamine is derived from other sources in the host. In rabbits, histamine and 5-hydroxytryptamine (5-HT) are both present in high concentrations in platelets, and since thrombocytopenia is a common feature of trypanosomiasis[73] this could be the major source. If this hypothesis proves to be correct the mechanism of release could well be via an immunological reaction on the surface of the platelet as described for 5-HT.[74]

Histamine release has also been reported in malaria[75,76] and *Babesia* infections.[77]

IV. 5-HYDROXYTRYPTAMINE AND TRYPANOSOMIASIS

A. Pharmacology

5-HT is synthesized by hydroxylation of the essential amino acid tryptophan to form 5-hydroxytryptophan which is subsequently decarboxylated to form the amine. The enzymes involved in these reactions are tryptophan hydroxylase and aromatic amino acid decarboxylase. Aspects of the metabolism of tryptophan and its importance in trypanosomiasis have been discussed by Seed (see Chapter 1). Much of the 5-HT in the body is found in the mucosa of the gastrointestinal tract and within blood platelets. Like histamine, the concentration varies markedly between different tissues and hosts. Many of its pharmacological actions are similar to histamine and it has been implicated in the pathogenesis of asthma, inflammation, and various immune reactions.[25] It is a potent vasoconstrictor, although skeletal and coronary vessels are dilated. It is a powerful bronchoconstrictor and contracts many smooth muscle preparations. It is probably involved as a neurotransmitter in tryptaminergic neurones in the central nervous system.

B. Release in Trypanosomiasis

Despite extensive studies on the metabolism of indole amines in trypanosome infections (see Chapter 1), surprisingly little is known about 5-HT release during infections. In goats infected with *T. vivax*, 5-HT levels in the blood decrease during temperature peaks when the parasitemia is at its highest.[50,52] A correlation was shown to exist between parasitemia, pyrexia, decreases in blood 5-HT, and platelet aggregation. Decreases in whole blood 5-HT levels have also been reported in cattle infected with *T. vivax*[51] and rabbits infected with *T. brucei*.[48] There is evidence to suggest that 5-HT release results from an immunological reaction on the surface of platelets. 5-HT can be released from platelets by addition of *T. vivax* antigen and antibody directed against this antigen, but not by either component alone.[74] It has also been shown that a single injection of dead *T. vivax* antigen into endotoxin-sensitized rabbits caused no changes in either blood 5-HT levels or temperature, but that a second injection 10 days later caused both a pyrexia and fall in blood 5-HT levels. No endogenous pyrogen was detected in trypanosomes[48] which could explain the pyrexia.

Marked thrombocytopenia, caused by platelet aggregation, is a common feature of trypanosomiasis.[73,78] In some species platelet-containing microthrombi have been described,[48,51,79] as well as fibrin-containing thrombi.[18,51,80,81] During this aggregation and microthrombus formation 5-HT is likely to be released and since only falls in whole blood 5-HT have been seen it implies rapid metabolism of this autocoid. It would be of considerable interest to measure plasma 5-HT levels during trypanosome infections.

V. CATECHOLAMINES AND TRYPANOSOMIASIS

A. Pharmacology

The starting points in the synthesis of the catecholamines are the essential amino acids phenylalanine and tyrosine. Synthesis of noradrenaline involves dopa and dopamine as intermediates. Noradrenaline is converted to adrenaline by the enzymes phenethanolamine-*N*-methyltransferase. Two major enzymes are involved in the catabolism of catecholamines mono-amine oxidase and catechol-*o*-methyltransferase. Catecholamines are mainly stored in nervous tissue and the adrenal medulla, and when released prepare the host for emergencies — the fear-fright syndrome. As a response to catecholamine release the heart rate is increased, blood is transferred from the viscera to skeletal muscle, blood sugar is raised, pupils become dilated, and hair becomes erect.

B. Release in Trypanosomiasis

Catecholamine release from the adrenal medulla is greatly increased in conditions of physical stress. Such conditions are found in the successive crises that occur in trypanosomiasis, and it has been suggested that depletion of adrenaline and noradrenaline from the adrenal medulla may be the cause of the observed cardiovascular collapse.[15] Despite their obvious importance little attention has been paid to the catecholamines in trypanosomiasis. No evidence of adrenaline depletion was found in the adrenal glands of mice acutely infected with *T. brucei* or in rabbits with chronic infections.[70,71] However, in the rabbit some depletion of noradrenaline in the heart was seen. Metadrenalines which are known to be important metabolites of catecholamines in the rabbit are increased in the urine following an infection with *T. brucei*, but concentrations are very variable and difficult to interpret.[71] Thus, currently, it is not known whether there is an increased turnover of catecholamines in trypanosomiasis. Increased release of sympathomimetic amines from nerves does occur during trypanosomiasis and is responsible for the vasoconstriction demonstrated in the central artery of the ear of the rabbit.[82]

VI. OTHER BIOLOGICALLY ACTIVE SUBSTANCES

A number of other substances, which are known to have biological activity, are released or activated during trypanosome infections. In most cases their role in the pathogenesis of the disease has not been investigated.

A. Lysosomal Enzymes

Phagocytic cells, mainly of the mononuclear series, are known to accumulate in the vicinity of tissues and blood vessels in trypanosome infections.[18,83] These cells contain hydrolytic enzymes within the lysosomes including lysozyme, acid phosphatase, lipase, cathepsin, acid ribonuclease, β-glucuronidase, aminopeptidase, succinic dehydrogenase, neuraminidase, hyaluronidase, aryl sulfatase, and various esterases and proteases.[84] These lysosomal enzymes can be released either with or without destruction of the cell and have the potential to destroy all cell components and organelles. Possible pathways by which these enzymes may contribute towards the pathogenesis of trypanosomiasis include increasing leakage from vessels by direct action on the vascular endothelium, activation of the kallikrein-kinin system, chemotactic effects on granulocytes, and destruction of connective tissue.

B. Products of Complement Activation

Many authors have demonstrated activation of complement in trypanosomiasis of man,[85] cattle,[86-89] monkeys,[90] rabbits,[58] rats,[91] and mice.[92,93] Both the alternative and classical pathways appear to be involved. In addition, immunoconglutinins, autoantibodies directed against new antigenic determinants on fixed complement components, have been detected in humans,[94] sheep,[95] rabbits,[96-98] and rats[99] infected with trypanosomes. However, in cattle infected with *T. congolense* no increase was found.[100] These studies provide additional evidence for complement activation in most species. Complement activation leads to the formation of a number of fragments with known biological activity which could be involved in the disease process.[101] Both C3a and C5a are capable in vivo and in vitro of degranulating mast cells causing the liberation of their biogenic amines, causing vasoconstriction and enhancement of vascular permeability within the microcirculation and are chemotactic for neutrophils and other leukocytes.[102] The trimolecular complex C567 is also known to be chemotactic, while a low molecular weight cleavage product of C3, distinct from C3a, has been shown to mobilize neutrophils and monocytes. These substances would certainly be produced in trypanosomiasis, but their significance in the pathogenesis of the disease is unknown at present.

C. Fibrin-Fibrinogen Degradation Products (FDP)

Plasmin degrades both fibrin and fibrinogen in a stepwise manner to smaller fragments, some of which have biological properties.[103,104] These include potentiation of biogenic amines and peptides[105] and increasing vascular permeability.[106] In rabbits infected with *T. brucei* significant increases in FDP occur in the plasma with a peak 14 to 21 DPI.[106] At the same time plasminogen concentrations decrease, which is indicative of activation. FDP were also detected in the urine of rabbits late in the infection, probably as a result of glomerular damage, allowing the filtration of larger molecular weight substances.[107] Raised FDP levels are present in human trypanosomiasis[108,109] and this, combined with the thrombocytopenia,[73] suggests that disseminated intravascular coagulation is occurring. The mechanism by which plasminogen is activated in trypanosomiasis is unknown although circulating immune complexes may well be responsible.

VII. PATHOLOGICAL CONSEQUENCES OF AUTOCOID RELEASE

Although histamine, 5-HT, adrenaline, bradykinin, and acetylcholine have no direct effect on trypanosomes,[110] it is probable that their release does affect the pathogenesis of the disease, especially early in the infection.

A. Hypotension

Hypotension is an important feature of trypanosomiasis of the rabbit.[61,111] Changes in blood pressure were detected as early as 10 DPI and it is apparent that kallikrein, activated by immune complexes, mediates the reaction.[61] No changes in heart rate or cardiac output were seen but a significant fall in total peripheral resistance occurred.[72,111] These results, combined with the known increase in viscosity,[112,113] would account for the observed blood stasis and microthrombus formation.[83] Although hypotension has been reported in humans with trypanosomiasis,[114,115] it does not appear to be a consistent feature of the disease, neither has any attempt been made to explain its etiology.

B. Capillary Permeability

Increased capillary permeability can readily be demonstrated in experimental trypanosomiasis by intravenous injection of particulate material. The most comprehensive study has been undertaken by Edeghere[116,117] who extended the observations of Goodwin.[15,19,82,83] The major conclusion was that the permeability changes were consistent with that seen by injecting autocoids rather than that induced by substances that cause nonspecific tissue damage.[118-120] Histamine, 5-HT, and bradykinin all cause gaps to appear between endothelial cells, especially in the venules, and this is the picture seen in trypanosomiasis.

Several mechanisms may be involved in causing permeability changes. Autocoids released as a result of immune complex activation or the complexes themselves may act directly on the endothelial cells or, alternatively, the vascular permeability factor of trypanosomes[121] or proteases released from dead or dying organisms my be responsible.[20] Another interesting possibility has recently been suggested.[122,123] *T. congolense* binds to erythrocytes and endothelial cells of the microvasculature and damage to erythrocytes may occur after antibody and complement are bound to the cell. Increased permeability of mesenteric vessels of mice was demonstrated by Evans blue dye studies and it was postulated that the endothelial cells were damaged by bystander lysis. Bystander lysis occurs when the active C567 complex of complement, formed in the fluid phase, is transferred to an adjacent biological membrane in close proximity to an unrelated complement fixing site. No evidence of attachment of *T. brucei* to vessel walls has been demonstrated.[82,83]

Permeability changes also occur in the glomerulus of the kidney resulting in proteinuria and a negative water balance.[15] Renal insufficiency was demonstrated by a steady loss of serum albumin and calcium and increase in urea and creatinine in tissue fluids and serum of infected rabbits.[124] Two types of renal lesion have been described, a proliferative glomerulonephritis,[90,125-128] probably resulting from deposition of IgM, IgG, C3, and trypanosome antigen in the glomerulus, and tubular atrophy,[126] similar to that seen in tissue ischemia.

C. Smooth Muscle Contractility

A comparison of passive and active tensions of the caudal artery of both control rats and rats infected with *T. brucei* has been made.[129] Passive tensions were similar in both groups of rats, but there was a significant increase in active tension in the infected group. Active tension relates to contractility resulting from a stimulus, in this case by increasing the potassium ion concentration, while passive tension is a characteristic of the connective tissue content. The authors suggested that this change in the contractile properties of the muscle may have been due to an alteration in muscle membrane potentials induced by released autocoids.

D. Chemotaxis

Chemotaxis, which is the determined directional response of a cell or organism towards chemical substances in the environment, is an important mechanism for recruiting cells. Those substances which exert a direct stimulatory effect on cells are termed cytotaxins, and those which induce the formation of cytotaxins, cytotaxigens.[130] Many of the chemicals discussed above are known to be cytotaxins and these include components of the kallikrein-kinin systems, complement fragments and breakdown products of fibrin and fibrinogen. Using a modified Boyden technique, Cook[131] has shown that complexes of trypanosomes and antibody but not trypanosomes alone were chemotactic for mouse peritoneal exudate cells.

At present no information is available which, if any, of the autocoids are involved in chemotaxis in trypanosomiasis. However, accumulation of mononuclear cells at sites of inflammation is not entirely protective. Some cells die, releasing their lysosomal enzymes, while others attach to vessel walls causing changes in blood flow patterns, microthrombus formation, blood stasis, and tissue anoxia.[83,117]

5-HT, but not histamine, will enhance attachment of trypanosomes to mouse peritoneal exudate cells in vitro,[132] an essential prerequisite for phagocytosis. It is possible that this reaction is mediated via lipid receptors present on macrophages,[133] but its significance in host protection remains to be determined.

VIII. THE PATHOGENESIS OF TRYPANOSOMIASIS

One important conclusion can be drawn from the above discussions. There is no doubt that autocoids are released in all pathogenic trypanosome infections so far examined. The species of host may well determine the relative amounts of the different autocoids released, but more extensive data are required before a definite conclusion can be reached. The greatest amounts of autocoids are released early in chronic infections at a time when pathological changes in the host are beginning to occur. Although this is only circumstantial evidence that autocoids are involved in the pathogenesis of the disease, it is known that kallikrein directly causes the hypotension seen in the rabbit.[61] At least two mechanisms are known to cause kinin release in trypanosomiasis: one which occurs very early in 4 to 5 DPI, but about which little is known, and a second about 10 DPI involving the activation of Hageman factor by immune complexes. It seems quite probable that histamine and 5-HT are released from tissue stores, particularly platelets, by immune complexes.

Circulating immune complexes have been detected in the blood of many species including man,[134-136] rabbits,[57,58,62] rats,[127] and mice,[137-139] and deposition in the tissues has been reported in monkeys,[90] rabbits,[128,140] and mice.[137,138,141] Many biological properties have been assigned to immune complexes,[142] several of which probably contribute to the pathogenesis of the disease. In addition to release of autocoids, immune complexes are probably responsible for plasminogen activation[106] and are one of the mechanisms by which complement is activated.[58,83-93] The distribution of immune complexes within the body can be markedly influenced by complement. The size of the complex is greatly increased when complement is bound leading to its removal in the reticuloendothelial system or deposition in the glomerulus or other tissues. Since decomplementation inhibits the formation of B memory cells,[143] immune complex activation of complement may contribute to the immunosuppression, which is an important feature of the disease.[144,145]

The formation of immune complexes on the surface of various cell types in trypanosomiasis potentially has very serious consequences. Such reactions may be direct or involve complement receptors present on the cells.[142] Thrombocytopenia[73,78] and anemia[146] will result from immunocytoadherence to platelets and erythrocytes. Immune complexes can also be bound to lymphocytes, cells of the macrophage series, and polymorphonuclear cells and could play roles in modulating antibody synthesis, phagocytosis, and tissue destruction by lysosomal enzymes.[142]

In order for immune complexes to be formed in trypanosomiasis, proliferation of B lymphocytes, leading to polyclonal synthesis of antibodies, must first occur.[23,145,147] The antibody response primarily consists of macroglobulins including free light chains and 7s IgM molecules.[148] One of the features of the disease is the production of a large number of autoantibodies[149-155] which will contribute to the circulating immune complexes,[156] the increased plasma protein and hyperviscosity,[113] as well as possibly causing pathological changes in the tissues against which the autoantibody is directed.

Figure 7 attempts to summarize some of the possible mechanisms contributing to the pathogenesis of the disease. This diagram is certainly an oversimplification since many interrelationships exist which have not been shown. Perhaps the most important pathological effect of autocoid release will turn out to be the increased vascular permeability which they induce along with other factors. Once there is free movement of molecules between the blood and tissue compartments of the body, intense inflammatory reactions occur[15,17,18,21,157] which will exacerbate the release of autocoids, mobilize inflammatory cells, and result in edema.

It is not intended that the reader should conclude from this review that the release of autocoids and their pathological sequelae answer all the questions regarding the pathogenesis of trypanosomiasis. Nevertheless, it does appear that immune complex formation and subsequent autocoid release early in the infection constitutes an important key to the development of pathology. A detailed study of the formation and constituents of immune complexes at all stages of the infection is required and urgent attempts need to be made to devise effective methods of preventing the release of all autocoids in trypanosomiasis.

ACKNOWLEDGMENTS

The original work described in this chapter was undertaken with grants from the U.K. Ministry of Overseas Development. I wish to thank Dr. Ian Wright for his constructive criticism of this chapter.

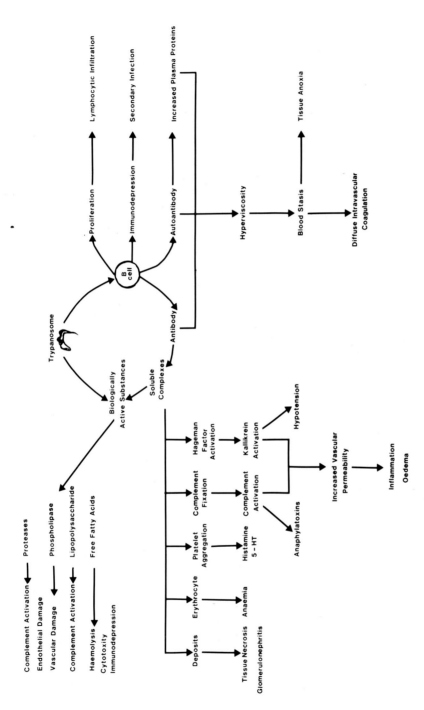

FIGURE 7.   Suggested mechanisms of the pathogenesis of African trypanosomiasis with particular reference to the role played by immune complexes and polyclonal B cell proliferation. This diagram represents a simplification as many interactions will occur.

REFERENCES

1. **Goodwin, L. G. and Richards, W. H. R.,** Pharmacologically active peptides in the blood and urine of animals infected with *Babesia rodhaini* and other pathogenic organisms, *Br. J. Pharmacol. Chemother.,* 15, 152, 1960.
2. **Dukelsky, O.,** Ueber die Neutralisierung des Anaphylatoxins durch Salvarsan in Verbindung mit der Pathogenese der Todesfalle bei Tryanosomenerkrankungen, *Z. Immunitaetsforsch. Exp. Ther.,* 42, 113, 1925.
3. **Dale, H. H.,** Local vasodilator reactions. Histamine cont., acetylcholine, conclusion, *Lancet,* 1, 1285, 1929.
4. **Mackie, F. P.,** The Jarisch-Herxheimer reaction in trypanosomiasis with a note on the morular cells of Mott, *Trans. R. Soc. Trop. Med. Hyg.,* 28, 377, 1935.
5. **Fiennes, R. N. T.-W.,** The cattle trypanosomiases: some considerations of pathology and immunity, *Ann. Trop. Med. Parasitol.,* 44, 42, 1950.
6. **Stephan, O. and Esquibel, A.,** Methodo de premunicao contra a "tristeza" usado no posto zootechnico de São Paulo, *Archos. Inst. Biol. Def. Agric. Anim. São Paulo,* 2, 183, 1929.
7. **Willett, K. C.,** Sleeping sickness in East Africa and its treatment, *East Afr. Med. J.,* 32, 273, 1955.
8. **Robertson, D. H. H.,** The treatment of sleeping sickness (mainly due to *Trypanosoma rhodesiense*) with melarsoprol. I. Reactions observed during treatment, *Trans. R. Soc. Trop. Med. Hyg.,* 57, 122, 1963.
9. **Whittle, H. C. and Pope, H. M.,** The febrile response to treatment in Gambian sleeping sickness, *Ann. Trop. Med. Parasitol.,* 66, 7, 1972.
10. **Boreham, P. F. L. and Wright, I. G.,** The release of pharmacologically active substances in parasitic infections, in *Progress in Medicinal Chemistry,* Vol. 13, Ellis, G. P. and West, G. B., Eds., North-Holland, Amsterdam, 1976, 159.
11. **de Raadt, P. and Seed, J. R.,** Trypanosomes causing disease in man in Africa, in *Parasitic Protozoa, Taxonomy, Kinetoplastids and Flagellates of Fish,* Vol. 1, Kreier, J. P., Ed., Academic Press, New York, 1977, 175.
12. **Maegraith, B. G., Devakul, K., and Leithead, C. S.,** Action of noradrenaline in medical shock in *Plasmodium knowlesi* malaria, *Trans. R. Soc. Trop. Med. Hyg.,* 50, 311, 1956.
13. **Maegraith, B., Gilles, H. M., and Devakul, K.,** Pathological processes in *Babesia canis* infections, *Z. Tropenmed. Parasitol.,* 8, 485, 1957.
14. **Fiennes, R. N. T.-W.,** Pathogenesis and pathology of animal trypanosomiases, in *The African Trypanosomiases,* Mulligan, H. W., Ed., George Allen and Unwin, London, 1970, 729.
15. **Goodwin, L. G.,** The pathology of African trypanosomiasis, *Trans. R. Soc. Trop. Med. Hyg.,* 64, 797, 1970.
16. **Ormerod, W. E.,** Pathogenesis and pathology of trypanosomiasis in man, in *The African Trypanosomiases,* Mulligan, H. W., Ed., George Allen and Unwin, London, 1970, 587.
17. **Hutt, M. S. R. and Wilks, N. E.,** African trypanosomiasis (sleeping sickness), in *Pathology of Protozoal and Helminthic Diseases with Clinical Correlation,* Marcial-Rojas, R. A., Ed., Williams & Wilkins, Baltimore, 1971, 57.
18. **Losos, G. J. and Ikede, B. O.,** Review of pathology of disease in domestic and laboratory animals caused by *Trypanosoma congolense, T. vivax, T. brucei, T. rhodesiense* and *T. gambiense, Vet. Pathol.,* 9 (Suppl.,) 1, 1972.
19. **Goodwin, L. G.,** The African scene: mechanisms of pathogenesis in trypanosomiasis, in *Trypanosomiasis and Leishmaniasis with Special Reference to Chagas Disease,* CIBA Foundation Symp. No. 20 (New Series), Elliott, K., O'Connor, M., and Wolstenholme, G. E. W., Eds., Elsevier, Amsterdam, 1974, 107.
20. **Tizard, I., Nielsen, K. H., Seed, J. R., and Hall, J. E.,** Biologically active products from African trypanosomes, *Microbiol. Rev.,* 42, 661, 1978.
21. **Boreham, P. F. L.,** The pathogenesis of African and American trypanosomiasis, in *Biochemistry and Physiology of Protozoa,* Vol. 2, 2nd ed., Levandowsky, M. and Hutner, S. H., Eds., Academic Press, New York, 1979, 429.
22. **Henson, J. B. and Noel, J. C.,** Immunology and pathogenesis of African animal trypanosomiasis, *Adv. Vet. Sci. Comp. Med.,* 23, 161, 1979.
23. **Greenwood, B. M. and Whittle, H. C.,** The pathogenesis of sleeping sickness, *Trans. R. Soc. Trop. Med. Hyg.,* 74, 716, 1980.
24. **Goodman, L. S. and Gilman, A., Eds.,** *The Pharmacological Basis of Therapeutics: A Text Book of Pharmacology, Toxicology and Therapeutics for Physicians and Medical Students,* 6th ed., Macmillan, New York, 1980, sect. 5.
25. **Bowman, W. C. and Rand, M. J.,** *Textbook of Pharmacology,* 2nd ed., Blackwell Scientific, Oxford, 1980, chap. 12.

26. **Goodwin, L. G.,** Vasoactive amines and peptides: their role in the pathogenesis of protozoal infections, in *Pathophysiology of Parasitic Infections,* Soulsby, E. J. L., Ed., Academic Press, New York, 1976, 161.

27. **Wright, I. G.,** The kallikrein-kinin system and its role in the hypotensive shock syndrome of animals infected with the haemoprotozoan parasites *Babesia, Plasmodium* and *Trypanosoma, Gen. Pharmacol.,* 10, 319, 1979.

28. **Timofeev, B. A.,** Role of the kinin system and cryofibrinogen process in the pathogenesis of animal protozoan diseases (in Russian), *S. Kh. Biol.,* 16, 652, 1981.

29. **Regoli, D. and Barabe, J.,** Pharmacology of bradykinin and related kinins, *Pharmacol. Rev.,* 32, 1, 1980.

30. **Schachter, M.,** Kallikreins (kininogenases) — a group of serine proteases with bioregulatory action, *Pharmacol. Rev.,* 31, 1, 1980.

31. **Ogston, D. and Bennett, B.,** Surface-mediated reactions in the formation of thrombin, plasmin and kallikrein, *Br. Med Bull.,* 34, 107, 1978.

32. **Coleman, R. W.,** Formation of human plasma kinin, *N. Engl. J. Med.,* 291, 509, 1974.

33. **Murano, G.,** The "Hageman" connection: interrelationships of blood coagulation, fibrino(geno)lysis, kinin generation, and complement activation, *Am. J. Hematol.,* 4, 409, 1978.

34. **Regoli, D.,** Vascular receptors for polypeptides, *Trends Pharmacol. Sci.,* 3, 286, 1982.

35. **Margolius, H. S.,** Kallikreins, kinins and the kidney: what's going on in there?, *J. Lab. Clin. Med.,* 91, 717, 1978.

36. **Katori, M., Iwanaga, S., Komiya, M., Han, Y. N., Suzuki, T., and Ohishi, S.,** Structure and a possible physiological function of a fragment ("histidine-rich peptide") released from a bovine plasma high molecular weight kininogen by plasma kallikrein, in *Kininogenases 3,* Haberland, G. L., Rohen, J. W., Blumel, G., and Huber, P., Eds., Schattauer, New York, 1975, 11.

37. **Voorheis, H. P.,** The effect of *Trypanosoma brucei* (S-42) on host carbohydrate metabolism: liver production and peripheral tissue utilisation of glucose, *Trans. R. Soc. Trop. Med. Hyg.,* 63, 122, 1969.

38. **Newton, B. A.,** The metabolism of African trypanosomes in relation to pathogenic mechanisms, in *Pathogenicity of Trypanosomes,* Losos, G. and Chouinard, A., Eds., International Development Research Centre, Ottawa, 1979, 17.

39. **van den Ingh, T. S. G. A. M.,** Pathomorphological changes in *Trypanosoma brucei brucei* infection in the rabbit, *Zentralbl. Veterinaermed. Reihe B,* 24, 773, 1977.

40. **Richards, W. H. G.,** Pharmacologically active substances in the blood, tissues and urine of mice infected with *Trypanosoma brucei, Br. J. Pharmacol. Chemother.,* 24, 124, 1965.

41. **Boreham, P. F. L.,** Pharmacologically active peptides in the tissues of the host during chronic trypanosome infections, *Nature (London),* 212, 190, 1966.

42. **Goodwin, L. G. and Boreham, P. F. L.,** Pharmacologically active peptides in trypanosome infections, in *Hypotensive Peptides,* Erdos, E. G., Back, N., and Sicuteri, F., Eds., Springer-Verlag, New York, 1966, 545.

43. **Bhattacharya, B. K., Sen, A. B., and Talwalkar, V.,** Pharmacologically active substances in the plasma of guinea-pig infected with *Trypanosoma evansi, Arch. Int. Pharmacodyn. Ther.,* 156, 106, 1965.

44. **Tella, A. and Maegraith, B. G.,** Studies on bradykinin and bradykininogen in malaria, *Ann. Trop. Med. Parasitol.,* 60, 304, 1966.

45. **Wright, I. G.,** Kinin, kininogen and kininase levels during acute *Babesia bovis* (= *B. argentina*) infection of cattle, *Br. J. Pharmacol.,* 61, 567, 1977.

46. **Wright, I. G., Goodger, B. V., and Mahoney, D. F.,** Virulent and avirulent strains of *Babesia bovis*: the relationship between parasite protease content and pathophysiological effect of the strain, *J. Protozool.,* 28, 118, 1981.

47. **Boreham, P. F. L.,** Immune reactions and kinin formation in chronic trypanosomiasis, *Br. J. Pharmacol. Chemother.,* 32, 493, 1968.

48. **van den Ingh, T. S. G. A. M., Schotman, A. J. H., van Duin, C. Th. M., Busser, E. J. M., ten Hoedt, E., and de Neys, M. H. H.,** Clinico-pathological changes during *Trypanosoma brucei brucei* infection in the rabbit, *Zentralbl. Veterinaermed. Reihe B,* 24, 787, 1977.

49. **Boreham, P. F. L.,** Kinin release and the immune reaction in human trypanosomiasis caused by *Trypanosoma rhodesiense, Trans. R. Soc. Trop. Med. Hyg.,* 64, 394, 1970.

50. **Veenendaal, G. H., van Miert, A. S. J. P. A. M., van den Ingh, T. S. G. A. M., Schotman, A. J. H., and Zwart, D.,** A comparison of the role of kinins and serotonin in endotoxin induced fever and *Trypanosoma vivax* infections in the goat, *Res. Vet. Sci.,* 21, 271, 1976.

51. **van den Ingh, T. S. G. A. M., Zwart, D., van Miert, A. S. J. P. A. M., and Schotman, A. J. H.,** Clinico-pathological and pathomorphological observations in *Trypanosoma vivax* infection in cattle, *Vet. Parasitol.,* 2, 237, 1976.

52. **Zwart, D. and Veenendaal, G. H.,** Pharmacologically active substances in *T. vivax* infections, in *Pathogenicity of Trypanosomes,* Losos, G. and Chouinard, A., Eds., International Development Research Centre, Ottawa, 1979, 111.

53. **Ferreira, S. H. and Vane, J. R.,** Half-lives of peptides and amines in the circulation, *Nature (London)*, 215, 1237, 1967.

54. **Boreham, P. F. L.,** *In vitro* studies on the mechanism of kinin formation by trypanosomes, *Br. J. Pharmacol.,* 34, 598, 1968.

55. **Boreham, P. F. L.,** Kallikrein — its release and possible significance in trypanosomiasis, *Ann. Soc. Belge Med. Trop.,* 57, 191, 1977.

56. **Wright, I. G. and Boreham, P. F. L.,** Studies on urinary kallikrein in *Trypanosoma brucei* infections of the rabbit, *Biochem. Pharmacol.,* 26, 417, 1977.

57. **Boreham, P. F. L. and Parry, M. G.,** The role of kallikrein in the pathogenesis of African trypanosomiasis, in *Current Concepts in Kinin Research,* Haberland, G. L. and Hamberg, U., Eds., Pergamon Press, Oxford, 1979, 85.

58. **Parry, M. G.,** Kallikrein and Its Activation in Experimental *Trypanosoma brucei* Infections of Rabbits, Ph.D. thesis, University of London, 1980.

59. **Movat, H. Z., DiLorenzo, N. L., Mustard, J. F., and Helmel, G.,** Activation of Hageman and a vascular permeability factor in serum by AG-AB precipitates, *Fed. Proc. Fed. Am. Soc. Exp. Biol.,* 25, 682, 1966.

60. **Boreham, P. F. L. and Goodwin, L. G.,** The release of kinins, as the result of an antigen-antibody reaction in trypanosomiasis, in *Bradykinin and Related Kinins, Cardiovascular, Biochemical and Neural Actions,* Sicuteri, F., Rocha e Silva, M., and Back, N., Eds., Plenum Press, New York, 1970, 539.

61. **Boreham, P. F. L. and Wright, I. G.,** Hypotension in rabbits infected with *Trypanosoma brucei, Br. J. Pharmacol.,* 58, 137, 1976.

62. **Boreham, P. F. L.,** Pharmacologically active substances in *T. brucei* infections, in *Pathogenicity of Trypanosomes,* Losos, G. and Chouinard, A., Eds., International Development Research Centre, Ottawa, 1979, 114.

63. **Musoke, A. J. and Barbet, A. F.,** Activation of complement by variant-specific surface antigen of *Trypanosoma brucei, Nature (London),* 270, 438, 1977.

64. **Venkatesan, S., Bird, R. G., and Ormerod, W. E.,** Intracellular enzymes and their localization in slender and stumpy forms of *Trypanosoma brucei rhodesiense, Int. J. Parasitol.,* 7, 139, 1977.

65. **Movat, H. Z., Steinberg, S. G., Habal, F. M., and Ranadive, N. S.,** Demonstration of kinin-generating enzyme in the lysosomes of human polymorphonuclear leukocytes, *Lab. Invest.,* 29, 669, 1973.

66. **Nustad, K.,** Localization of kininogenase in the rat kidney, *Br. J. Pharmacol.,* 39, 87, 1970.

67. **Keiser, H. R., Geller, R. G., Margolius, H. S., and Pisano, J. J.,** Urinary kallikrein in hypertensive animal models, *Fed. Proc. Fed. Am. Soc. Exp. Biol.,* 35, 199, 1976.

68. **Rocha e Silva, M., Ed.,** *Handbook of Experimental Pharmacology, Vol. 18, Histamine and Antihistamines, Part 1, Histamine. Its Chemistry: Metabolism and Physiological and Pharmacological Actions,* Springer-Verlag, Berlin, 1966, chap. 1.

69. **Black, I W., Duncan, W. A. M., Durant, C. J., Genellin, C. R., and Parsons, E. M.,** Definition and antagonism of histamine H_2-receptors, *Nature (London),* 236, 385, 1972.

70. **Yates, D. B.,** Pharmacology of trypanosomiasis, *Trans. R. Soc. Trop. Med. Hyg.,* 64, 167, 1970.

71. **Yates, D. B.,** Summary of work carried out on pharmacology of African sleeping sickness between 1967—1970, *Trans. R. Soc. Trop. Med. Hyg.,* 65, 238, 1971.

72. **Yates, D. B.,** Involvement of Biogenic Amines, Enzymes and the Cardiovascular System in the Pathology of Trypanosomiasis in Laboratory Animals, Ph.D. thesis, University of London, 1978.

73. **Davies, C E.,** Thrombocytopenia: a uniform complication of African trypanosomiasis, *Acta Trop.,* 39, 123, 1982.

74. **Slots, J. M. M., van Miert, A. S. J. P. A. M., Akkerman, J. W. N., and de Gee, A. L. W.,** *Trypanosoma brucei* and *Trypanosoma vivax,* antigen-antibody complexes as a cause of platelet serotonin release *in vitro* and *in vivo, Exp. Parasitol.,* 43, 211, 1977.

75. **Maegraith, B. G. and Onabanjo, A. O.,** The effects of histamine in malaria, *Br. J. Pharmacol.,* 39, 755, 1970.

76. **Srichaikul, T., Archararit, N., Siriasawakul, T., and Viriyapanich, T.,** Histamine changes in *Plasmodium falciparum* malaria, *Trans. R. Soc. Trop. Med. Hyg.,* 70, 36, 1976.

77. **Wright, I. G.,** Biogenic amine levels in acute *Babesia bovis* infected cattle, *Vet. Parasitol.,* 4, 393, 1978.

78. **Davis, C.E., Robbins, R. S., Weller, R. D., and Braude, A. I.,** Thrombocytopenia in experimental trypanosomiasis, *J. Clin. Invest.,* 53, 1359, 1974.

79. **van den Ingh, T. S. G. A. M., Zwart, D., Schotman, A. J. H., van Miert, A. S. J. P. A. M., and Veenendaal, G. H.,** The pathology and pathogenesis of *Trypanosoma vivax* infection in the goat, *Res. Vet. Sci.,* 21, 264, 1976.

80. **van Dijk, J. E., Zwart, D., and Leeflang, P.,** A contribution to the pathology of *Trypanosoma simiae* infection in pigs, *Zentralbl. Veterinaermed. Reihe B,* 20, 374, 1973.

81. **Morrison, W. I., Murray, M., Sayer, P. D., and Preston, J. M.,** The pathogenesis of experimentally induced *Trypanosoma brucei* infection in the dog. I. Tissue and organ damage, *Am. J. Pathol.,* 102, 168, 1981.

82. **Goodwin, L. G. and Hook, S. V. M.,** Vascular lesions in rabbits infected with *Trypanosoma (Trypanozoon) brucei, Br. J. Pharmacol. Chemother.,* 32, 505, 1968.

83. **Goodwin, L. G.,** Pathological effects of *Trypanosoma brucei* on small blood vessels in rabbit ear-chambers, *Trans. R. Soc. Trop. Med. Hyg.,* 65, 82, 1971.

84. **Hirschhorn, R.,** Lysosomal mechanisms in the inflammatory process, in *The Inflammatory Process,* Vol. 1, 2nd ed., Zweifach, B. W., Grant, L., and McCluskey, R. T., Eds., Academic Press, New York, 1974, 259.

85. **Greenwood, B. M. and Whittle, H. C.,** Complement activation in patients with Gambian sleeping sickness, *Clin. Exp. Immunol.,* 24, 133, 1976.

86. **Kobayashi, A. and Tizard, I. R.,** The response to *Trypanosoma congolense* infection in calves. Determination of immunogobulins IgG1, IgG2, IgM and C3 levels and the complement fixing antibody titres during the course of infection, *Z. Tropenmed. Parasitol.,* 27, 411, 1976.

87. **Nielsen, K. H., Sheppard, J., Tizard, I. R., and Holmes, W. L.,** Experimental bovine trypanosomiasis: changes in the catabolism of serum immunoglobulins and complement components in infected cattle, *Immunology,* 35, 817, 1978.

88. **Rurangirwa, F. R., Tabel, H., Losos, G., and Tizard, I. R.,** Haemolytic complement and serum C3 levels in zebu cattle infected with *Trypanosoma congolense* and *Trypanosoma vivax* and the effect of trypanocidal treatment, *Infect. Immun.,* 27, 832, 1980.

89. **Tabel, H., Losos, G. J., and Maxie, M. G.,** Experimental bovine trypanosomiasis *(Trypanosoma vivax* and *T. congolense).* II. Serum levels of total protein, albumin, hemolytic complement, and complement component, C3, *Tropenmed. Parasitol.,* 31, 99, 1980.

90. **Nagle, R. B., Ward, P. A., Lindsley, H. G., Sadun, E. H., Johnson, A. J., Berkaw, R. E., and Hildebrandt, P. K.,** Experimental infections with trypanosomes. VI. Glomerulonephritis involving the alternate pathway of complement activation, *Am. J. Trop. Med. Hyg.,* 23, 15, 1974.

91. **Lambert, P. H. and Galvao Castro, B.,** Role de la response immune dans la pathologie de la trypanosomiase Africaine (resume), *Ann. Soc. Belge Med. Trop.,* 57, 267, 1977.

92. **Jarvinen, J. A. and Dalmasso, A. P.,** *Trypanosoma musculi:* infections in normocomplementemic, C5-deficient, and C3 depleted mice, *Infect. Immun.,* 16, 557, 1977.

93. **Shirazi, F. M., Holman, M., Hudson, K. M., Klaus, G. G. B., and Terry, R. J.,** Complement (C3) levels and the effect of C3 depletion in infections of *Trypanosoma brucei* in mice, *Parasite Immunol.,* 2, 155, 1980.

94. **Lachmann, P. J.,** Conglutinin and immunoconglutinin, *Adv. Immunol.,* 6, 479, 1967.

95. **Kobayashi, A., Soltys, M. A., and Woo, P. T. K.,** Comparative studies in the laboratory diagnosis of experimental *Trypanosoma congolense* infection in sheep, *Ann. Trop. Med. Parasitol.,* 70, 53, 1976.

96. **Ingram, D. G., Barber, H., McLean, D. M., Soltys, M. A., and Coombs, R. R. A.,** The conglutination phenomenon. XII. Immuno-conglutinin in experimental infections of laboratory animals, *Immunology,* 2, 268, 1959.

97. **Ingram, D. G. and Soltys, M. A.,** Immunity in trypanosomiasis. IV. Immunoconglutinin in animals infected with *Trypanosoma brucei, Parasitology,* 50, 231, 1960.

98. **Pautrizel, R., Duret, J., Tribouley, J., and Ripert, Ch.,** Application de la réaction conglutination au diagnostic sérologique des trypanosomoses, *Bull. Soc. Pathol. Exot.,* 55, 391, 1962.

99. **Rickman, W. J. and Cox, H. W.,** Association of autoantibodies with anaemia, splenomegaly and glomerulonephritis in experimental African trypanosomiasis, *J. Parasitol.,* 65, 65, 1979.

100. **Tizard, I. R., Mittal, K. R., and Nielsen, K.,** Depressed immunoconglutinin responses in calves experimentally infected with *Trypanosoma congolense, Res. Vet. Sci.,* 28, 203, 1980.

101. **Barkas, T.,** Biological activities of complement, *Biochem. Soc. Trans.,* 6, 798, 1978.

102. **Hugli, T. E. and Muller-Eberhard, H. J.,** Anaphylatoxins: C3a and C5a, *Adv. Immunol.,* 26, 1, 1978.

103. **Triantaphyllopoulos, D. C. and Triantaphyllopoulos, E.,** Physiological effects of fibrinogen degradation products, *Thromb. Diath. Haemorrh.,* 39(Suppl.), 175, 1970.

104. **Gaffney, P. J.,** Breakdown products of fibrin and fibrinogen: molecular mechanisms and clinical implications, *J. Clin. Pathol.,* 33(Suppl. 14), 10, 1980.

105. **Barnhart, M. I.,** The inflammatory process: biochemical parameters of exudative proteins, *Tice's Pract. Med.,* 5, 1, 1969.

106. **Boreham, P. F. L. and Facer, C. A.,** Fibrinogen and fibrinogen/fibrin degradation products in experimental African trypanosomiasis, *Int. J. Parasitol.,* 4, 143, 1974.

107. **Boreham, P. F. L. and Facer, C. A.,** Fibrinogen and fibrinogen/fibrin degradation products in the urine of rabbits infected with *Trypanosoma (Trypanozoon) brucei, Z. Parasitenkd.,* 52, 257, 1977.

108. **Greenwood, B. M. and Whittle, H. C.,** Coagulation studies in Gambian trypanosomiasis, *Am. J. Trop. Med. Hyg.,* 25, 390, 1976.

109. **Robins-Browne, R. M. and Schneider, J.,** Coagulation disturbances in African trypanosomiasis, in *Medicine in a Tropical Environment,* Gear, J. H. S., Ed., Balkema, Rotterdam, 1977, 565.

110. **Boreham, P. F. L.,** The effect of histamine, 5-hydroxytryptamine, adrenaline, acetylcholine and bradykin on the infectivity of trypanosomes, *Rep. East Afr. Trypan. Res. Org.,* 72, 1966.

111. **Yates, D. B.,** Changes in blood pressure, cardiac output and rate, and the response to lower body negative pressure (LBNP) in trypanosome-infected rabbits, *Br. J. Pharmacol.,* 64, 397P, 1978.

112. **Boreham, P. F. L.,** Physiopathological changes in the blood of rabbits infected with *Trypanosoma brucei, Rev. Elev. Med. Vet. Pays Trop.,* Suppl., 279, 1974.

113. **Facer, C. A.,** Blood hyperviscosity during *Trypanosoma (Trypanozoon) brucei* infections of rabbits, *J. Comp. Pathol.,* 86, 393, 1976.

114. **Sicé, A.,** La Trypanosomiase Humaine en Afrique Intertropicale, Vigot, Paris, 1937, 86.

115. **Buyst, H.,** The diagnosis of sleeping sickness in a district hospital in Zambia, *Ann. Soc. Belge Med. Trop.,* 55, 551, 1975.

116. **Edeghere, H. U. F. I.,** Vascular changes in experimental African trypanosomiasis, *Parasitology,* 79, IX, 1979.

117. **Edeghere, H. U. F. I.,** Morphological and Ultrastructural Changes in Small Blood Vessels of Rabbits Infected with *Trypanosoma brucei,* Ph.D. thesis, University of London, 1980.

118. **Majno, G. and Palade, G. E.,** Studies on inflammation. I. The effect of histamine and serotonin on vascular permeability: an electron microscopic study, *J. Biophys. Biochem. Cytol.,* 11, 571, 1961.

119. **Majno, G., Palade, G. E., and Schoefl, G. I.,** Studies on inflammation. II. The site of action of histamine and serotonin along the vascular tree: a topographical study, *J. Biophys. Biochem. Cytol.,* 11, 607, 1961.

120. **Majno, G., Shea, S., and Leventhal, M.,** Endothelial contraction induced by histamine-type mediators: an electron microscopic study, *J. Cell. Biol.,* 42, 647, 1969.

121. **Seed, J. R.,** *Trypanosoma gambiense* and *T. lewisi:* increased vascular permeability and skin lesions in rabbits, *Exp. Parasitol.,* 26, 214, 1969.

122. **Banks, K. L.,** Binding of *Trypanosoma congolense* to the walls of small blood vessels, *J. Protozool.,* 25, 241, 1978.

123. **Banks, K. L.,** Injury induced by *Trypanosoma congolense* adhesion to cell membranes, *J. Parisitol.,* 66, 34, 1980.

124. **Goodwin, L. G. and Guy, M. W.,** Tissue fluid in rabbits infected with *Trypanosoma (Trypanozoon) brucei, Parasitology,* 66, 499, 1973.

125. **Murray, M.,** The pathology of African trypanosomiasis, *Prog. Immunol. II,* 4, 181, 1974.

126. **Facer, C. A., Molland, E. A., Gray, A. B., and Jenkins, G. C.,** *Trypanosoma brucei:* renal pathology in rabbits, *Exp. Parasitol.,* 44, 249, 1978.

127. **Lindsley, H. B., Nagle, R. B., Werner, P. A., and Stechschulte, D. J.,** Variable severity of glomerulonephritis in inbred rats infected with *Trypanosoma rhodesiense,* correlation with immunoglobulin class-specific antibody responses to trypanosomal antigens and total IgM levels, *Am. J. Trop. Med. Hyg.,* 29, 348, 1980.

128. **Nagle, R. B., Dong, S., Guillot, J. M., McDaniel, K. M., and Lindsley, H. B.,** Pathology of experimental African trypanosomiasis in rabbits infected with *Trypanosoma rhodesiense, Am. J. Trop. Med. Hyg.,* 29, 1187, 1980.

129. **Greer, C. A., Cain, G. D., and Schottelius, B. A.,** Changes in vascular smooth muscle contractility associated with *Trypanosoma brucei* infections in rats, *J. Parasitol.,* 65, 825, 1979.

130. **Wilkinson, P. C.,** Leukocyte locomotion and chemotaxis: effects of bacteria and viruses, *Rev. Infect. Dis.,* 2, 293, 1980.

131. **Cook, R. M.,** The chemotactic response of murine peritoneal exudate cells to *Trypanosoma brucei, Vet. Parasitol.,* 7, 3, 1980.

132. **Cook, R. M.,** Studies on Phagocytic Activity in Experimental African Trypanosomiasis, Ph.D. thesis, University of London, 1977.

133. **Davey, M. J. and Asherson, G. L.,** Cytophilic antibody. I. Nature of the macrophage receptor, *Immunology,* 12, 13, 1967.

134. **Fruit, J., Santoro, F., Afchain, D., Duvallet, G., and Capron, A.,** Les immuncomplexes circulants dans la trypanosomiase africaine humaine et experimentale, *Ann. Soc. Belge Med. Trop.,* 57, 257, 1977.

135. **Whittle, H., Greenwood, B. M., and Mohammed, I.,** Immune complexes in Gambian sleeping sickness, *Trans. R. Soc. Trop. Med. Hyg.,* 74, 833, 1980.

136. **Lambert, P. H., Berney, M., and Kazyumba, G.,** Immune complexes in serum and in cerebrospinal fluid in African trypanosomiasis: correlation with polyclonal B cell activation and with intracerebral immunoglobulin synthesis, *J. Clin. Invest.,* 67, 77, 1981.

137. **Galvao-Castro, B., Hochmann, A., and Lambert, P. H.,** The role of the host immune response in the development of tissue lesions associated with African trypanosomiasis in mice, *Clin. Exp. Immunol.,* 33, 12, 1978.

138. **Poltera, A. A.,** Immunopathological and chemotherapeutic studies in experimental trypanosomiasis with special reference to the heart and brain, *Trans. R. Soc. Trop. Med. Hyg.,* 74, 706, 1980.

139. **Poltera, A. A., Hockmann, A., Rudin, W., and Lambert, P. H.,** *Trypanosoma brucei brucei:* a model for cerebral trypanosomiasis in mice — an immunological, histological and electronmicroscopic study, *Clin. Exp. Immunol.,* 40, 496, 1980.

140. **Boreham, P. F. L. and Kimber, C. D.,** Immune complexes in trypanosomiasis of the rabbit, *Trans. R. Soc. Trop. Med. Hyg.,* 64, 168, 1970.

141. **Murray, M., Lambert, P. H., and Morrison, W. I.,** Renal lesions in experimental trypanosomiasis, *Med. Mal. Infect.,* 5, 638, 1975.

142. **Nydegger, U. E.,** Biologic properties and detection of immune complexes in animal and human pathology, *Rev. Physiol. Biochem. Pharmacol.,* 85, 63, 1979.

143. **Klaus, G. G. B. and Humphrey, J. H.,** The generation of memory cells. I. The role of C3 in the generation of B memory cells, *Immunology,* 33, 31, 1977.

144. **Greenwood, B. M.,** Immunosuppression in malaria and trypanosomiasis, in *Parasites in the Immunized Host: Mechanisms of Survival,* CIBA Foundation Symp. No. 25 (New Series), Porter, R. and Knight, J., Eds., Elsevier, Amsterdam, 1974, 137.

145. **Urquhart, G. M.,** The pathogenesis and immunology of African trypanosomiasis in domestic animals, *Trans. R. Soc. Trop. Med. Hyg.,* 74, 726, 1980.

146. **Amole, B. O., Clarkson, A. B., and Shear, H. L.,** Pathogenesis of anaemia in *Trypanosoma brucei*-infected mice, *Infect. Immun.,* 36, 1060, 1982.

147. **Morrison, W. I., Murray, M., Sayer, P. D., and Preston, J. M.,** The pathogenesis of experimentally induced *Trypanosoma brucei* infection in the dog. II. Changes in the lymphoid organs, *Am. J. Pathol.,* 102, 182, 1981.

148. **Frommel, D., Perey, D.Y. E., Masseyeff, R., and Good, R. A.,** Low molecular weight immunoglobulin M in experimental trypanosomiasis, *Nature (London),* 228, 1208, 1970.

149. **Houba, V., Brown, K. N., and Allison, A. C.,** Heterophile antibodies, M-anti-globulins and immunoglobulins in trypanosomiasis, *Clin. Exp. Immunol.,* 4, 113, 1969.

150. **Boreham, P. F. L. and Facer, C. A.,** Autoimmunity in trypanosome infections. II. Anti-fibrin/fibrinogen (anti-F) autoantibody in *Trypanosoma (Trypanozoon) brucei* infections of the rabbit, *Int. J. Parasitol.,* 4, 601, 1974.

151. **Lindsley, H. B., Kysela, S., and Steinberg, A. D.,** Nucleic acid antibodies in African trypanosomiasis: studies in rhesus monkeys and man, *J. Immunol.,* 113, 1921, 1974.

152. **MacKenzie, A. R. and Boreham, P. F. L.,** Autoimmunity in trypanosome infections. I. Tissue autoantibodies in *Trypanosoma (Trypanozoon) brucei* infections of the rabbit, *Immunology,* 26, 1225, 1974.

153. **Kobayakawa, T., Louis, J., Izui, S., and Lambert, P. H.,** Autoimmune response to DNA, red blood cells, and thymocyte antigens in association with polyclonal antibody synthesis during experimental African trypanosomiasis, *J. Immunol.,* 122, 296, 1979.

154. **Mattern, P., Klein, F., Pautrizel, R., and Jongepier-Geerdes, Y. E. J. M.,** Anti-immunoglobulins heterophile agglutinins in experimental trypanosomiasis, *Infect. Immun.,* 128, 812, 1980.

155. **Wolga, J. I., Ribeiro, C. D., Gaillat, J., Stahl, J. P., Micoud, M., and Gentilini, M.,** Autoanticorps dans les trypanosomiases humanes africaines: anticorps antimuscle lisse au cours d'une maladie a *Trypanosoma gambiense, Bull. Soc. Pathol. Exot.,* 74, 676, 1981.

156. **Rose, L. M., Godman, M., and Lambert, P.-H.,** Simultaneous induction of an idiotype corresponding anti-idiotypic antibodies, and immune complexes during African trypanosomiasis in mice, *J. Immunol.,* 128, 79, 1982.

157. **Cook, R. M.,** Quantitation of acute phase protein Cx-reactive (CxRP) in rabbits infected with *Trypanosoma brucei, Vet. Parasitol.,* 5, 107, 1979.

Chapter 4

PHOSPHOLIPASES OF TRYPANOSOMES

Alan Mellors

TABLE OF CONTENTS

I. INTRODUCTION

Damage to lymphoid and reticular tissues is one of the most common manifestations of chronic trypanosomiasis. Denudement or hypertrophy of the blood endothelium is frequently observed.[1] Anemia and splenomegaly are also found in all infected species. Landsteiner and Raubitschek[2] showed that a suspension of *Trypanosoma equiperdum*, aged on ice overnight, could hemolyze erythrocytes. This gave impetus to a renewed search for trypanosomal toxins, originally reported by Laveran and Mesnil.[3] Much work was done on trypanosomal extracts which showed anaphylatoxin activities, for example, Novy et al.[4] showed that dead trypanosomal suspensions from five species, *T. b. brucei, T. equinum, T. equiperdum, T. evansi*, and *T. lewisi*, showed anaphylatoxin production within minutes of injection into rodents. It was felt, however, that anaphylatoxin production in vivo is of doubtful significance in the pathogenesis of trypanosomiasis. The complexity and variability of the toxic responses in animals gave rise to the view that trypanosomes are not toxigenic organisms.

A challenge to this view came from studies on a hemolytic factor produced in vivo in cattle infected with *T. congolense*.[5] The factor was transient and appeared at rare intervals of active trypanolysis. A similar hemolytic factor was reported in mice infected with *T. b. brucei*.[6] A hemolysin was also detected in suspensions of *T. b. brucei, T. gambiense, T. vivax*, and *T. congolense*;[7] the activity was associated with a protein of molar mass 100,000. Hemolytic activity is rarely observed in fresh trypanosomal suspensions, and it usually arises after autolysis of the suspension following incubation for several hours. For *T. congolense*[8] the incubation period is 9 to 10 hr at 20°C and a similar development of hemolytic activity is seen for *T. b. brucei*.[9] The hemolytic factors are lipid soluble, and the main components appear to be free fatty acids produced by the action of trypanosomal phospholipases on endogenous phosphatidylcholines. In autolyzing suspensions of *T. congolense* 3×10^9 organisms will generate 0.01 to 0.03 mg free fatty acid in 9 to 10 hr at 20°C. The principal fatty acids released are palmitic, stearic, and linoleic (each comprising 25% of the total free fatty acid), with lesser amounts of oleic and arachidonic acids.[10] While free fatty acids are potently surface active in vitro, sequestration by serum albumin and other proteins renders them inactive in vivo and they do not contribute directly to the anemia seen in cattle infected with *T. congolense*.[11]

It is likely that the phospholipases of the autolyzing trypanosomes are more important in the pathology of trypanosomiasis than the free fatty acids which they may generate.

II. PROPERTIES OF PHOSPHOLIPASES A_1 AND A_2

The phospholipases A (phospholipid acylhydrolases) are found to be widely distributed. Phospholipase A_2 is the best studied and is specific for the acylester bond at the C2 position of phospholipids. For phospholipases A_2, Ca^{2+} is usually essential for activity. The best studied phospholipases A_2 are those of snake and bee venoms, these being very soluble, very active, and remarkably stable to heat or other means of denaturation. The stability is apparently due to six or seven disulfide bridges commonly found in these enzymes.[12] Several isozymes of molecular mass about 14,000 are found in each venom. In each case Ca^{2+} is required for activity, the optimum pH is 8.0 to 8.5, and activity is much greater against micellar rather than monomolecular substrates. The venom phospholipases A_2 generally do not hemolyze red blood cells unless another polypeptide factor is present, which presumably modifies the surface pressure or charge or the membrane structure in some way.[13] The effectiveness of venom phospholipases at disrupting cellular functions without necessarily causing widespread cell lysis is illustrated by β-bungarotoxin. This presynaptic toxin has a phospholipase activity which is essential for toxicity. It appears to act by releasing free fatty acids in the synapses and causing inhibition of mitochondrial oxidative phosphorylation.[14,15]

Snake venoms frequently contain phospholipase inhibitors in addition to other enzymes and neurotoxins.

Another rich source of phospholipase A_2 is the màmmalian pancreas. The porcine pancreatic phospholipase A_2 has been well studied.[16] It is similar to the venom enzymes in size, stability, and Ca^{2+} requirement. The pancreatic enzyme occurs as a zymogen in the pancreatic juice. In the duodenum, the enzyme is activated by trypsin, which removes seven amino acid residues from the N terminus. Whereas the zymogen can degrade monomeric substrate molecules, the activated enzyme can also digest ordered phospholipid micelles. The bovine active enzyme has a molecular weight of 14,000. Its peptide chain consists of 123 amino acids and the sequence shows a great deal of homology with other phospholipases A_2 (Fleer et al.[17]). The enzyme has 14 cysteine residues in seven disulfide bridges and no free sulfhydryl groups. Although 71% of all residues of phospholipase A_2 from bovine, porcine, and equine sources are conserved, bovine phospholipase A_2 differs from the others in its total number of residues and by substitutions at positions 20 and 33. The three-dimensional structure of porcine prophospholipase has been elucidated,[18] but attempts to obtain suitable crystals of the active form of this enzyme were unsuccessful.

Intracellular digestive enzymes, in contrast to the extracellular (i.e., pancreatic) digestive enzymes which are inactive within the cell by being present as zymogen, are controlled by containment within lysosomes. Both phospholipase A_1 and A_2 have been demonstrated and partially characterized in rat liver lysosomes.[19,20] These enzymes have a pH optimum close to 4.0, and are inhibited by Ca^{2+}. The lysosomal phospholipase A_1 has a molecular weight of approximately 55,000. These enzymes are, thus, considerably different from the snake venom and pancreatic phospholipases A_2 which have an alkaline pH optimum and require Ca^{2+}. The phospholipases A_1 isolated from rat and calf brain[21] and human brain[22] show similar properties and are probably lysosomal in origin. Phospholipases A_1 have been purified from a number of other sources inluding *Escherichia coli* membranes.[23] Such enzymes generally show a wider substrate specificity than phospholipase A_2, showing activity against such substrates as mono- and diglycerides as well as diacyl phospholipids. Purified phospholipase A_1often shows both phospholipase A_1 and lysophospholipase 1 activity. Lysophospholipases are frequently present in high activity compared to other phospholipases, presumably to allow efficient removal of toxic lysophospholipids, but have only been purified from a few sources, including beef liver,[24] *E. coli*,[25] and *Corticium centrifugum*.[26]

III. TRYPANOSOMAL PHOSPHOLIPASE A_1

Phospholipase activity was detected in autolyzing suspensions of *T. congolense* by the use of ^{32}P-labeled phosphatidylcholine as substrate.[27] The use of the specifically labeled substrates 1-acyl-2-[^{14}C]-linoleoyl-*sn*-glycero-3-phosphocholine (abbreviation: 2-[^{14}C]-acyl PC) and phosphocholine (abbreviation: 1-[^{3}H]-acyl PC) showed that the *T. congolense* enzyme is a phospholipase A_1 (EC.3.1.1.32) that cleaves the 1-acyl ester bond of phosphatidylcholines and does not attack the 2-acyl bond.[23] Only low levels of phospholipase A_2 activity, no phospholipase C, and phospholipase D activities were detected in four species examined: *T. congolense, T. b. brucei, T. theileri,* and *T. lewisi.*

While phosphatidylcholines specifically labeled in the 2-acyl fatty acid only are commercially available and are convenient substrates for phospholipase A_2, the substrates of choice for phospholipase A_1 assay, with radiolabel in the 1-acyl moiety, are not commercially available. 1-[^{3}H]-Acyl PC can be prepared from egg yolk phosphatidylcholine by hydrolysis of the latter using *Rhizopus arrhizus* lipase to yield 2-acyl-*sn*-glycero-3-phosphocholine[29] and the immediate reacylation of this product using (9,10-^{3}H) palmitic acid and rat liver microsomes, to give 1-[^{3}H]-acyl PC.[30] This substrate can be isolated from the reaction mixture by thin-layer chromatography, and the specificity of the radiolabeled fatty acylation at the 1-acyl position can be checked by enzyme cleavage (snake venom phospholipase A_2 or *R. arrhizus* lipase).[28] The advantage of this substrate for assay of phospholipase A_1 is that the only labeled product is ³H-palmitate liberated from the 1 position of the phosphatidylcholine, and this can be largely separated from unhydrolyzed 1-[³H]-acyl PC in the reaction mixture by extraction with hexane to ethanol (5:4 v/v).[31] A similar simple method of phospholipase A_1 assay is now possible using commercially available di[¹⁴C-palmitoyl]phosphatidylcholine (Amersham) if no phospholipase A_2 activity is present in the biological sample.

A. *T. congolense*

The phospholipase A_1 activity of *T. congolense* is maximal at pH 6 and requires surface-active agents but not Ca^{2+} for activity.[28] Linoleate (0.5 mM) is an effective activator. Detergent activation of phospholipases is a common phenomenon and usually involves a change in the structure and size of substrate micelles. Sodium dodecylsulfate (0.02 mM) is a less effective activator. The specific activity in *T. congolense* suspensions at pH 6.0 in the presence of 0.5 mM linoleate is 10 nmol min⁻¹ mg⁻¹ protein.

B. *T. b. brucei*

Suspensions of *T. b. brucei* (Shinyanga III) show the highest phospholipase A_1 levels reported for whole organisms. In the presence of 0.125% Triton® X-100, at pH 7.0, the specific activity of *T. b. brucei* suspensions is 145 nmol min⁻¹ mg⁻¹ protein. This exceeds by three orders of magnitude the level found in *E. coli*[32] and is much greater than reported levels for other prokaryote or eukaryote cells. The *T. b. brucei* phospholipase A_1 is more active against phosphatidylcholines than against phosphatidylethanolamines and the enzyme shows lysophospholipase 1 activity in that it hydrolyzes the acyl bond of 1-acyl-*sn*-glycero-3-phosphocholine[31] (see below). The Km for the substrate 1-palmitoyl-2-acyl-*sn*-glycero-3-phosphocholine is about 2.4×10^{-4} M. The pH dependence curves for the *T. b. brucei* phospholipase A_1 consistently show two maxima at pH 6.5 and 8, and activity over a wide range from pH 5.5 to 8.5. The enzyme is strongly activated by the detergent Triton® X-100 (0.1% w/v), but other detergents tested, including linoleate, showed little or no activation. Again the detergent effect appears to be on the substrate micellar structure, and this is borne out by the lack of detergent effect on the lysophospholipase action against a more soluble substrate, 1-acyl-LPD. Reagents which alkylate thiol groups have an inhibitory effect on the phospholipase A_1 and storage, assay, and purification of the enzyme is best carried out in the presence of 2 mM dithiothreitol. Like the other trypanosomal phospholipases A_1 the enzyme from *T. b. brucei* does not have any metal ion requirement. Calcium ions do not activate the hydrolysis, unlike the phospholipases A_2, from many sources which require Ca^{2+} for substrate binding.[33,34] When sonicated fresh *T. b. brucei* are centrifuged at 100,000 g for an hour, most of the recovered enzyme activity is found in the supernatant. The *T. b. brucei* phospholipase A_1 has been chromatographed on DEAE-cellulose and Sephacryl® 200 to give 160-fold purification,[31] but octyl-agarose, a hydrophobic gel, is much more efficient for the separation of the enzyme and other hydrophobic proteins from the other trypanosomal supernatant proteins including the variable surface glycoproteins (VSG). Octyl-agarose gels retain the hydrophobic proteins which can be eluted with buffers containing detergents, 0.1% (v/v) Triton® X-100 with 0.01% deoxycholate. Recovery of the phospholipase A_1 from the column is over 90% with a 60-fold increase in specific activity.[45] Further purification on DEAE-cellulose gives 60% of the original phospholipase A_1 with a 390-fold increase in specific activity over that of the trypanosomal supernatant. Electrophoresis of this material on polyacrylamide gels in the presence of sodium dodecyl sulfate shows one major band of protein with a molecular mass of 26,000. Nondenaturing polyacrylamide gel electrophoresis shows that the major band corresponds to phospholipase A_1 activity.[31]

C. *T. b. brucei* Lysophospholipase 1

During the course of measurements of trypanosomal phospholipase A_1 activity it was noted that lysophospholipase 1 activity was also present in that the substrate 1-acyl-*sn*-glycero-3-phosphocholine was hydrolyzed to release a free fatty acid. Lysophospholipase activity is frequently found in preparations containing phospholipase A_1 activity, but has been purified from only a few sources including bovine liver,[24] *E. coli*,[25] and *C. centrifugum*.[26] The properties of the lysophospholipase 1 activity in *T. b. brucei* were compared to those of the phospholipase A_1 to determine if the same enzyme is responsible for the two activities.[31] Throughout chromatography of the phospholipase A_1 there was co-chromatography of the lysophospholipase 1 activity. A constant ratio of the two activities of about 10:1 for the phospholipase A_1 to lysophospholipase 1 activity was found. Both activities were found to be similarly inhibited by the thiol reagents *N*-ethylmaleimide and *p*-chloromercuribenzoate. Similar patterns of heat stability were seen but the pH dependence and the effect of detergents are essentially different for the two activities. The lysophospholipase 1 activity is optimal at pH 8.5 and has a much narrower pH range for activity than the phospholipase A_1. Detergents inhibited lysophospholipase 1 while activating substantially the phospholipase A_1 action, again suggesting that the detergents function to activate substrate micelles, an effect which probably is not significant for the strongly surface-active lysophosphatidylcholine substrate. The Km for the lysophospholipase 1 activity is 0.15 mM using 1-palmitoyl-*sn*-glycero-3-phosphocholine as substrate. It is likely that the lysophospholipase 1 activity of *T. b. brucei* is due to the same enzyme that catalyzes phospholipase A_1 activity. In *T. congolense* there are also two activities, phospholipase A_1 and lysophospholipase 1, in about the same ratio as that found for *T. b. brucei*.

D. *T. theileri*

The nonpathogenic *T. theileri* species has a phospholipase A_1 activity which is maximal at pH 6.75 and which shows activation in the presence of 0.1% Triton® X-100.[28] Under these conditions the specific activity of the enzyme in *T. theileri* was about 30 nmol min^{-1} mg^{-1} protein. No significant phospholipase A_1 was detected in this species, or in *T. congolense* or *T. b. brucei*, though low levels of phospholipase A_1 might be masked by high levels of A_1 activity.

E. *T. lewisi*

Another nonpathogenic stercorarian species, *T. lewisi*, shows very low levels of phospholipase A_1. This activity is optimal at pH 5.0 and, thus, resembles mammalian lysosomal phospholipases.[19,20] The enzyme is mildly activated by sodium dodecyl sulfate at 0.2 mM but inhibited at higher detergent concentrations. The activity under optimal conditions is about 1 nmol min^{-1} mg^{-1} protein. Unlike the *T. congolense* enzyme which is similarly activated by sodium dodecylsulfate, the *T. lewisi* phospholipase A_1 is not activated by linoleate.[28] In the presence of 5 mM calcium some phospholipase A_2 activity was detected in *T. lewisi*, whereas no such activity was seen for the species *T. congolense*, *T. b. brucei*, or *T. theileri*. None of the trypanosomal phospholipase A_1 enzymes studied showed any metal ion activator requirement.

F. *T. musculi*

Low levels of phospholipase A_1 and of lysophospholipase 1 activity have been detected in *T. musculi*, but no characterization of these activities has been attempted.

IV. METABOLIC ROLE OF TRYPANOSOMAL PHOSPHOLIPASES

Since only a few of the pathogenic or nonpathogenic *Trypanosoma* species have been examined, it is premature to draw conclusions regarding the role of the trypanosomal phospholipases. It is interesting that the salivarian trypanosome *T. b. brucei* which invades the tissue spaces has a very high phospholipase A_1 content. The only forms of this organism that have been examined are the trypomastigotes which undergo striking changes in their morphology, especially in the form of their mitochondria. Since phospholipases are frequently associated with membrane remodeling, the primary role of the *T. b. brucei* phospholipase A_1 could be in the development of pleomorphs.

It may be useful to examine the levels of phospholipase A_1 in the procyclic forms of *T. b. brucei*. Lower levels of phospholipase A_1 in stercorarian or hematic trypanosomes suggest a possible role for the enzyme in crossing the reticuloendothelial barrier of the mammalian host or the gut wall of the insect vector. However, more comparative study is necessary to test these hypotheses.

To determine if the phospholipase A_1 found in *T. b. brucei* is released into the host's tissue fluids during infection, tissue fluid was collected from plastic cages implanted subcutaneously in infected rabbits.[36] High levels of phospholipase A_1 were found in the tissue fluid at times of peak parasitemia. The phospholipase A_1 activity appeared in the tissue fluid about 7 days after infection, and the level of enzyme rose and fell with the waves of parasitemia. The phospholipase A_1 levels were much greater in the tissue fluid than could be explained by the numbers of intact trypanosomes found in the fluid. Assuming that the *T. b. brucei* organisms in the tissue fluid have the same phospholipase A_1 activity as the same strain cultured in rats, then only about 5 to 10% of the phospholipase A_1 is located in intact organisms, and the remainder is free and has been secreted by living trypanosomes or results from lysis of dead trypanosomes. Much lower activities of phospholipase A_1 were found in the blood plasma from infected animals even when high blood counts of *T. b. brucei* were observed. Plasma from infected rabbits at 20 to 40 days postinfection showed a marked inhibition of phospholipase A_1, probably due to neutralizing antibodies.[36] No significant increases in plasma phospholipase A_1 activity indicative of rabbit leukocyte proliferation were observed. At high parasitemia the infected rabbits displayed respiratory distress, a symptom of trypanosomiasis in other species including man.[37] This may be the result of the hydrolysis by trypanosomal phospholipases of alveolar phospholipids or of lung surfactant.

One possible role for the trypanosomal phospholipase A_1 is in the generation of membrane-active products from phospholipids. The generation of free fatty acids is unlikely to be significantly cytolytic in vivo since these lipids are effectively sequestered by the circulating serum albumin. However, localized damage might arise in the reticuloendothelial or in the lymphoid system. Fatty acids have been shown to be immunosuppressive in vitro and in vivo,[38] and immunosuppression is characteristic of African trypanosomiases, such that infected hosts frequently die of secondary infections.[41] It is unlikely that direct intravascular hemolysis of erythrocytes by free fatty acids is the cause of the severe hemolytic anemia observed in infected animals and humans, since the clinical hemolysis is apparently extravascular in origin.[39]

The role of the other phospholipase A_1 product, the 2-acyl lysophospholipid in the metabolism, or pathological effects of *Trypanosoma* have not been studied. Much is known about the effects of 1-acyl lysophospholipids on membranes and living cells, for these compounds are potent membrane-active fusogenic agents.[40] It has been shown that gradients of the natural stereoisomer L-1-acyl-lysophosphatidylcholine are chemotactic for lymphoblastoid cells.[41] The generation of large amounts of 2-acyl lysophosphatidylcholine (2-acyl LPC) or similar 2-acyl lysophospholipids might disrupt this chemotactic response. When 1-acyl lysophospholipids are generated in vivo by endogenous phospholipase A_2 action on membrane phospholipids, these membrane-active compounds are rapidly reacylated by a very active scavenging enzyme in cell membranes, 1-acyl lysophosphatidylcholine:acyl CoA acyl transferase (EC.2.3.1.23).[42] The product of trypanosomal phospholipase A_1 action (2-

acyl LPC) may interfere with this reacylation and with the process of membrane repair and membrane fluidity modulations. It is not known whether reacylation of the 2-acyl LPC occurs in trypanosome-infected hosts at a rate which will remove this metabolite, but it has been shown in rabbit lymphocyte microsomal membranes that two acyl transferase activities exist which will reacylate the 1-acyl LPC and the 2-acyl LPC isomers at similar rates.[43]

Apart from the possible harmful effects of free fatty acids and lysophospholipids, the direct attack by the trypanosomal phospholipases A_1 on the membrane lipids of the host could be pathologically important. The snake, arthropod, and insect venom phospholipases A_2, while much more localized in their actions, contribute significantly to the toxicity of these venoms by promoting the diffusion of the toxic agents.[44] The production of phospholipase A_1 throughout the hematic system and the tissue spaces in *T. b. brucei* infection will have consequences in all tissues, but especially in the reticuloendothelial and the lymphoid systems.

REFERENCES

1. **Fiennes, R. N. T.-W.,** Pathogenesis and pathology of African trypanosomiasis, in *The African Trypanosomiases,* Mulligan, H. W., Ed., Allen and Unwin, London, 1970, chap. 38.
2. **Landsteiner, K. and Raubitschek, H. H.,** Beobachtungen über Hämolyse und Hämagglutination, *Centralbl. Bakt. Abb. Orig.,* 45, 660, 1907.
3. **Laveran, A. and Mesnil, F.,** Recherche morphologiques et expérimentales sur le trypanosome du nagana ou maladie de la mouche tsétsé, *Ann. Inst. Pasteur,* 16, 1, 1902.
4. **Novy, F. G., De Kruif, P. H., and Novy, R. K.,** Anaphylatoxin and anaphylaxis: trypanosome anaphylatoxin, *J. Infect. Dis.,* 20, 461, 1917.
5. **Fiennes, R. N. T.-W.,** Hematological studies in trypanosomiasis of cattle, *Vet. Rec.,* 66, 423, 1954.
6. **Ikede, B. O., Lule, M., and Terry, R. J.,** Anemia in trypanosomiasis: mechanisms of erythrocyte destruction in mice infected with *Trypanosoma congolense* or *T. brucei, Acta Trop.,* 34, 53, 1977.
7. **Huan, C. N.,** Pathogenesis of the anemia in African trypanosomiasis: characterization and purification of a hemolytic factor, *J. Suisse Med.,*47,1582, 1975.
8. **Tizard, I. R. and Holmes, W. L.,** The generation of toxic activity from *Trypanosoma congolense, Experientia,* 32, 1533, 1976.
9. **Tizard, I. R., Sheppard, J., and Nielsen, K.,** The characterization of a second class of hemolysins from *Trypanosoma brucei, Trans. R. Soc. Trop. Med. Hyg.,* 72, 198, 1978.
10. **Tizard, I. R., Nielsen, K., Mellors, A., and Assoku, R. K. G.,** Biologically active lipids generated by autolysis of *Trypanosoma congolense,* in *Recent Advances in the Study of the Pathogenesis of African Trypanosomiasis,* Losos, G. and Chouinard, A., Eds., International Development Research Centre, Ottawa, 1979, 103.
11. **Tizard, I. R., Holmes, W. L., and Nielsen, K.,** Mechanisms of the anemia in trypanosomiasis: studies on the role of the hemolytic fatty acids derived from *Trypanosoma congolense, Tropenmed. Parasitol.,* 29, 108, 1978.
12. **Van den Bosch, H.,** Phosphoglyceride metabolism, *Ann. Rev. Biochem.,* 43, 243, 1974.
13. **McMurray, W. C. and Magee, W. L.,** Phospholipid metabolism, *Ann. Rev. Biochem.,* 41, 129, 1972.
14. **Strong, P. N., Goerke, J., Obert, S. G., and Kelly, R. B.,** β-Bungarotoxin, a pre-synaptic toxin with enzymatic activity, *Proc. Natl. Acad. Sci. U.S.A.,* 73, 178, 1976.
15. **Wernicke, J. F., Vakar, A. D., and Howard, B. D.,** The mechanism of action of β-bungarotoxin, *J. Neurochem.,* 25, 483, 1975.
16. **De Haas, G. H., Postema, N. M., Niewenhuizen, W. N., and Van Deenen, L. L. M.,** Purification and properties of phospholipase A from porcine pancreas, *Biochim. Biophys. Acta,* 159, 103, 1968.
17. **Fleer, E. A. M., Verheij, H. M., and De Haas, G. H.,** The primary structure of bovine pancreatic phospholipase A_2, *Eur. J. Biochem.,* 82, 262, 1978.
18. **Volwerk, I., Peterson, W. A., and De Haas, G. H.,** Histidine at the active site of phospholipase A_2, *Biochemistry,* 13, 1450, 1974.
19. **Mellors, A. and Tappel, A. L.,** Hydrolysis of phospholipids by a lysosomal enzyme, *J. Lipid Res.,* 8, 479, 1967.

20. **Waite, M., Griffin, H. D., and Fransom, R.,** The phospholipases A of lysosomes, in *Lysosomes in Biology and Pathology,* Vol. 5, Dingle, J. T. and Dean', R. T., Eds., North-Holland, Amsterdam, 1976, 257.

21. **Gatt, S.,** Purification and properties of phospholipase A₁ from rat and calf brain, *Biochim. Biophys. Acta,* 159, 304, 1968.

22. **Cooper, M. F. and Webster, G. R.** The differentiation of phospholipase A₁ and A₂ in rat and human nervous tissue, *J. Neurochem.,* 17, 1543, 1970.

23. **Proulx, P., Nantel, G., and Baraff, G.,** Partial purification of a lipolytic enzyme from *Escherichia coli, Can. J. Biochem.,* 56, 319, 1978.

24. **De Jong, J. G. N., Van den Bosch, H., Rijken, D., and Van Deenen, L. L. M.,** Studies on lysophospholipases, *Biochim. Biophys. Acta,* 369, 50, 1974.

25. **Doi, O. and Nojima, S.,** Lysophospholipase of *Escherichia coli, J. Biol. Chem.,* 250, 5208, 1975.

26. **Vehara, S., Hasegawa, K., Tada, M., Murata, M., Suzuki, T., and Iwai, K.,** Purification and properties of lysophospholipase produced by *Corticium centrifugum, Agric. Biol. Chem.,* 41, 1567, 1977.

27. **Tizard, I. R., Mellors, A., Holmes, W. L., and Nielsen, K.,** The generation of phospholipase A and hemolytic fatty acids by autolysing suspensions of *Trypanosoma congolense, Tropenmed. Parasitol.,* 29, 127, 1978.

28. **Hambrey, P. N., Mellors, A., and Tizard, I. R.,** The phospholipases of pathogenic and non-pathogenic *Trypanosoma* species, *Mol. Biochem. Parasitol.,* 2, 177, 1981.

29. **Nishijima, M., Akamatsu, Y., and Nojima, S.,** Purification and properties of a membrane-bound phospholipase A₁ from *Mycobacterium phlei, J. Biol. Chem.,* 249, 5658, 1974.

30. **Albright, F. R., White, D. A., and Lennartz, W. J.,** Studies on enzymes involved in the catabolism of phospholipids in *Escherichia coli, J. Biol. Chem.,* 248, 3968, 1973.

31. **Sage, L., Hambrey, P. N., Werchola, G. M., Mellors, A., and Tizard, I. R.,** Lysophospholipase 1 in *Trypanosoma brucei, Tropenmed. Parasitol.,* 32, 215, 1981.

32. **Scandella, C. J. and Kornberg, A.,** A membrane-bound phospholipase A₁ purified from *Escherichia coli, Biochemistry,* 10, 4447, 1971.

33. **Hughes, A.,** The action of snake venoms on surface films, *Biochem. J.,* 29, 437, 1935.

34. **Wells, M. A.,** A kinetic study of the phospholipase A₂ (*Crotalus adamanteus*) catalyzed hydrolysis of 1,2-dibutyryl-sn-glycero-3-phosphorylcholine, *Biochemistry,* 11, 1030, 1972.

35. **Uehara, S., Hasegawa, K., and Iwai, K.,** Purification and properties of phospholipase A₁ produced by *Corticium centrifugum, Agric. Biol. Chem.,* 43, 517, 1979.

36. **Hambrey, P. N., Tizard, J. R., and Mellors, A.,** Accumulation of phospholipase A₁ in tissue fluid of rabbits infected with *Trypanosoma brucei, Tropenmed. Parasitol.,* 31, 439, 1980.

37. **Lebras, M., Longy, P., Roussy, P., Delmas, M., and Maretti, G.,** Trypanosomiase humaine africaine: découvert exceptionnelle par pneumopathie aigue à rechutes, *Nouv. Presse Med.,* 8, 1098, 1979.

38. **Meade, C. J. and Mertin, J.,** The mechanism of immunoinhibition by arachidonic and linoleic acid: effects on the lymphoid and reticulo-endothelial systems, *Int. Arch. Allergy Appl. Immunol.,* 48, 203, 1975.

39. **Apted, Fl. C.,** Clinical manifestations and diagnosis of sleeping sickness in the African trypanosomiases, in *The African Trypanosomiases,* Mulligan, H. W., Ed., Allen and Unwin, London, 1970, 661.

40. **Lucy, J. A.,** The fusion of biological membranes, *Nature (London),* 227, 814, 1970.

41. **Hoffman, R. D., Kligerman, M., Sundt, T. M., Anderson, N. D., and Shin, H. S.,** Stereospecific chemoattraction of lymphoblastic cells by gradients of lysophosphatidylcholine, *Proc. Natl. Acad. Sci. U.S.A.,* 79, 3285, 1982.

42. **Lands, W. E. M. and Hart, P.,** Metabolism of glycerolipids. VI. Specificities of acyl coenzyme A: phospholipid acyltransferases, *J. Biol. Chem.,* 240, 1905, 1965.

43. **Ferber, E. and Resch, K.,** Phospholipid metabolism of stimulated lymphocytes: activation of acyl-CoA:lysolecithin acyltransferases in microsomal membranes, *Biochim. Biophys. Acta,* 296, 335, 1973.

44. **Condrea, E. and De Vries, A.,** Venom phospholipase A: a review, *Toxicon,* 2, 261, 1965.

45. **Mellors, A., et al.,** in preparation.

Chapter 5

IMMUNOBIOLOGY OF AFRICAN TRYPANOSOMIASIS IN LABORATORY RODENTS

Greg J. Bancroft and Brigette A. Askonas

TABLE OF CONTENTS

I. INTRODUCTION

African trypanosomes cause serious disease in man and cattle in Africa and are of considerable economic and social importance. However, much recent work has dealt with rodent models of infection to allow more detailed analysis of the confrontation between the parasite and the immune system. In such models of trypanosomiasis there are two major features by which the parasite evades the host's immune control. First is the phenomenon of antigenic variation, in which the surface glycoprotein coat of the organism is altered.[1] This results in a continuous progression of noncross-reactive antigenic variants being presented to the host. As one wave of parasitemia is controlled by specific antibodies, the next wave of variant parasites arises, to which the host must respond for survival. The second feature of this infection is a generalized depression of immune competence which affects responses to both parasite-related and -unrelated (heterologous) antigens. Immune dysfunction during the course of trypanosome infection is particularly acute, and, in view of the variation in parasite surface antigens, is of particular importance for the outcome of the disease. Impaired immune responsiveness is a feature of many infections including those caused by viruses,[2] bacteria,[3] and metazoan[4] or protozoan[5] parasites. It is, therefore, of general importance to understand the cellular and molecular basis of immunosuppression during infection, and African trypanosomes provide a strong model for such work. This review is concerned with the alterations of the immune system induced by trypanosomes and will focus on infections with the subspecies of *Trypanosoma brucei* (*T. brucei, T. rhodesiense, T. gambiense*) and with *T. congolense, T. musculi,* and *T. lewisi* will be discussed in another chapter of this edition (see Chapter 10).

Many facets of immune function during trypanosomiasis have been studied and will be discussed in greater detail in particular sections of this paper. In general, the function of almost all lymphoid cells is adversely affected by the infection. B and T cells are stimulated to proliferate and the polyclonal production of immunoglobulins (Ig) increases, but the cells become refractory to selection by antigen and, thus, antigen-specific immune responses are defective. The effects on antibody production have been extensively studied and here the normal control signals regulating the amplification of a response and its subsequent shut off are disturbed. In some instances there may be a paradoxical duality in the effects of the parasite with a transient period of enhanced antibody responses preceding the more characteristic generalized depression of antibody formation to specific antigens. Such work has generally used common heterologous antigens such as foreign erythrocytes and haptenated proteins, but the suppressive effects also apply to antiparasite responses (see Section IV.D). Severe changes in lymphoid organs are associated with trypanosome infection and may contribute to the suppression observed later in infection. Also, the activity of regulatory T-cell populations and the phenotype and function of host macrophages are altered. Macrophages appear to be at least one of the key target cells for the action of trypanosomes, since after ingestion of the parasite they can mediate immunosuppression in vivo in normal mice.

Thus, many changes occur due to infection with trypanosomes, each having some influence on the function of the host's immune system; while each area is discussed in the individual sections of this paper, it is clear that immunomodulation by the trypanosome is the result of all these complex changes. Another important point in studying this system is how the characteristics of the infection are reflected in these disturbances. African trypanosomes are extracellular protozoa, and in mice *T. brucei* and *T. congolense* replicate in the spleen during the early stages of infection. It is noticeable that spleen cell function is affected early in infection while responses in the lymph nodes are still normal and only decrease later when the infection is more widespread. The presence of the parasite in the lymphoid organ examined has considerable bearing on whether changes are observed.

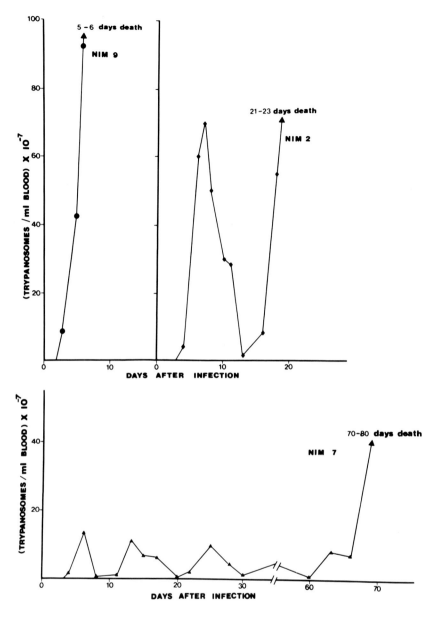

FIGURE 1.   Course of infection of (CBA × C57Bl/6)F₁ mice with three clones of *T. brucei* differing in virulence. Experimental details are described by Sacks et al.[54]

The virulence of trypanosome strains and individual clones within a strain can vary from acute to chronic, leading either to rapid death or repeated waves of parasitemia over prolonged periods of time. For our studies four clones of *T. brucei* have been selected. We describe these here since all the work from our laboratory is based on these clones; and they represent the spectrum of infections seen in the mouse models of trypanosomiasis which we will discuss (Figure 1). Clone NIM 2 was derived from strain *T. b. brucei* S42 and causes acute infection. One wave of parasitemia is controlled by our standard mouse strain (CBA × C57Bl/6)F₁, while the second wave of parasitemia is uncontrolled and leads to death within 25 to 30 days. Clone NIM 6 is slightly less virulent than NIM 2 (not shown). NIM 9 is from a different isolate and induces a lethal uncontrolled parasitemia (death by day 6 to 7), while NIM 7 causes a more chronic infection and (CBA $\times$ C57Bl/6)F_1 mice survive for 80 to 120 days.

II. HOST GENOTYPE AND THE COURSE OF TRYPANOSOME INFECTION

The mechanisms determining resistance or susceptibility to trypanosome infection are complex in view of the extensive changes in the host immune system induced by the parasite. Since African trypanosomes have the ability to vary their surface glycoprotein coat, survival of the host depends on its continued ability to mount an adequate antibody response. Several studies have examined the course of parasitemia following infection of mice with various strains of *T. b. brucei*, *T. congolense*, or *T. rhodesiense*. A continuous spectrum of relative resistance can be observed, but mice inevitably succumb to the parasite at various times after infection, unlike the resistance shown by some cattle (N'dama) in Africa.[6] C57Bl/6 mice were found to be most resistant to all three trypanosome species tested while other mouse strains varied in susceptibility and survival times.[7-9] In general, an inverse correlation was noted between the host's parasite load or parasitemia and survival time. However, a number of differences occurred in the strains of mice showing intermediate resistance to infection with the three species of trypanosomes, and even between different clones within one strain. For example, Grosskinsky[10] found that *T. brucei* clone NIM 2 was more virulent in DBA/2 mice than in (CBA $\times$ C57Bl)F_1 and other mouse strains, and led to death within 10 days. On the other hand, clone NIM 6, which is only slightly less virulent than clone NIM 2 in other mouse strains and was derived from NIM 2 in (CBA $\times$ C57B1)F_1 mice, results in a less virulent infection in DBA/2 mice than in the above F_1 mice. No NIM 6 parasites are detected for more than 2 weeks in the blood of DBA/2 mice, but they eventually die at the same time. This would suggest some specific resistance for individual organisms.

Resistance to trypanosomes was not linked to H-2 when parasitemia levels and survival times were compared in mice varying in haplotype[7] or in congenic mice on the resistant C57Bl/10 background.[8] In many, but not every, instance, resistance was dominant in F_1 mice.[7-10] A comparison of Biozzi high or low responder mice selected with foreign RBC or Salmonella showed only minor differences in survival time, although the height of the first parasitemia wave varied significantly.[10] Relative resistance has been associated with rapid antibody responses and effective control of the first parasite wave,[11] but in DBA/2, for example, more efficient control of early parasitemia with antibody appears to predispose to earlier death with a recurrent wave of parasites. However, this phenomenon may relate to the immunosuppressive activity of macrophages after uptake of antibody-coated trypanosomes (see Section VI).

Present views would suggest that, in general, inheritance of resistance to trypanosomes is under polygenic control, although it is occasionally partially specific for individual organisms.[11] Further analyses are required to pinpoint the most important factor(s) in each model. In addition to variations in the virulence of parasite clones, trypanosomes can also vary in growth rate. Genetic regulation by the host will relate to control of the first wave of parasitemia (by immune mechanisms as well as nonimmune, nonantigen-specific pathways) and the effect of the parasite on the immune system which shows some variation in kinetics in different strains of mice. Thus, for example, Selkirk and Sacks[12] compared the inhibition of antibody responses to a thymus-independent antigen (DNP-Ficoll) following infection with clone NIM 7 (causing a chronic infection) of (CBA/H $\times$ C57Bl/6)F_1 vs. C3H/He mice (survival 90 to 100 days and 28 to 34 days, respectively). In C3H mice the IgM response is inhibited by 85% on day 5 and nonexistent by day 20, while the more resistant F_1 mice show only a 50% inhibition of IgM response on day 20. The height of the first wave of parasites is similar in both mouse strains, clearly indicating that the same parasite load can have a differential effect. More commonly, parasitemia and changes on lymphoid cell populations correlate.[13] It is not surprising, in view of the many alterations induced by the parasite in MØ and lymphocyte function (see later sections), that the influence of host genotype on the outcome of infection is not as clear-cut in trypanosomiasis as in other virus and parasite infections.[14]

III. ALTERATIONS IN LYMPHOID ARCHITECTURE

A major feature of many protozoal infections is the alteration of cellularity and architecture of various lymphoid organs. In view of the importance of lymphocyte recirculation and the interaction between lymphoid cells, macrophages, follicular dendritic cells, etc., it is to be expected that these changes will interfere with normal immune function. The changes induced by African trypanosomes are severe, particularly in the later stages of infection, and, in general, parallel the disturbances seen with other protozoa such as *Plasmodia* or *Toxoplasma*.[5] Alterations in the size of lymphoid organs are an obvious finding in rodent trypanosomiasis with, characteristically, splenomegaly, lymphadenopathy, and thymic atrophy occurring.[15] In the spleen and lymph nodes this is a reflection of marked hyperplasia of lymphoid and mononuclear cells.

In mice infected with *T. brucei*, B cell areas of the spleen are enlarged, with increases in large lymphoid cells and immature and mature plasma cells.[16] The periarteriolar lymphatic sheaths (T cell areas) have reduced numbers of small lymphocytes and are infiltrated with macrophages and plasmablasts.[17] Also, there is an increase in plasma cells seen in the cords of the red pulp. The number of T cells ($Ig^- \theta^+$) increases transiently in the spleen just prior to the peak of parasitemia, followed several days later by increases in B cells ($Ig^+ \theta^-$) and, more substantially, of null cells ($Ig^- \theta^-$).[18] This is reflected in the 10- to 40-fold enhancement of DNA synthesis of spleen cells from infected mice in vitro. As shown by a combination of autoradiography and immunofluorescence this involves all three cell populations but with a predominant effect on null cells.[18]

Later in infection similar changes occur in the lymph nodes, with replacement of the paracortical (T cell) areas with plasma cells and lymphoblasts, and general increases in large lymphoid cells in the organ.[16] Infection also causes a leukopenia in the peripheral blood which is interrupted by a transient leukocytosis temporally associated with the parasitemia wave.[19] In addition to effects on cells in the periphery, severe changes are also found in the bone marrow. Disruption of the marrow is evident histologically within a few days of infection, and as the first wave of parasitemia occurs, the yield of nucleated cells is severely reduced. Cell numbers remain low for several days but partially recover after the subpatent period. In parallel, the spleen colony forming units of the marrow, predominantly precursors of the erythrocyte and granulocyte lineages, are depleted and, subsequently, show partial restoration during the subpatent period.[19]

Extensive studies on more chronic infection with *T. congolense* in mice have been performed by Morrison and colleagues.[13] The general observations of lymphoid hyperplasia are again present, but are seen to be influenced by the genotype of the host. Thus, relatively resistant mouse strains had lower levels of parasitemia and less marked B and null cell changes in the spleen than susceptible mice. Initially, in the spleen there is marked cell proliferation in the white pulp and red pulp. The stimulation to the latter is such that in the later stages of infection over half of the spleen cells obtained from these mice are nucleated erythroid cells.[20] This is clearly an important consideration when attempting to measure the function of cells obtained from infected spleens. The red pulp continues to enlarge in the later stages of infection but the lymphoid components undergo a gradual reduction, with the disappearance of plasma cells from the red pulp and, to a lesser extent, the periarteriolar regions.

With *T. congolense*, alterations in the lymph nodes occur later than in the spleen and are generally less severe. The initial increase in cellularity is more restricted to the B cell dependent follicular areas, and severe lymphoid depletion is not observed later in the infection.[21] The differences between disruption of the spleen and lymph nodes are a general finding in rodent trypanosomiasis and presumably reflect the distribution of the organism in the host.

The changes in lymphoid organs during infection are clear, but their contribution to altered immune competence of the host is less defined. Suppression of immune responses cannot be simply accounted for by gross cell death, as marked proliferation of many cell types occurs during the infection. Only later in infection does depletion of lymphoid cells occur. Interestingly, the severe effects of the parasite on the lymphoid system are not necessarily terminal. Mice rescued from lethal infection by trypanocidal drugs show gradual recovery of lymphoid organ structure and function therefore, immunosuppression is not due to a complete loss of responsive lymphoid cells and their precursors[16,19,22] (see later sections). The disruption of lymphoid organs will have some effect on host responses, but it is a feature which cannot be considered in isolation. In the following sections we will outline the many other influences of the infection which may also contribute to the altered responsiveness of the host.

IV. B CELL FUNCTION

A. Polyclonal B Cell Stimulation

The earliest indications that host B cell function was altered in African trypanosomiasis came from studies on serum agglutinin and immunoglobulin (Ig) levels in infected humans. Marked elevation of serum IgM in infected individuals is a prominent feature of the infection and has been known for many years (see review by Greenwood and Whittle).[23] Raised IgM, as well as free Ig light chains,[24] are also found in the cerebrospinal fluid, apparently produced by plasma cells within the central nervous system.[25] In fact, enhanced IgM in the presence of moderately raised CSF protein levels is considered as highly diagnostic for the later stage of this infection. Similar changes in serum Ig are present in a number of animal models of trypanosomiasis including cattle,[26,27] rabbits,[28,29] and monkeys.[30]

In the mouse, serum levels of IgM and IgG are increased many-fold following infection with *T. rhodesiense, T. congolense, T. gambiense, T. brucei*, or *T. equiperdum*.[21,31-35] Spleen cells of *T. brucei*-infected mice show in vitro, also, significantly enhanced release of both IgM and IgG.[36] Thus, a hallmark of trypanosomiasis is an elevation of IgM, and also IgG in some hosts. Enhancement of other Ig classes such as IgA and IgE is not extensively documented, but apparently does not occur in *T. congolense*-infected cattle.[27]

Changes in Ig levels occur at, or slightly after, the initial increase in parasite load, and are paralleled by histological and in vitro evidence of B cell activation in lymphoid tissues[16,36] (see also Section III). Enhanced Ig levels are observed in both acute and chronically infected mice[33] and remain high after the initial parasite stimulus and also during the prepatent period or after the administration of trypanocidal drugs when blood parasites are below measurable levels.[33] Since IgM has a short half-life, this continued elevation may reflect the presence of parasites in the lymphoid organs maintaining the stimulus to B cells. Prolonged elevation of serum IgM is also present in human infections.[37,38] However, some variations in serum IgM that relate to the fluctuating parasite load have been reported with *T. congolense* (cattle)[27] and *T. equiperdum*.[33]

Studies on the specificity of Ig molecules induced by trypanosomiasis have led to the conclusion that the trypanosome-mediated B cell stimulus is polyclonal and not antigen specific. Only a small proportion of Ig molecules induced are antibodies directed against the parasite. This was observed initially by Henderson-Begg[39] who documented raised levels of serum heterophile agglutinins in human *T. gambiense* infections. Later, Corsini and associates[36] found that less than 10% of Ig secreted in vitro by spleen cells from *T. brucei*-infected mice could be absorbed by homologous parasites.

Similarly, *T. brucei*-infected, nonimmunized mice had increased numbers of splenic antibody-forming cells to a variety of heterologous antigens including SRBC, pneumococcal polysaccharide (SIII), and hapten-coated erythrocytes,[31,40] and increases in T15-idiotype-bearing antibodies to phosphorylcholine.[35] At the same time anti-idiotypic antibodies directed against the T15 idiotype are enhanced. The supernatant from sonicated trypanosomes does not inhibit these antihapten antibody-forming cells, while the relevant heterologous hapten does.[40] Once more, specific antibodies to the parasite surface glycoprotein showed no evidence of any cross-reaction with the commonly used antigens.[41] Thus, all the data support the concept of a nonantigen-specific stimulation by the trypanosomes. Stimulation of B cell activity is also seen in CBA/N mice which have abnormal B cell maturation and are unable to respond to nonmitogenic T cell-independent antigens.[32,42] Infection of CBA/N mice with *T. rhodesiense* stimulates the production of IgG_3 antibodies, overcoming the usual defect in the production of this isotype in this mouse strain.[43]

This polyclonal stimulus of B cells is also reflected in enhanced autoimmune humoral responses in rabbits,[44] mice,[45] rats,[46] monkeys, and man.[47] Some of these antibodies appear to have rheumatoid factor-like activity,[30,45,48] but this is not found in every experimental infection.[48] Other studies, particularly in rabbits, have illustrated the induction of autoantibodies to a number of host tissue antigens. These include liver, brain, kidney, and heart, as well as thymocytes, erythrocytes, complement (C3b), and fibrin/fibrinogen products (e.g., see Mackenzie and Boreham[49] and Kobayakawa et al.[50] and review by Mansfield[15]). The involvement of such autoantibodies in the pathogenesis of trypanosome infection is still uncertain.

B. Suppression of Mitogen Responses

At the time of the polyclonal increase in circulating antibody molecules, trypanosome infection leads to unresponsiveness of splenic B lymphocytes in vitro to mitogens such as bacterial lipopolysaccharide (LPS). In normal spleen cells LPS induces B cell proliferation and secretion of Ig, but in *T. brucei*-infected mice both features were almost totally absent by 12 days after infection with clone NIM 2.[36] Cell depletion experiments suggested this was due to suppressive macrophages and T cells (see also later sections), but in the later stages of infection the intrinsic B cell potential to respond to LPS appeared lost. Similar suppression of LPS activation occurs in *T. congolense* infection of mice.[51] The loss of responsiveness cannot be explained by dilution of B cells in the spleen through an increase in null and T cells. Similar numbers of B cells were present in control and infected spleen cell cultures when assayed by fluorescent staining with antibody to Ig. The mitogen response in the spleen was found to be most severely affected, while B cell stimulation in the lymph nodes was not reduced until much later in the infection.[51] This is a reflection of the early presence of parasites in the spleen and their much later appearance in lymph nodes. This differential effect on lymphoid tissues can also be seen in primary in vitro B cell responses to antigen and the generation of suppressive cells in spleen vs. lymph nodes. In *T. rhodesiense* infection, induction of antibodies to sheep erythrocytes is already suppressed in the spleen 3 days after infection, whereas lymph node cells show enhanced responses until day 15, after which time antibodies fall below normal levels.[52] Suppressive cells in the spleen show similar kinetics, but they are not found in the lymph nodes of infected mice.

C. Suppression of Specific Antibody Responses

In addition to the stimulation of nonspecific B cell proliferation and maturation and the loss of mitogen responsiveness described above, trypanosomiasis also affects antigen-specific

B cell responses. The polyclonal B cell activation is associated only very transiently with enhanced antigen-specific B cell responses in chronic infections, but with highly virulent clones of trypanosomes this phase is not detectable. The most striking consequence of infection is a profound suppression of immunocompetence in the host. In the initial studies of Goodwin and colleagues,[53] this was seen as a severe reduction of serum agglutinin formation to a primary challenge of sheep erythrocytes in infected mice and rabbits. Suppression of antibody production to such heterologous antigens has also been confirmed at the cellular level. For instance, the generation of both IgM and IgG PFC in spleen is reduced by over 95% if SRBC are given to infected mice around the time of overt parasitemia.[16,31,54] As well as such changes in responses to T-dependent (TD) antigens, antibody production to T-independent (TI) antigens is also altered, although the reduction of TI responses is more variable. Murray and collaborators[16] found that *T. brucei*-infected mice were unable to respond to LPS, and in another mouse strain/parasite combination giving a more chronic *T. brucei* infection, the anti-DNP-Ficoll PFC response was reduced from day 5 postinfection until death 80 days later.[12] On the other hand, Mansfield and Bagasra,[55] examining a semiacute *T. rhodesiense* infection in mice, reported an enhanced response to TNP-Ficoll throughout 30 days of the infection, and to within a few days of death. This is the only example of normal or enhanced antibody production over a prolonged period of an experimental infection with trypanosomes.

Thus, an apparent paradox exists, in that during infection the parasites induce a polyclonal, antigen-independent increase in B cell proliferation and maturation, while the host is unable to mount a specific response to heterologous (i.e., nonparasite-related) antigens given at this time. The extent of dysfunction depends on the virulence of the parasite clone, the timing of antigen administration in relation to the stage of infection, and the host genetics. Hudson and colleagues[31] first demonstrated that antibody production was actually enhanced if SRBC were injected within several days of initiating an infection with *T. brucei* S42 but then depressed if given at or after the first wave of parasitemia. The phenomenon of enhanced primary responses to heterologous antigens during the early stages of infection is also seen with *T. cruzi* and murine malaria (see review by Bancroft and Askonas[5]) Although the suppressive effects of experimental trypanosome infection are observed in many cases, whether or not a transient period of enhancement occurs is influenced by the host/parasite model studied. For instance, Selkirk and Sacks[12] observed a short period of enhanced IgM production to DNP-Ficoll in (CBA × C57Bl)F$_1$ mice infected with a chronic *T. brucei* clone (NIM 7). Yet in the same experiment, more susceptible C3H mice already had suppressed responses when given antigen at the same time after infection. Also, in studying trypanosomes of varying virulence, acute and semiacute clones often have no apparent enhancement and show only suppression of responses to heterologous antigens.[151]

The data obtained with *T. brucei* infections indicate that transient enhancement, followed by more prolonged suppression of B cell activity to T-dependent[31] and T-independent antigens, occurs.[12] By contrast, in *T. rhodesiense*-infected mice the antigen used affects the results. Mansfield and Bagasra[55] found a transient enhancement with the T-dependent antigen SRBC, followed by suppression, while the TNP-Ficoll response, which is T independent, was enhanced until a few days prior to death. These authors assign suppression to alterations in T and B cell interaction rather than impaired B cell function. In our view, varied effects exerted by different trypanosome populations may be assigned to the parasite load, strain, and genetics of the host.

The studies described above have dealt with the modulation of primary responses to heterologous antigens. Trypanosomiasis also impairs the secondary antibody response, as seen in mice infected with *T. brucei*. The spleens of mice primed with DNP-KLH and infected several months later are depleted of TI and TD memory B cells as shown by adoptive transfer.[32] Also, the activity of T helper memory cells declines during infection and is lost by 2 weeks after infection with clone NIM 2[32] (see also Section V).

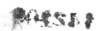

D. Antibody Responses to the Parasite

Infection of humans, cattle, or experimental animals with African trypanosomes is almost invariably fatal, due to the inability of the host to achieve a state of sterile immunity. Immune responses to the parasite do occur, but host survival depends on continued antibody responses to successive waves of variant parasites. The immune system does affect the course of infection, as lethally irradiated or B cell-deprived mice are unable to limit the proliferation of the parasite and die with an uncontrolled parasitemia.[56] T cell function is not an important facet of this response, at least with *T. brucei* and *T. rhodesiense*, since athymic mice, producing only IgM antibodies to the parasite, are capable of controlling parasite replication and become resistant to subsequent challenge with homologous organisms.[57] However, T cells are responsive to the organism as seen in the T helper cell-dependent production of IgG antibodies in euthymic, infected mice[57] and the antigen-specific proliferation of primed T cells to parasite antigens.[58] These observations, together with the transfer of protection by immune serum,[59] implicate the production of clone-specific antibodies to the parasite as the major determinant of immunity. This immunity is effective against individual parasite clones, but does not afford complete protection to the animal. (For a more extensive review of this area see Mansfield[15].)

Antibodies against the parasite are primarily directed against the variant surface glyco-protein (VSG) and protection against the homologous clone is acquired by immunization with purified VSG.[60] The kinetics of the parasitemia wave is influenced by the production of antibodies to external determinants of the VSG and by the differentiation of the trypan-osomes from slender, rapidly dividing parasites to stumpy forms.[41] Induction of anti-VSG antibodies is present in infections with pleomorphic (slender/stumpy) strains but not in mice infected with monomorphic (slender) *T. brucei*. This is thought to reflect the release of parasite membrane fragments containing VSG determinants from degenerating stumpy forms but not monomorphic trypanosomes.[41,61]

The majority of studies on the suppression of immune responses have used common heterologous antigens (Section IV.C) rather than the parasite, since these experiments are hampered by the availability of defined parasite antigens and quantitative tests. However, the suppression of antiparasite responses during infection has been reported. Sacks and Askonas[62] compared the effect of infection with an acute (NIM 2) and a chronic (NIM 7) *T. brucei* clone on the antibody responses to a noncross-reactive third parasite clone (NIM 6). At the time of the first parasite wave, the acute clone had almost entirely suppressed the IgG and even the IgM antitrypanosome response, whereas the chronic parasite was considerably less suppressive. Also, when mice were examined for their responses to successive parasite waves of a chronic infection, IgG antibody was rapidly suppressed but IgM responses to the parasite declined more gradually as the infection progressed.

The greater susceptibility to suppression of IgG rather than IgM is a general finding and can be seen with both parasite and heterologous antigen responses in infection and with different parasite fractions.[62,63] During a chronic infection with *T. brucei*, IgG responses to heterologous antigens are rapidly lost while IgM production shows a more gradual reduction. When this residual activity is artificially abrogated by cyclophosphamide treatment, the parasitemia is no longer controlled and death follows.[64] Altogether the data would suggest that residual IgM production is sufficient to control the waves of variant trypanosomes. It should be noted that in extremely acute infections resulting in death within 7 to 10 days, suppression of antibody production to parasite or heterologous antigens has not been demonstrated.[41,66] The rapidity of death does not permit a sufficient interval between infection and antigen challenge.

Thus, in the murine model of *T. brucei*[62] and as recently shown with *T. rhodesiense*,[65] suppression of responses can extend to antibodies directed against the parasite itself and in intensity, this is influenced by the virulence of the infecting organisms. It is further suggested that the severity of trypanosome-induced suppression is reflected in the course of infection seen in trypanosome strains of differing virulence. Mechanisms responsible for B cell dysfunction in the infection will be covered in the general discussion (Section IX and Sections V and VI).

V. T CELL FUNCTION

It is unlikely that effector T cells play a role in attacking the extracellular trypanosomes in infected hosts, but changes in regulatory T cells undoubtedly have a profound effect on immune function during the infection. T cells in mice have been primed by subcutaneous administration of live *T. brucei*[67] or by immunization with irradiated *T. rhodesiense*[57] and, subsequently, these cells will proliferate specifically in the presence of trypanosome antigens in vitro. However, this proliferative ability is short lived during infection, and priming is abolished if infection precedes immunization with irradiated parasites by as few as 3 days.[68] This inability of primed T cells to proliferate in the presence of antigen was attributed to infection-induced immunosuppressive events mediated possibly by defective macrophages and suppressive T cells. This dysfunction could be reversed by the trypanocidal drug Berenil.[68] Cell-mediated hypersensitivity against the parasite has been detected in rabbits infected with *T. brucei* or *T. rhodesiense,* but dead organisms did not induce this response.[69] Interestingly, there was a cross-reaction between the two trypanosome strains. In mice, killed *T. rhodesiense* resulted in delayed skin reactions and after two sensitizations survival was reported, possibly through priming of T helper cells.[10]

T cells are not associated with all B cell or MØ changes observed in trypanosomiasis. The course of parasitemia with *T. brucei* or *T. rhodesiense* in nude mice does not greatly differ from that in normal mice.[57,71] If anything, nu/nu mice control the first wave of parasitemia better, presumably because of their activated reticuloendothelial system, but then succumb to subsequent waves of parasites. B lymphocyte function is also suppressed in athymic nude mice following *T. brucei* infection[71] and changes in Ia expression of MØ from nu/nu hosts parallel those observed in normal infected mice.[72] There is an early but transient increase in T cell proliferation in the spleen of euthymic mice, but T cell numbers are less affected than B or null cells during the course of infection.[18]

There is no doubt, however, that T cell function is greatly affected in rodent trypanosomiasis. As infection progresses, all types of T cell responses decline, with the possible exception of delayed skin reactions. Earlier work by Mansfield and Wallace[73] showed a reduction in skin sensitization to mycobacterial proteins (PPD) in rabbits infected with *T. congolense*. In contrast, more virulent *T. brucei* infections of mice did not lead to a decline in delayed skin reaction to oxazolone[16,74] or DNFB.[36] Whether these contrasting observations reflect assay methods or a species difference is not clear.

However, many other T cell functions become defective subsequent to trypanosome infection. The rapid depression of in vitro mitogen responses by spleen cells from infected mice to Con A or PHA has been documented by several investigators, e.g., after *T. equiperdum,*[75] *T. brucei,*[36,76] and *T. congolense*[77] infection. T helper cell memory is lost during the course of *T. brucei* infection as assayed in vivo[32] by adoptive cell transfer. Other antigen-specific T cell responses have been assayed generally in vitro, but spleen cells from infected mice show a clear loss of proliferative responses to allogeneic cells (mixed lymphocyte reactions[32,77]), and the generation of alloreactive cytotoxic T cells is depressed.[77,78] Also, *T. congolense*-infected mice show prolonged allograft survival compared to normal mice.[77] The loss of T cell function thus parallels that of B cell responsiveness during the course of infection.

Another feature associated with rodent trypanosomiasis is the generation in the spleen of suppressive T cells that are not antigen specific. These suppressive cells have so far only been demonstrated in tissue culture, and have been shown to affect in vitro responses of T and B cells to mitogens and heterologous antigens (see below). Therefore, depression of some of the above-described T cell functions may be attributable to the effect of suppressive T cells as well as suppressive MØ (Section VI). Mixed lymphocyte reactions early after *T. brucei* infection can be partially restored by nylon purification of T cells, which tends to remove at least some of the more adherent suppressive T cells,[36] and by removal of the larger MØ by iron filings. However, late in infection even these maneuvers do not restore T cell reactivity.[36]

We have no evidence that the parasite acts directly on T cells. Trypanosome membrane fractions have been shown to stimulate T cell proliferation in vitro both in man[79] and mouse.[152] On the other hand, highly purified T cell populations do not respond to trypanosome membrane fractions on their own, but their proliferative ability is restored in the presence of peripheral blood monocytes in man.[80] Similarly in mice, B cell-depleted T and null cells are stimulated to proliferate in the presence of trypanosomal membranes, but a macrophage-free T cell population does not respond.[152] Once more it looks as though macrophages are a target cell for the parasite and mediate signals leading to T cell proliferation and functional changes.

Several studies have examined suppressive activity by spleen cells from infected mice on in vitro responses of normal spleen cells to B or T cell mitogens or on antigen-specific B cell responses. In general, it was found that such suppressive events could be attributed to more than one cell type. Removal of T cells by treatment with antibody to Thy-1 and complement partially depleted suppressive function, and this led to the conclusion that suppressive T cells were involved. In addition, splenic non-T cells adherent to plastic were also found to suppress T and B cell responses and this implicated suppressive MØ (see Wellhausen and Mansfield[81] and Section VI).

The T cells that suppress normal responses in vitro are still rather ill defined. Jayawardena and colleagues[82] found that the spleen cells suppressing antibody responses to SRBC or DNP-Ficoll in vitro arise within 6 days of *T. brucei* infection of mice, are insensitive to antilymphocyte serum, are lost after adult thymectomy, and bear the Lyt $1^+,2^+,3^+$ phenotype. Earlier in infection (up to day 4) suppressive activity of spleen cells appears masked by transiently enhanced T helper cell (Lyt $1^+,2^-,3^-$) activity. Similarly, *T. congolense* infection of mice by day 14 generates spleen cells with the ability to suppress responses by normal T or B cells to mitogens or allogeneic cells.[83] One difficulty is that not all Thy 1^+ cells in the spleens of infected mice are readily lysed by anti-Thy-1 and complement and weak Thy-1^+ cells could not be removed[83] and appear to represent the suppressive cells.

In trypanosomiasis, there is no evidence that antigen-specific suppressive T cells are generated,[15] and it is not clear how the antigen-nonspecific T suppressor cells arise. Lectins such as Con A stimulate T suppressor cells, and most probably the mitogenic stimulus of T cells in infection is responsible for the appearance of suppressive T cells in the spleen.

VI. CHANGES IN MACROPHAGE PHENOTYPE AND FUNCTION

Macrophages are central cells in the action and regulation of the immune network. This is in view of their function as phagocytic and antigen-presenting cells, and their release of mediators, expression of surface receptors, and interaction with T and B cells (see reviews by Unanue[84] and Nathan et al.[85]). Trypanosomiasis, like many other infections, is accompanied by a multitude of changes in macrophage (MØ) function and populations. Furthermore, recent studies suggest that such alterations have considerable influence on immune function.

During infection, increased numbers of macrophages are found in many organs, particularly where trypanosomes are present, including the liver, spleen, lymph nodes, and bone marrow.[17,19-21] Microscopically, the MØ have the appearance of activated cells and often contain cellular debris. Macrophages are also stimulated to divide in the peritoneal cavity of infected mice, as seen in the case of *T. brucei*.[19] The majority of studies on MØ have used cells harvested from the peritoneal cavity of infected mice because of the difficulty of obtaining pure spleen MØ.

A. Uptake of Parasites by Macrophages

Normal macrophages have some difficulty in taking up trypanosomes; although some of the parasites attach to the MØ, they are not internalized (e.g., Grosskinsky[10]). However, in the presence of parasite-specific antibodies,[86] internalization and degradation of the trypanosome takes place.[87] Radiolabeled parasites have been used for studying the clearance of trypanosomes from the circulation.[88] This is predominantly due to antibody-mediated phagocytosis occurring to a large part in the liver, and can be observed in infected hosts or normal mice passively immunized with hyperimmune serum.[89] The control of infection by nude mice which do not produce IgG antiparasite antibodies suggests that IgM antibody is sufficient for opsonization of the trypanosomes[57] (see Section IV.D). Also, IgG antibody formation is suppressed early in infection, while the host can seemingly control the parasitemia waves as long as some IgM can still be formed.[62,64]

In the studies of MacAskill and colleagues[89] in complement-depleted mice, passive immunization of uninfected hosts required C3. However, in mice deprived of T cells and with C3 levels reduced to less than 10% with Cobra venom factor, the course of parasitemia is the same as that in infected, normal mice and successive parasite waves are controlled.[90] Since phagocytosis does occur, and as no IgM receptors on MØ have been described, there must be sufficient C left or produced by the MØ to permit opsonization of IgM parasites via the C receptor.

B. Changes in Macrophage Surface and Mediator Release

Macrophages from trypanosome-infected mice show the same signs of activation that result from other stimulants such as BCG.[91] A panel of assays was used to examine various parameters of peritoneal MØ activation following infection of (CBA × C57B1)F$_1$ mice with *T. brucei* clone NIM 6. A clear reduction in mannose receptors, Fc receptors, and the MAC 1 and F4/80 surface markers occurs by day 4, reaching the lowest level by day 9,[72] after the first peak of parasitemia has been controlled and the parasites in the body fluids have been cleared by the phagocytic cells. Then follows a prepatent period and during this time surface receptor and marker expression returns to normal. On the other hand, receptor-mediated phagocytosis is enhanced during infection[92] and the expression of Ia by MØ rises.[72] Ia levels remain high even during the prepatent period in our hands,[72] while in *T. rhodesiense* infection Ia has been reported to decline.[93] Ia also increases in nu/nu mice infected with *T. brucei*, and, thus, Ia appearance appears to be T cell independent.[72] Since nu/nu mice possess Thy-1$^+$ precursor cells, the question arises whether infection leads to maturation of functional T cells. In our experiments using young nu/nu mice it has not been possible to demonstrate functional T cells following infection (unpublished observations). However, an increase in θ$^+$ Ig$^-$ cells has been reported in the spleens of athymic mice infected with *T. congolense*.[13] The same changes in MØ properties are characteristic of BCG and other infections with the only difference being that, in general, appearance of Ia molecules on mouse peritoneal cells tends to be T dependent.[91] Recent work has suggested that interferons can lead to enhanced Ia expression by MØ,[94,95] and since interferon is released during infection (see Section VII), this may contribute to the MØ changes observed. It is not yet known whether MØ themselves release interferon during the infection.

The effect of infection on antigen presentation has not been studied extensively, but during a chronic trypanosome infection of mice with *T. brucei*, there appeared no change in antigen-presenting ability of MØ for an anti-SRBC response 3 weeks after infection.[17] Alternatively, during infection with *T. rhodesiense,* MØ presentation of *Listeria* to T cells is defective, and this has been temporally correlated with the decrease in Ia expression by MØ in this system.[93]

Not only are there changes in surface properties of MØ from infected mice, but the release of mediators also shows drastic alterations. Plasminogen activator is released by MØ following infection and the ability to secrete the oxygen metabolites H_2O_2 and O_2^- after stimulation with phorbol myristate acetate is enhanced.[72] MØ are also active in secreting prostaglandins (PG); during a *T. brucei* infection, the ratio of $PGE_2/PGF_{1\alpha}$ is reversed, so that peritoneal macrophages secrete far more PGE_2 than normally.[96] Maximum release of PGE_2 by macrophages from infected mice occurs at the height of parasitemia induced by *T. brucei* clone NIM6. During the prepatent period PGE_2 returns to normal levels, while later in the infection it is below that of normal controls.[96] This is another facet that will affect immune function of the host since prostaglandins are thought to inhibit different lymphoid activities[97] and modulate MØ Ia expression.[98]

We have also examined the influence of infection and the resultant uptake of parasites by macrophages on secretion of IL-1, a product known to influence T and B cell function.[84] In the standard assay measuring the co-mitogenesis of IL-1 and PHA on thymocytes, supernatants from normal macrophages have no activity (Figure 2). In contrast, macrophages taken from *T. brucei*-infected mice, when a considerable parasite load is present, are stimulated to secrete large amounts of IL-1. Such MØ supernatants are also strongly mitogenic when incubated with thymocytes alone. The release of IL-1 by MØ can be further increased by the addition of LPS.[153] Macrophages taken from mice several days prior to death also have increased IL-1 release; however, this cannot be enhanced by LPS, suggesting the cells cannot be stimulated further in the final stages of infection. The importance of the increase in IL-1 secretion is not yet known, but its presence may be reflected in the T cell proliferation observed in the infection, and conceivably have some influence on host B cell function. Similar enhancement of IL-1 is also observed in mice infected with *Listeria,*[99] BCG,[100] and malaria.[101]

The multiple phenotypic changes occurring in MØ during trypanosomiasis are similar to those in other infections and are summarized in Figure 3. The mechanisms underlying these changes are as yet ill defined, and the chemical nature of the active parasite product responsible for inducing MØ activation is not yet characterized (see also Section VIII).

C. Macrophage Mediate Immunosuppression in Trypanosomiasis

MØ have been implicated for some years in the modulation of immune responsiveness by trypanosomes. In earlier work it was found that a plastic adherent fraction of spleen cells from infected mice would actively suppress antibody or mitogen responses in vitro. About 40% of spleen cells adhere to plastic, and, therefore, this represents a mixed cell population, and in many early studies no further characterization of the suppressive cell type was undertaken. However, it then became clear that suppression could be T cell independent and this directed attention to the MØ as a potential suppressive cell type. Spleen cells from *T. rhodesiense*-infected nude (nu/nu) mice suppressed the LPS response of normal spleen cell cultures[102] and infected nu/nu mice developed defective LPS responses.[71,102] As there is no evidence to date that the infection leads to maturation of T precursor cells in nu/nu mice, these findings imply a T cell-independent suppressor cell. In the experiments of Wellhausen and Mansfield,[103] the suppressive cell type was radiation resistant, but suppressor function was blocked by silica or heat treatment. Suppression in this system was not reversible by indomethacin and could not be attributed to prostaglandin release.[103] On the other hand, suppression was resistant to lysis by anti-Thy-1, anti-Lyt-2, or anti-Ig and C', implicating MØ involvement.[15]

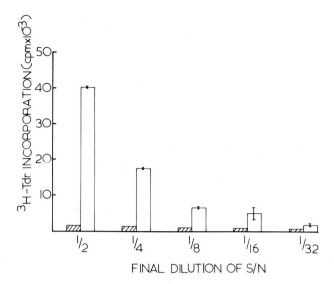

FIGURE 2. Release of IL-1 by macrophages from mice infected with *T. brucei*. (CBA × BALB/c)F$_1$ mice were infected with *T. brucei* clone NIM 2 for 7 days. The supernatant of peritoneal macrophages was assayed for IL-1 secretion by the proliferation of thymocytes in vitro.[100,153] ▨▨ Normal mice; ☐ infected mice.

TRYPANOSOMES AND MACROPHAGE FUNCTION

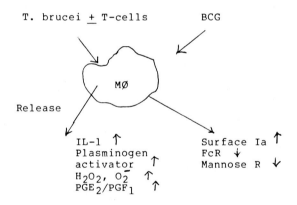

FIGURE 3. Summary of macrophage changes in phenotype and mediator release resulting from *T. brucei* infection of (CBA × C57Bl/6)F$_1$ mice. Details are described by Grosskinsky et al.[72]

More direct evidence for MØ-mediated changes of immune responsiveness comes from cell transfer experiments. Peritoneal exudate cells, after uptake of trypanosomes in the presence of antibodies and following removal of T cells by anti-Thy-1 and C′, on transfer to normal mice inhibited a primary IgG antibody response to SRBC in vitro.[104] Again the duality of trypanosome effect can be observed. If antigen is given on the day of MØ transfer, there is a transient enhancement, while antigen given 4 days later results in suppressed antibody response. Further evidence for the parasite acting via an intermediate cell such as the macrophage rather than directly on lymphoid cells comes from other in vitro data. Trypanosome membrane preparations that are active in vivo[54] stimulate human peripheral blood T cells to proliferate in vitro only in the presence of monocytes.[156] At present we

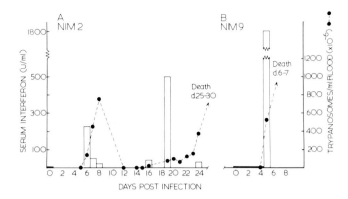

FIGURE 4.   Serum interferon levels in mice infected with two clones of
T. brucei varying in virulence. For details see Bancroft et al.[118] – – – –
Parasitemia; ☐ interferon level in serum.

have no evidence for direct interaction between *T. brucei* components and lymphoid cells
(see Section VIII). This contrasts with the data obtained on trypanosome-derived substances
from *T. musculi* which bind to host cells and are associated with immunosuppression.[105]

Activation of macrophages during infection is not restricted to African trypanosomes, but
has also been described in other parasite infections, for example, *Plasmodia*,[106] *T. cruzi*,[107]
and *T. gondii*.[108] It needs to be resolved whether macrophages are immunodepressive because
they release a parasite product or because of their activated state. Since immune dysfunction
accompanies so many different infections and also follows administration of bacterial products, e.g., LPS of *E. coli*,[109] a general pathway relating to changes in MØ phenotype and
mediator release is a more likely cause of poor immune function. Macrophages, though
lacking specific recognition mechanisms for antigen, play a central role in regulation of the
immune network and in cell-cell interaction with T and B cells,[84] and we suggest that African
trypanosomes can interfere with the normal activity of the immune system by activation of
MØ.

VII. INTERFERON AND NATURAL KILLER CELLS

A. Trypanosome-Induced Interferons

Since the initial discovery of interferon (IFN) induction by viruses,[110] it has become
apparent that a large number of other agents have similar effects. Raised interferon levels
in vivo or in vitro have been reported with bacteria or their products, foreign or neoplastic
cells, and synthetic polyribonucleotides.[111,112] In addition, the intracellular protozoa *Toxoplasma*,[113,114] *Plasmodium berghei*,[115] and *Trypanosoma cruzi*[116] can also enhance IFN production in vivo. With the extracellular African trypanosomes, infection of mice with *T.
brucei* clearly augments serum IFN levels[117,118] as does *T. equiperdum*.[119] In our studies,
mice infected with *T. brucei* clone NIM2 parasites (Figure 4A) show enhancement of serum
IFN once parasites are detectable in the blood. IFN returns to control levels after the first
wave of parasitemia. The subsequent wave of parasite replication also enhances IFN, but
again only transiently, although the parasite burden continues to increase until the death of
the host several days later. In infection with the acute clone NIM 9, no stimulation is present
during the prepatent period, but as parasites appear in the blood, serum IFN is rapidly
enhanced[118] (Figure 4B).

The interferons produced by this infection are a mixture of α/β and γ (immune) IFN as
determined by neutralization with anti-interferon sera. The IFN-γ is probably a reflection
of the mitogenic pressure of the parasite on T cells,[18] since in other systems this class of
IFN is seen to be a T cell product.[120] The α/β IFN is less readily explained, perhaps resulting

from the stimulation of null cells[18] and macrophages[72] which is known to occur during the infection.

Infection with *T. brucei* clearly stimulates the interferon system, but it is less certain whether this IFN has any effect on either the trypanosome or the host. Previous experiments have demonstrated the immunomodulatory actions of interferons in vivo and in vitro, and it was interesting to see if IFN generation was a means by which the parasite could affect host immune function. Injection of normal mice with lethally irradiated but intact parasites is known to suppress primary antibody responses to heterologous antigens in a similar fashion to a normal infection[121] (see also Section VIII). However, this treatment has no effect on serum IFN levels for up to a week after infection, although it induces a severe reduction in PFC to SRBC.[118] This suggests that the presence of parasite-induced serum IFN is not a prerequisite for suppression of antibody responses, although it is present around the same time. The more severe effects of an infection are required for IFN generation by *T. brucei*, and by altering the form of contact between parasite and host, loss of antibody responses can be separated from IFN stimulation at least in this model.

B. Effect of Exogenous Interferon on Infection

The influence of exogenous IFN and IFN inducers on protozoan infections has yielded variable results in studies on intracellular[122,123] and extracellular organisms. Injection of mice with polyinosinic:polycytidilic acid (poly I:C) has no effect on mortality or parasitemia in infections with *T. equiperdum* or *T. duttoni*.[124,125] In contrast, Herman and Baron[124] found that several doses of poly I:C given before and after infection of mice with *T. congolense* significantly reduced mortality.[124] Interestingly, this was dependent on the organism used for infection, in that parasites stably resistant or sensitive to the influence of poly I:C were isolated after serial passage of trypanosomes in mice. In this model it is believed that poly I:C acted through the immune system, rather than by a direct effect of the interferon on parasite replication. Poly I:C also influences the course of infection with *T. brucei* clone NIM 2. Mice injected 1 day before and several days after infection show a clear decrease in parasite load during the entire first parasitemia wave. A similar course of injections with murine IFN α/β (10^4 U per injection) did not alter the peak parasite load, but clearly decreased the initial wave of parasitemia and, as with poly I:C, enhanced the clearance of blood parasites to end the first wave.[154] However, despite such changes in parasitemia profile, neither poly I:C nor IFN α/β altered the mortality of the host.

C. Natural Killer Cells

One of the innate defense mechanisms exhibited in unsensitized hosts is the phenomenon of naturally occurring cell-mediated cytotoxicity. In studies of antigen-specific cytotoxicity against tumors, cells from normal individuals unexpectedly showed significant killing of novel tumor targets. This has since been ascribed to a subpopulation of lymphoid cells called natural killer (NK) cells found in normal members of many species, but particularly well documented for mice and man.[126] NK cells have been implicated as an important early defense mechanism against neoplasia and some infectious diseases, especially those of viral etiology (reviewed by Herberman and Ortaldo[127]).

More recently, their involvement in protozoal infections has been questioned, with some results suggesting a link between NK cell activity and host susceptibility to malaria and Babesia infection.[128,129] Furthermore, modulation of NK cell function, as measured against tumor cell targets, has been described in mice infected with *T. gondii*,[130] *Plasmodium yoelli*,[131] and *T. cruzi*.[132] From preliminary experiments, splenic NK cell activity against YAC tumor cells is also altered in mice infected with *T. brucei*. Killing remains at control levels during the early stages of infection and up to the time of peak parasitemia (days 6 to 7). At this time serum interferon levels are raised (this section), but no enhancement of NK activity has been observed. In contrast, NK activity from day 9 onwards is severely reduced, often to less than 20% of control values.[154] This loss of activity is seen at the time of considerable trypanosome-induced disruption of splenic architecture and cellularity, but is not entirely due to dilution of NK cells by other cell types as total activity per spleen is also reduced. To date there is no evidence of a transferable suppressor cell acting in the system as previously described for carrageenan-induced suppression of NK cell function.[133] Also, the inhibition of killing is not accounted for by poor viability of effector cells taken late in infection, or by nonspecific inhibition of the cytotoxic assay, by large numbers of red cells present in spleen cell suspensions from infected mice. Further experiments are required before any conclusions are drawn as to the mechanisms responsible for this change and its importance to the host.

VIII. THE SEARCH FOR ACTIVE PARASITE PRODUCTS

The multiple effects of trypanosome infection on the host raise important questions regarding the nature of the active parasite product(s) and as to whether these act directly on various lymphoid cell populations or via intermediary target cells. Research efforts have not been restricted to mediators of the immunological sequelae of infection, but have been aimed also at the neurological and hematological disruption that occurs (see review by Tizard[134] and Chapter 4 in this book). That parasite-associated products can interfere with immune responses has already been documented for the metazoan parasites *Trichinella* and *Schistosoma*,[135] and the intracellular protozoa *Trypanosoma cruzi* and *Plasmodium*[136,137] (see review by Bancroft and Askonas[5]).

The search for the active component(s) of African trypanosomes has used two types of assay systems to test the ability of parasite fractions, first, to alter antibody production by normal cells in vivo or in vitro and, second, to provide a mitogenic stimulus for lymphocytes in vitro (for summary of results obtained with *T. brucei* see Figure 5). The first type of approach has been used in our laboratory where it was shown that infection-induced suppression of antibody production in vivo could be mimicked by injection of killed but intact *T. brucei* organisms into normal mice.[121] This activity was associated with crude parasite membrane fractions.[63,121] A relatively small quantity of material was sufficient, and therefore, suppression could not be attributed to a gross antigen overload of the lymphoid and reticuloendothelial systems. The crude membrane fractions from our *T. brucei* clones almost completely inhibited the IgG response to SRBC, whereas depression of the IgM response was less rapid, dose dependent, and varied with the virulence of the parasite clones from which it was derived. Thus, the extent of inhibition of IgM production correlated with the virulence of the parasite clone (Figure 6) indicating that *T. brucei* membrane fractions varied intrinsically in their immunosuppressive ability. This could not be attributed to the differences in the variant surface glycoprotein (VSG) of the clones, since in crude or purified form VSG has no apparent activity in vivo,[63] and internal as well as external parasite membranes had a similar effect.

Macrophages have been implicated as potential intermediary cells between the parasite and its effect on the host[104] (see Section VI). A soluble fraction from homogenized *T. brucei* on its own has no effect on antibody responses to SRBC in vivo but can induce depressed antibody formation following interaction with syngeneic peritoneal macrophages. Further fractionation of this supernatant on Sepharose 4B identified the active component as a complex of trypanosome lipids, protein, and glycoproteins eluting in the exclusion volume of the column. This complex mediated three major features of infection with different kinetics, namely, polyclonal stimulation of splenic B cells, as well as early enhancement and subsequent suppression of antigen-specific B cell responses. When the lipid was extracted from this complex, mixed with macrophages, and the suspension injected into normal mice,

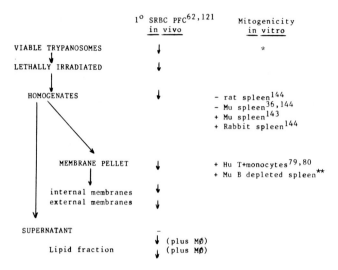

FIGURE 5. Active *T. brucei* fractions. Superscripts refer to the reference concerned. ↓ — Inhibition of responsiveness in vivo; + — symbol: mitogenic response; − — symbol: no effect; * — symbol: no effect on mouse spleen cells (unpublished observation); ** — symbol.[152]

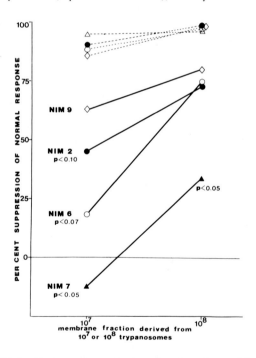

FIGURE 6. Crude membrane fractions from four clones of *T. brucei* varying in virulence from acute to chronic differ intrinsically in their ability to suppress antibody responses. Mice were primed with SRBC 4 days after injection of trypanosome membranes, and 6 days later the splenic PFC-anti-SRBC response was assayed. Each point is the arithmetic mean (five mice per group). —— IgM PFC; – – – – IgG PFC. (Reprinted from Sacks, D. L., Selkirk, M., Ogilvie, B. M., and Askonas, B. A., *Nature (London)*, 283, 476, 1980. With permission.)

partial suppression of the anti-SRBC response occurred, but this was less severe than that seen with intact organisms or parasite membranes.[63] Some lipid species can inhibit primary antibody responses or be mitogenic to normal spleen cells in other systems,[138,139] but further work is needed to see if pure lipid components are responsible for the modulatory effects of trypanosomes seen in these assays. Previously, lipid components of trypanosomes have been assigned B cell mitogenic properties in vitro. Assoku and Tizard[140] reported that autolysates of *T. congolense* stimulated proliferation of spleen cells from athymic nude mice in vitro; free fatty acids were released from such autolysates and the mitogenicity of the crude autolysates could be mimicked by addition of purified fatty acids to the culture.[141] The importance of such lipids in the immunological and hematological features of the infection is an interesting problem, but, as previously stated, their effects would be expected to occur locally since free fatty acids readily bind to host serum albumin and are inactivated.

The mitogenic or immunosuppressive properties of trypanosome membranes have been clearly demonstrated in vivo, but similar effects on mouse spleen cells in vitro have been more difficult to observe. However, recently Beer[152] has demonstrated stimulation of mouse spleen cells depleted of B lymphocytes by *T. brucei* membranes. The activity of this parasite membrane fraction on human peripheral blood cells in vitro was monocyte dependent and directed at T cells rather than B cells.[79,80] Thus, in our hands the polyclonal B cell stimulation in vivo has not been replicated in vitro with the same parasite fraction. This indicates further the complexity of the link between parasite components and the changes in immunological function which occur, and we have no evidence that the parasite can act directly on B cells.

Overall, the literature on suppression or enhancement of immune responses or lymphocyte proliferation by trypanosomes or their components in vitro is controversial. Results from different laboratories vary and a range of tissue culture conditions and parasite preparations have been used and probably account for this variability. At present the studies relating to T cell vs. B cell activation do not permit definitive conclusions. Wellhausen and Mansfield[81] found that addition of low numbers of viable *T. rhodesiense* augmented in vitro PFC responses with suppression occurring only with excessive numbers of organisms, presumably by interference with the culture conditions and cell viability. Similarly, whole trypanosomes did not inhibit mouse spleen cell responses to Con A or LPS except possibly at very high parasite numbers.[76,155]

The large increase in null cells and B cells in the spleen and lymph nodes of infected mice (see Section I) would suggest the presence of mitogenic substances in the parasite and that the effects on immune responsiveness parallel those induced by polyclonal stimulators such as LPS.[74,109,142] In other laboratories, mitogenic effects on B cells by trypanosome homogenates have been reported. Spleen cells from normal and athymic, nude mice were stimulated in vitro[143] and homogenates of *T. brucei* and *T. congolense* were mitogenic to non-PHA responsive cells (presumably B cells) in rabbit spleen and peripheral blood.[144] Notably, this effect was not observed with spleen cells of rats, guinea pigs, or mice.

Moulton and Coleman[145] have described a soluble suppressor substance isolated from the spleens of deer mice infected with *T. brucei*. This crude supernatant inhibited primary B cell responses to SRBC both in vivo and in vitro. The effect was further reflected in histological evidence of reduced germinal center development and lower numbers of mature plasma cells in the red pulp of mice given the suppressive factor. It should be noted that, as with the serum suppressor substance of *T. cruzi*,[136] it is not known whether the active component is of parasite origin or derived indirectly from lymphoid cells or macrophages after contact with the organism.

Thus, further work is required to help our understanding of the action of parasite products. We favor the view that trypanosome products do not act directly on lymphoid cells, but via an intermediary cell.

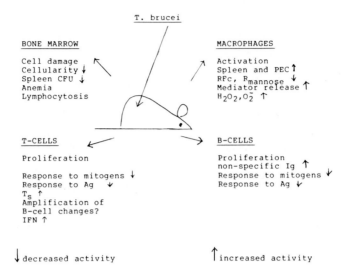

FIGURE 7.   Summary of the trypanosome-induced changes in the immune system.

IX. DISCUSSION AND CONCLUSIONS

It is evident that African trypanosomes cause havoc in the immune system by inducing multiple changes in the lymphoid organs. In rodents, almost every lymphoid cell subpopulation is affected and immune responses to both parasite-related and -unrelated antigens are depressed (see Figure 7 for summary). Immunosuppression and deficient responses to superinfection not only accompany rodent trypanosomiasis[74] but have been observed both in cattle[15,146] and man;[147] antibody responses to vaccines are inhibited, and the hosts may die of secondary infections if they survive the trypanosomal invasion. Trypanosome infection in cattle and humans is being discussed in detail in another chapter of this book.

A feature of trypanosomiasis is the duality of its action on the immune system. Early in infection T and B cells are polyclonally stimulated to divide and B cell maturation is reflected by enhanced serum levels of Ig. In relatively chronic infection this stimulation is associated with a very transient enhancement of specific antibody responses and T-helper activity, soon to be followed by profound immunosuppression. This occurs rapidly in acute infections and whether enhancement occurs is influenced by the timing of antigen administration, the antigen used, and the host-parasite combination studied. During infection, specific IgG antibody production is more rapidly shut off than IgM production, and there are indications that IgM antibody suffices for control of parasitemia. No totally resistant rodent strain has been discovered, but the relatively resistant C57B1/6 mice show less immune dysfunction than more susceptible mouse strains with the same parasitemia level. In general, the parasite load is another factor which affects the course of infection, in as far as low parasite loads are associated with less profound immune changes. Also, the virulence of the infecting organisms can be correlated with the severity of immunosuppression, and since the antiparasite response is also disturbed, this will influence the outcome of the infection. In addition, local effects are associated with the presence of the parasite in different lymphoid organs, as seen in delayed immune suppression in lymph nodes as compared to the spleen which is the site of early trypanosome replication in the rodent models.

While many of the lymphoid changes that we describe are apt to contribute to the immune dysfunction, the mechanisms inducing defective immune responsiveness remain ill defined and large gaps exist in our understanding of the host-parasite interactions and biology of trypanosomes. Are the suppressive MØ and T cells sufficient to cause profound immune dysfunction, or are there additional reasons why antigen-specific selection of the relevant clones fails in an organ where T and B cells are proliferating? The disruption of the splenic architecture will play a role and, in addition, proliferating T cells and B cells may be out of phase and unable to collaborate for antibody production, as suggested by Thomas and Calderon.[148] The end result is that the polyclonal parasite-induced stimuli to the cells dominate. Antigen nonspecific Ig levels remain high during the course of infection, at times when no antigen-specific response remains. At first it had been suggested that this lack of specific responsiveness was a consequence of a parasite-derived B cell mitogen and the polyclonal exhaustion of antigen-specific B cells due to extensive cell proliferation. However, the rapidity of the immunosuppression induced by virulent clones argues against clonal exhaustion as the only mechanism, and we can conclude only that the lymphoid cells become refractory to normal control signals and antigen, in addition to the role played by suppressive MØ and T cells (see Sections V and VI).

Several other questions still remain open. Does the parasite or its products act directly on lymphoid cells or indirectly via an intermediary cell, and what is the nature of the parasite product(s) which exerts such profound effects on the immune system? Parasite activity in vivo appears to be associated with internal and external membranes of the trypanosomes while the surface glycoprotein per se has been excluded. In our hands we find no evidence of a direct interaction between parasite products and lymphoid cells from experiments with parasite fractions in vitro. We, therefore, favor the view that parasites act via intermediary cell types important in immune regulation, and that MØ, after uptake of trypanosomes in the presence of antibodies, are at least one of the key intermediary cells for parasite activity. It has been demonstrated that during trypanosomiasis, MØ are activated and change the expression of surface receptors as well as the release of mediators (Section VI) in parallel to alterations observed in other infections such as BCG[91] and malaria.[149] Clarke and associates[149] have pointed out that after activation, MØ may be important in causing bone marrow depression, hypergammaglobulinemia, and splenomegaly through the release of IFN, lymphocyte activating factor, and many other mediators. With its central role in immune homeostasis and interaction with T cells, in particular,[84] the macrophage would provide a common pathway for immunosuppression that accompanies so many different infections, be they bacterial,[3] viral,[2] or parasitic.[4,5] Better defined microbial products (e.g., LPS of *E. coli*) and so-called adjuvants show similar kinetics of polyclonal enhancement, followed by depression of immune responses, to that observed in African trypanosomiasis.[150] Although the latter infection causes particularly acute immunosuppression, there may be nothing unique associated with this parasite. Investigation of immune dysfunction in this system will hopefully yield more information on common mechanisms by which microorganisms or their products interact with the immune system.

ACKNOWLEDGMENTS

We are most grateful to Rachel Woodward for her patience in typing the manuscript. GJB gratefully acknowledges the financial support of the Hackett Foundation of the University of Western Australia.

REFERENCES

1. **Vickerman, K.,** Antigenic variation in trypanosomes, *Nature (London),* 273, 613, 1978.
2. **Notkins, A. L., Mergenhagen, S., and Howard, R.,** Effect of virus infections on the function of the immune system, *Ann. Rev. Microbiol.,* 24, 525, 1970.
3. **Schwab, J.,** Suppression of the immune response by microorganisms, *Bacteriol. Rev.,* 39, 121, 1975.
4. **Mitchell, G. F.,** Response to infection with metazoan and protozoan parasites, *Adv. Immunol.,* 28, 451, 1979.
5. **Bancroft, G. J. and Askonas, B. A.,** Regulation of antibody production in protozoal infections, *Clin. Immunol. Allergy,* 2, 511, 1982.
6. **Murray, P. K., Murray, M., Morrison, W. I., Wallace, M., and McIntyre, W. I. M.,** Trypanosomiasis in N'dama and Zebu cattle, in *Proc. Int. Scientific Council for Trypanosomiasis Research and Control,* 15th Meeting, The Gambia, 1977, 470.
7. **Clayton, C. E.,** *Trypanosoma brucei:* influence of host strain and parasite antigenic type on infections in mice, *Exp. Parasitol.,* 44, 202, 1978.
8. **Morrison, W. I. and Murray, M.,** *Trypanosoma congolense:* inheritance of susceptibility to infection in inbred strains of mice, *Exp. Parasitol.,* 48, 364, 1979.
9. **Greenblatt, H. C., Rosenstreich, D. I., and Diggs, C. L.,** Genetic control of natural resistance to *Trypanosoma rhodesiense* in mice, in *Genetic Control of Natural Resistance to Infections and Malignancy — Perspectives in Immunology,* Skamene, E., Kingshavin, P., and Landy, M., Eds., Academic Press, New York, 1980, 89.
10. **Grosskinsky, C. M.,** Cellular Mechanisms of Immunosuppression in African Trypanosomiasis, Ph.D. thesis, National Institute for Medical Research, Mill Hill, London, 1981.
11. **Whitelaw, D. D., MacAskill, J. A., Holmes, P. H., Jennings, F. W., and Urquhart, G. M.,** Genetic resistance to *Trypanosoma congolense* infections in mice, *Infect. Immun.,* 27, 701, 1980.
12. **Selkirk, M. E. and Sacks, D. L.,** Trypanotolerance in inbred mice: an immunological basis for variation in susceptibility to infection with *Trypanosoma brucei, Tropenmed. Parasitol.,* 31, 435, 1980.
13. **Morrison, W. I., Roelants, G. E., Mayor-Withey, K. S., and Murray, M.,** Susceptibility of inbred strains of mice to *Trypanosoma congolense:* correlation with changes in spleen lymphocyte populations, *Clin. Exp. Immunol.,* 32, 25, 1978.
14. **Rosentreich, D. L., O'Brien, A. D., Groves, M. G., and Taylor, B. A.,** Genetic control of resistance to infection in mice, in *The Molecular Basis of Microbial Pathogenicity,* Smith, H., Skehel, J. J., and Turner, M. J., Eds., Verlag Chemie, Weinheim, 1980, 101.
15. **Mansfield, J. M.,** Immunology and immunopathology of African trypanosomiasis, in *Parasitic Diseases, The Immunology,* Vol. 1, Mansfield, J. M., Ed., Marcel Dekker, New York, 1982, 167.
16. **Murray, P. K., Jennings, F. W., Murray, M., and Urquhart, G. M.,** The nature of the immuno-suppression in *Trypanosoma brucei* infections in mice. II. The role of the T and B lymphocytes, *Immunology,* 27, 825, 1974.
17. **Murray, P. K., Jennings, F. W., Murray, M., and Urquhart, G. M.,** The nature of immunosuppresion in *Trypanosoma brucei* infections in mice. I. The role of the macrophage, *Immunology,* 27, 815, 1974.
18. **Mayor-Withey, K. S., Clayton, C. E., Roelants, G. E., and Askonas, B. A.,** Trypanosomiasis leads to extensive proliferation of B, T and null cells in spleen and bone, *Clin. Exp. Immunol.,* 34, 359, 1978.
19. **Clayton, C. E., Selkirk, M. E., Corsini, C. A., Ogilvie, B. M., and Askonas, B. A.,** Murine trypa-nosomiasis: cellular proliferation and functional depletion in the blood, peritoneum and spleen related to changes in bone marrow stem cells, *Infect. Immun.,* 28, 824, 1980.
20. **Morrison, W. I., Murray, M., and Bovell, D. L.,** Response of the murine lymphoid system to a chronic infection with *Trypanosoma congolense, Lab. Invest.,* 45, 547, 1981.
21. **Morrison, W. I., Murray, M., and Hudson, C. A.,** The response of the murine lymphoid system to a chronic infection with *Trypanosoma congolense.* II. The lymph nodes, thymus and liver, *J. Pathol.,* 138, 273, 1982.
22. **Roelants, G. E., Pearson, T. W., Morrison, W. I., Mayor-Withey, K. S., and Lundin, L. B.,** Immune depression in trypanosome-infected mice. IV. Kinetics of suppression and alleviation by the trypanocidal drug Berenil, *Clin. Exp. Immunol.,* 37, 457, 1979.
23. **Greenwood, B. M. and Whittle, H. C.,** The pathogenesis of sleeping sickness, *Trans. R. Soc. Trop. Med. Hyg.,* 74, 716, 1980.
24. **Greenwood, B. M. and Whittle, H. C.,** Production of free light chains in Gambian trypanosomiasis, *Clin. Exp. Immunol.,* 20, 437, 1975.
25. **Greenwood, B. M. and Whittle, H. C.,** Cerebrospinal fluid IgM in patients with sleeping sickness, *Lancet,* 2, 525, 1973.
26. **Luckins, A. J.,** The immune response of cattle to infection with *Trypanosoma congolense* and *T. vivax, Ann. Trop. Med. Parasitol.,* 70, 133, 1976.

27. **Nielson, K., Sheppard, J., Holmes, W., and Tizard, I.**, Experimental bovine trypanosomiasis. Changes in serum immunoglobulins, complement and complement components in infected animals, *Immunology,* 35, 817, 1978.

28. **Frommel, D., Percy, D. Y. E., Masseyeff, R., and Good, R. A.**, Low molecular weight immunoglobulin M in experimental trypanosomiasis, *Nature (London),* 228, 1208, 1970.

29. **Mattern, P., Klein, F., Poutrizel, R., and Jongepier-Geerdes, Y. E. J. M.**, Anti-immunoglobulins and heterophil agglutinins in experimental trypanosomiasis, *Infect. Immun.,* 128, 812, 1980.

30. **Houba, V., Brown, K. N., and Allison, A. C.**, Heterophile antibodies, M antiglobulins and immuno-globulins in experimental trypanosomiasis, *Clin. Exp. Immunol.,* 4, 113, 1969.

31. **Hudson, K. M., Byner, C., Freeman, J., and Terry, R. J.**, Immunodepression, high IgM levels and evasion of the immune response in murine trypanosomiasis, *Nature (London),* 264, 256, 1976.

32. **Askonas, B. A., Corsini, A. C., Clayton, C. E., and Ogilvie, B. M.**, Functional depletion of T- and B-memory cells and other lymphoid cell subpopulations during trypanosomiasis, *Immunology,* 36, 313, 1979.

33. **Baltz, T., Baltz, D., Giroud, C., and Pautrizel, R.**, Immune depression and macroglobulinaemia in experimental subchronic trypanosomiasis, *Infect. Immun.,* 32, 979, 1981.

34. **Finerty, J. F., Rosenberg, Y. J., Kendrick, L., McKelvin, R. P., and Hansen, C. T.**, The use of CBA/N and nude mice to study the regulation of B cell activation following infection with *Trypanosoma rhodesiense*, in *Proc. 3rd Int. Workshop on Nude Mice,* in press.

35. **Rose, L. M., Goldman, M., and Lambert, P.-H.**, Simultaneous induction of an idiotype, corresponding anti-idiotypic antibodies, and immune complexes during African trypanosomiasis in mice, *J. Immunol.,* 128, 79, 1982.

36. **Corsini, A. C., Clayton, C., Askonas, B. A., and Ogilvie, B. M.**, Suppressor cells and loss of B cell potential in mice infected with *Trypanosoma brucei, Clin. Exp. Immunol.,* 29, 122, 1977.

37. **Binz, G.**, Observations on levels of immunoglobulin M in confirmed cases of *Trypanosoma rhodesiense* infection in the Lambwe valley, *Bull. WHO,* 47, 751, 1972.

38. **Whittle, H. C., Greenwood, B. M., Bidwell, D. E., Bartlett, A., and Voller, A.**, IgM and antibody measurement in the diagnosis and management of Gambian trypanosomiasis, *Am. J. Trop. Med. Hyg.,* 26, 1129, 1977.

39. **Henderson-Begg, A.**, Heterophile antibodies in trypanosomiasis, *Trans. R. Soc. Trop. Med. Hyg.,* 40, 331, 1946.

40. **Kobayakawa, T., Louis, J., Izui, S., and Lambert, P. H.**, Autoimmune responses to DNA, red blood cells and thymocyte antigens in association with polyclonal antibody synthesis during experimental African trypanosomiasis, *J. Immunol.,* 122, 296, 1979.

41. **Sendashonga, C. N. and Black, S. J.**, Humoral responses against *Trypanosoma brucei* variable surface antigen are induced by degenerating parasites, *Parasite Immunol.,* 4, 245, 1982.

42. **Gasbarre, L. C., Finerty J. F., and Louis, J. A.**, Non-specific immune responses in CBA/N mice infected with *Trypanosoma brucei, Para. Immunol.,* 3, 273, 1981.

43. **Rosenberg, Y. J.**, Isotype-specific T-cell regulation of immunoglobulin expression, *Immun. Rev.,* 67, 33, 1982.

44. **Muschel, L. H., Simonton, L. A., Wells, P. A., and Fife, E. H., Jr.**, Occurrence of complement fixing antibodies reactive with normal tissue constituents in normal and disease states, *J. Clin. Invest.,* 40, 517, 1961.

45. **Popham, A. M. and Dresser, D. W.**, Rheumatoid factors in mice: nonspecific activators of heterophile rheumatoid factor production, *Immunology,* 41, 579, 1980.

46. **Rickman, L. J. and Cox, H. W.**, Immunologic reactions associated with anaemia, thrombocytopaenia and coagulopathy in experimental African trypanosomiasis, *J. Parasitol.,* 66, 28, 1980.

47. **Lindsley, H. B., Kysela, S., and Steinberg, A. D.**, Nucleic acid antibodies in African trypanosomiasis: studies in rhesus monkeys and man, *J. Immunol.,* 113, 1921, 1974.

48. **Klein, F., Mattern, P., Kornmann, V. D., and Bosch, H. J.**, Experimental induction of rheumatoid factor-like substances in animal trypanosomiasis, *Clin. Exp. Immunol.,* 7, 851, 1970.

49. **Mackenzie, A. R. and Boreham, P. F. L.**, Autoimmunity in trypanosome infections. I. Tissue auto-antibodies in *Trypanosoma (Trypanozoan) brucei,* infections in the rabbit, *Immunology,* 26, 1225, 1974.

50. **Kobayakawa, T., Louis, J., Izui, S., and Lambert, P. H.**, Autoimmune responses to DNA, red blood cells and thymocyte antigens in association with polyclonal antibody synthesis during experimental African trypanosomiasis, *J. Immunol.,* 122, 296, 1979.

51. **Roelants, G. E., Pearson, T. W., Tyrer, H. W., Mayor-Withey, K. S., and Lundin, L. B.**, Immune depression in trypanosome-infected mice. II. Characterization of the spleen cell types involved, *Eur. J. Immunol.,* 9, 195, 1979.

52. **Wellhausen, S. R. and Mansfield, J. M.**, Lymphocyte function in experimental African trypanosomiasis. III. Loss of lymph node cell responsiveness, *J. Immunol.,* 124, 1183, 1980.

53. **Goodwin, L. G., Green, D. G., Guy, M. W, and Voller, A.,** Immunosuppression during trypanosomiasis, *Br. J. Exp. Pathol.,* 53, 40, 1972.
54. **Sacks, D. L., Selkirk, M., Ogilvie, B. M., and Askonas, B. A.,** Intrinsic immunosuppressive activity of different trypanosome strains varies with parasite virulence, *Nature (London),* 283, 476, 1980.
55. **Mansfield, J. M. and Bagasra, O.,** Lymphocyte function in experimental African trypanosomiasis. I. B cell responses to helper T cell-independent and -dependent antigens, *J. Immunol.,* 120, 759, 1978.
56. **Campbell, G. H., Esser, K. M., and Weinbaum, F. I.,** *Trypanosoma rhodesiense* infection in B-cell-deficient mice, *Infect. Immun.,* 18, 434, 1977.
57. **Campbell, G. H., Esser, K. M., and Phillips, S. M.,** *Trypanosoma rhodesiense* infection in congenitally athymic (nude) mice, *Infect. Immun.,* 20, 714, 1978.
58. **Louis, J. A., Lima, G. M. C., and Engers, H. D.,** Murine T lymphocyte responses specific for the protozoan parasites *Leishmania tropica* and *Trypanosoma brucei, Clin. Immunol. Allergy,* 2, 597, 1982.
59. **Seed, J. R. and Gam, A. A.,** Passive immunity to experimental trypanosomiasis, *J. Parasitol.,* 52, 1134, 1966.
60. **Cross, G. A. M.,** Identification, purification and properties of clone-specific glycoprotein antigens constituting the surface coat of *Trypanosoma brucei, Parasitology,* 71, 393, 1975.
61. **Black, S. J., Hewett, R. S., and Sendashonga, C. N.,** *Trypanosoma brucei* variable surface antigen is released by degenerating parasites but not by actively dividing parasites, *Parasite Immunol.,* 4, 233, 1982.
62. **Sacks, D. L. and Askonas, B. A.,** Trypanosome-induced suppression of anti-parasite responses during experimental African trypanosomiasis, *Eur. J. Immunol.,* 10, 971, 1980.
63. **Sacks, D. L., Bancroft, G. J., Evans, W. H., and Askonas, B. A.,** Incubation of trypanosome-derived mitogenic and immunosuppressive products with peritoneal macrophages allows recovery of biological activities from soluble parasite fractions, *Infect. Immun.,* 36, 160, 1982.
64. **Hudson, K. M. and Terry, R. J.,** Immunodepression and the course of infection of a chronic *Trypanosoma brucei* infection in mice, *Parasite Immunol.,* 1, 317, 1979.
65. **Inverso, J. A. and Mansfield, J. M.,** Genetics of resistance to the African trypanosomes. II. Differences in virulence associated with VSSA expression among clones of *Trypanosoma rhodesiense, J. Immunol.,* 130, 412, 1983.
66. **MacAskill, J. A., Holmes, P. H., Jennings, F. W., and Urquhart, G. M.,** Immunological clearance of ^{75}Se-labelled *Trypanosoma brucei* in mice. III. Studies in animals with acute infections, *Immunology,* 43, 691, 1981.
67. **Gasbarre, L. C., Hug, K., and Louis, J. A.,** Murine T lymphocyte specificity for African trypanosomes. I. Induction of a T lymphocyte dependent proliferative response to *Trypanosoma brucei, Clin. Exp. Immunol.,* 41, 97, 1980.
68. **Gasbarre, L. C., Hug, K., and Louis, J.,** Murine T-lymphocyte specificity for African trypanosomes. II. Suppression of the T-lymphocyte proliferative response to *Trypanosoma brucei* by systemic trypanosome infection, *Clin. Exp. Immunol.,* 45, 165, 1981.
69. **Tizard, I. R. and Soltys, M. A.,** Cell-mediated hypersensitivity in rabbits infected with *Trypanosoma brucei* and *Trypanosoma rhodesiense, Infect. Immun.,* 4, 674, 1971.
70. **Finerty, J. F., Krehl, E. P., and McKelvin, R. L.,** Delayed type hypersensitivity in mice immunised with *Trypanosoma rhodesiense* antigens, *Infect. Immun.,* 20, 464, 1978.
71. **Clayton, C. E., Ogilvie, B. M., and Askonas, B. A.,** *Trypanosoma brucei* infection in nude mice: B-lymphocyte function is suppressed in the absence of T-lymphocytes, *Parasite Immunol.,* 1, 39, 1979.
72. **Grosskinsky, C. M., Ezekowitz, R. A. B., Berton, G., Gordon, S., and Askonas, B. A.,** Macrophage activation in murine African trypanosomiasis, *Infect. Immun.,* in press.
73. **Mansfield, J. M. and Wallace, J. H.,** Suppression of cell-mediated immunity in experimental African trypanosomiasis, *Infect. Immun.,* 10, 335, 1974.
74. **Urquhart, G. M., Murray, M., Murray, P. K., Jennings, F. W., and Bate, E.,** Immunosuppression in *Trypanosoma brucei* in rats and mice, *Trans. Soc. Trop. Med. Hyg.,* 67, 528, 1973.
75. **Moulton, J. E. and Coleman, J. L.,** Immunosuppression in deer mice with experimentally induced trypanosomiasis, *Am. J. Vet. Res.,* 38, 573, 1977.
76. **Jayawardena, A. N. and Waksman, B. H.,** Suppressor cells in experimental trypanosomiasis, *Nature (London),* 265, 539, 1977.
77. **Pearson, T. W., Roelants, G. E., Lundin, L. B., and Mayor-Withey, K. S.,** Immune depression in trypanosome-infected mice. I. Depressed T-lymphocyte responses, *Eur. J. Immunol.,* 8, 723, 1978.
78. **Mansfield, J. M., Wellhausen, S. R., and Bagasra, O.,** Loss of cytotoxic T-cell function in African trypanosomiasis, *Fed. Proc., Fed. Am. Soc. Exp.,* 39, 1053, 1980.
79. **Selkirk, M. E., Ogilvie, B. M., and Platts-Mills, T. A. E.,** Activation of human peripheral blood lymphocytes by a trypanosome derived mitogen, *Clin. Exp. Immunol.,* 45, 615, 1981.
80. **Selkirk, M. E., Wilkins, S. R., Ogilvie, B. M., and Platts-Mills, T. A. E.,** *In vitro* induction of human helper T-cell activity by *Trypanosoma brucei, Clin. Exp. Immunol.,* in press.

81. **Wellhausen, S. R. and Mansfield, J. M.,** Lymphocyte function in experimental African trypanosomiasis. II. Splenic suppressor cell activity, *J. Immunol.,* 122, 818, 1979.

82. **Jayawardena, A. N., Waksman, B. H., and Eardley, D. D.,** Activation of distinct helper and suppressor T-cells in experimental trypanosomiasis, *J. Immunol.,* 121, 622, 1978.

83. **Pearson, T. W., Roelants, G. E., Pinder, M., Lundin, L. B., and Mayor-Withey, K. S.,** Immune depression in trypanosome-infected mice. III. Suppressor cells, *Eur. J. Immunol.,* 9, 200, 1979.

84. **Unanue, E. R.,** The regulatory role of macrophages in antigenic stimulation. II. Symbiotic relationship between lymphocytes and macrophages, *Adv. Immunol.,* 31, 1, 1981.

85. **Nathan, C. F., Murray, H. W., and Cohn, Z. A.,** The macrophage as an effector cell, *N. Engl. J. Med.,* 303, 622, 1980.

86. **Takayanagi, T., Nakatake, Y., and Enriquez, G. L.,** Attachment and ingestion of *Trypanosoma gambiense* to the rat macrophage by specific antiserum, *J. Parasitol.,* 60, 336, 1974.

87. **Stevens, D. R. and Moulton, J. E.,** Ultrastructural and immunological aspects of the phagocytosis of *Trypanosoma brucei, Infect. Immun.,* 19, 972, 1978.

88. **Holmes, P. H., MacAskill, J. A., Whitelaw, D. P., Jennings, F. W., and Urquhart, G. M.,** Immunological clearance of Se[75]-labelled *Trypanosoma brucei* in mice. I. Aspects of the radiolabelling technique, *Immunology,* 36, 415, 1979.

89. **MacAskill, J. A., Holmes, P. H., Whitelaw, D. D., McConnell, I., Jennings, F. W., and Urquhart, G. M.,** Immunological clearance of ^{75}Se-labelled *Trypanosoma brucei* in mice. II. Mechanisms in immune animals, *Immunology,* 40, 629, 1980.

90. **Shirazi, M. F., Holman, M., Hudson, K., Klaus, G. G. B., and Terry, R. J.,** Complement (C3) levels and the effect of C3 depletion in infections of *Trypanosoma brucei* in mice, *Parasite Immunol.,* 2, 155, 1980.

91. **Ezekovitz, R. A. B., Austyn, J., Stahl, P. D., and Gordon, S.,** Surface properties of *Bacillus Calmette Guerin*-activated mouse macrophages, *J. Exp. Med.,* 154, 60, 1981.

92. **Fierer, J. and Askonas, B. A.,** *Trypanosoma brucei* infection stimulates receptor mediated phagocytosis by murine peritoneal macrophages, *Infect. Immun.,* 37, 1282, 1982.

93. **Bagasra, O., Schell, R. F., and LeFrock, J. L.,** Evidence for depletion of Ia[+] macrophages and associated immunosuppression in African trypanosomiasis, *Infect. Immun.,* 32, 188, 1981.

94. **Steeg, P. S., Moore, R. M., Johnson, H. H., and Oppenheim, J. J.,** Regulation of murine macrophage Ia antigen expression by a lymphokine with immune interferon activity, *J. Exp. Med.,* 156, 1780, 1982.

95. **Yoshie, O., Mellman, I. S., Broeze, R. J., Garcia-Blanco, M., and Lengyel, P.,** Interferon action: effects of mouse α and β interferons on rosette formation, phagocytosis and surface-antigen expression of cells of the macrophage-type line. RAW 309 Cr.1, *Cell. Immunol.,* 73, 128, 1982.

96. **Fierer, J., Salmon, J. A., and Askonas, B. A.,** African trypanosomiasis alters prostaglandin production by murine peritoneal macrophages, *J. Immunol.,* in press.

97. **Bray, M. A.,** Prostaglandins: fine tuning the immune system, *Immunol. Today,* 1, 65, 1980.

98. **Snyder, D. S., Beller, D. I., and Unanue, E. R.,** Prostaglandins modulate macrophage Ia expression, *Nature (London),* 299, 163, 1982.

99. **Unanue, E. R., Kiely, J.-M., and Calderon, J.,** The modulation of lymphocyte functions by molecules secreted by macrophages. II. Conditions leading to increased secretion, *J. Exp. Med.,* 144, 155, 1976.

100. **Meltzer, M. S. and Oppenheim, J. J.,** Bidirectional amplification of macrophage-lymphocyte interactions: enhanced lymphocyte activation factor production by activated adherent mouse peritoneal cells, *J. Immunol.,* 118, 77, 1977.

101. **Wyler, D. J., Oppenheim, J. J., and Koontz, L. C.,** Influence of malaria infection on the elaboration of soluble mediators by adherent mononuclear cells, *Infect. Immun.,* 24, 151, 1979.

102. **Mansfield, J. M., Levine, R. F., Dempsey, W. L., Wellhausen S. R., and Hansen, C. T.,** Lymphocyte function in experimental African trypanosomiasis. IV. Immunosuppression and suppressor cells in the athymic nu/nu mouse, *Cell. Immunol.,* 63, 210, 1981.

103. **Wellhausen, S. R. and Mansfield, J. M.,** Characteristics of the splenic suppressor cell-target cell interaction in experimental African trypanosomiasis, *Cell. Immunol.,* 54, 414, 1980.

104. **Grosskinsky, C. M. and Askonas, B. A.,** Macrophages as primary target cells and mediators of immune dysfunction in African trypanosomiasis, *Infect. Immun.,* 33, 149, 1981.

105. **Albright, J. W. and Albright, J. F.,** Inhibition of murine humoral responses by substances derived from trypanosomes, *J. Immunol.,* 126, 300, 1981.

106. **Roubin, R., Kennard, J., Foley, D., Zolla-Pazner, S.,** Markers of macrophage heterogeneity: altered frequency of macrophage subpopulations after various pathologic stimuli, *J. Retic. Soc.,* 29, 423, 1981.

107. **Nogueira, N. Gordon, S. J., and Cohn, Z.,** *Trypanosoma cruzi:* modification of macrophage function during infection, *J. Exp. Med.,* 146, 157, 1977.

108. **Murray, H. W. and Cohn, Z. A.,** Macrophage oxygen-dependent antimicrobial activity. III. Enhanced oxidative metabolism as an expression of macrophage activation, *J. Exp. Med.,* 152, 1596, 1980.

109. **Diamantstein, T., Keppler, W., Blitstein-Willinger, E., and Ben Efraim, S.,** Suppression of the primary immune response in vivo to sheep red blood cells by B cell mitogens, *Immunology,* 30, 401, 1976.

110. **Isaacs, A. and Lindenmann, J.,** Virus interference. I. The interferon, *Proc. R. Soc. London, Ser. B,* 147, 258, 1957.

111. **Finter, N. B.,** *Interferons and Interferon Inducers,* 2nd ed., Perkins, F. T. and Regamy, R. H., Eds., North-Holland, Amsterdam, 1973.

112. **Pestka, S.,** The interferons, in *Methods in Enzymology,* 78, Part A, 1981.

113. **Rytel, M. W. and Jones, T. C.,** Induction of interferon in mice infected with *Toxoplasma gondii, Proc. Soc. Exp. Biol. Med.,* 123, 859, 1966.

114. **Freshman, M. M., Merigan, T. C., Remington, J. S., and Brownlee, I. E.,** *In vitro* and *in vivo* antiviral action of an interferon-like substance induced by *Toxoplasma gondii, Proc. Soc. Exp. Biol. Med.,* 123, 862, 1966.

115. **Huang, K.-Y., Schultz, W. W., and Gordon, F. B.,** Interferon induced by *Plasmodium berghei, Science,* 162, 123, 1968.

116. **Sonnenfeld, G. and Kierzenbaum, F.,** Increased serum levels of an interferon-like activity during the acute period of experimental infection with different strains of *Trypanosoma cruzi, Am. J. Trop. Med. Hyg.,* 30, 1189, 1981.

117. **Martinotti, M. G., Forni, M., Del Monte, A. M., Giovarelli, M., Forni, G., and Landolfo, A.,** Immunedepression in *Trypanosoma brucei brucei* infected mice. Sequential histological and immunological findings, *Boll. Ist. Sieroter. Milan.,* 60, 288, 1981.

118. **Bancroft, G. J., Sutton, C. J., Morris, A. G., and Askonas, B. A.,** Production of interferons during experimental African trypanosomiasis, *Clin. Exp. Immunol.,* in press.

119. **Talas, M. and Glaz, E. T.,** Type I interferon induced by infection with *Trypanosoma equiperdum, J. Infect. Dis.,* 139, 595, 1979.

120. **Marcucci, F., Walker, M., Kirchner, H., and Krammer, P.,** Production of murine interferon by T cell clones from long term cultures, *Nature (London),* 291, 79, 1981.

121. **Clayton, C. E., Sacks, D. L., Ogilvie, B. M., and Askonas, B. A.,** Membrane fractions of trypanosomes mimic the immunosuppressive and mitogenic effects of living parasites on the host, *Parasite Immunol.,* 1, 241, 1979.

122. **Jahiel, R. I., Vilcek, J., and Nussenzweig, R. S.,** Exogenous interferon protects mice against *Plasmodium berghei* malaria, *Nature (London),* 227, 1350, 1970.

123. **Wyler, D. J., Liang, C. F., Downey, E., and Krim, M.,** Exogenous interferon administration in experimental leishmaniasis: *in vivo* and *in vitro* studies,

124. **Herman, R. and Baron, S.,** Immunologic mediated protection of *T. congolense* infected mice by polyribonucleotides, *J. Protozool.,* 18, 661, 1971.

125. **Glaz, E. T.,** Effect of low molecular weight inteferon inducers on *Trypanosoma equiperdum* infection of mice, *Ann. Trop. Med. Parasitol.,* 73, 83, 1979.

126. **Herberman, R. B. and Holden, H. T.,** Natural cell mediated immunity, *Adv. Cancer Res.,* 27, 305, 1978.

127. **Herberman R. B. and Ortaldo, J. R.,** Natural killer cells: their role in defences against disease, *Science,* 214, 24, 1981.

128. **Eugui, E. M. and Allison, A. C.,** Differences in susceptibility of various mouse strains to haemoprotozoan infections: possible correlation with natural killer activity, *Parasite Immunol.,* 2, 277, 1980.

129. **Ruebush, M. J., Hale, A. H., and McKinnon, K. P.,** *Proc. Am. Soc. Trop. Med. Hyg.,* in press.

130. **Kamiyama, T. and Hagiwara, T.,** Augmented followed by suppressed levels of natural cell mediated cytotoxicity in mice infected with *Toxoplasma gondii, Infect. Immun.,* 36, 628, 1982.

131. **Hunter, K. W., Jr., Folks, T. M., Sayles, P. C., and Strickland, G. C.,** Early enhancement followed by suppression of natural killer cell activity during murine malaria infections, *Immunol. Lett.,* 2, 209, 1981.

132. **Hatcher, F. M., Kuhn, R. E., Cerrone, M. C., and Burton, R. C.,** Increased natural killer cell activity in experimental American trypanosomiasis, *J. Immunol.,* 127, 1126, 1981.

133. **Hochmann, P. S., Cudkowicz, G., and Evans, P. D.,** Carrageenan-induced decline of natural killer activity. II. Inhibition of cytolysis by non-T, Ia negative suppressor cells activated *in vivo, Cell. Immunol.,* 61, 200, 1981.

134. **Tizard, I., Nielsen, K. H., Seed, J. R., and Hall, J. E.,** Biologically active products from African trypanosomes, *Microbiol. Rev.,* 42, 661, 1978.

135. **Capron, A. and Camus, D.,** Immunoregulation by parasite extracts, *Springer Semin. Immunopathol.,* 2, 69, 1979.

136. **Cunningham, D. S. and Kuhn, R. E.,** *Trypanosoma cruzi*-induced suppressor substance. I. Cellular involvement and partial characterization, *J. Immunol.,* 124, 2122, 1980.

137. **Khansari, N., Segre, M., and Segre, D.,** Immunosuppression in murine malaria: a soluble immunosuppressive factor derived from *Plasmodium berghei* infected blood, *J. Immunol.,* 127, 1889, 1981.

138. **Miller, H. C. and Esselman, W. J.,** Modulation of the immune response by antigen-reactive lymphocytes after cultivation with gangliosides, *J. Immunol.,* 115, 839, 1975.

139. **Ryan, J. and Shinitzky, M.,** Possible role for glycosphingolipids in the control of immune responses, *Eur. J. Immunol.,* 9, 171, 1979.

140. **Assoku, R. J. and Tizard, I. R.,** Mitogenicity of autolysates of *Trypanosoma congolense, Experientia,* 34, 127, 1978.

141. **Assoku, R. K. G., Hazlett, C. A., and Tizard, I.,** Immunosuppression in experimental African trypanosomiasis: polyclonal B-cell activation and mitogenicity of trypanosome derived saturated fatty acids, *Int. Arch. Allergy Appl. Immunol.,* 59, 298, 1979.

142. **Greenwood, B. M.,** Possible role of B cell mitogen in hypergammaglobulinaemia in malaria and trypanosomiasis, *Lancet,* 1, 435, 1974.

143. **Esuruoso, G. O.,** The demonstration *in vitro* of the mitogenic effects of trypanosomal antigen on the spleen cells of normal, athymic and cyclophosphamide treated mice, *Clin. Exp. Immunol.,* 23, 314, 1976.

144. **Mansfield, J. M., Craig, S. A., and Stelzer, G. T.,** Lymphocyte function in experimental African trypanosomiasis: mitogenic effects of trypanosome extracts *in vitro, Infect. Immun.,* 14, 976, 1976.

145. **Moulton, J. E. and Coleman, J. L.,** A soluble immunosuppressor substance in spleen in deer mice infected with *Trypanosoma brucei, Am. J. Vet. Res.,* 40, 1131, 1979.

146. **Ilemobade, A. A., Adegboye, D. S., Onovirau, O., and Chima, J. C.,** Immunodepressive effects of trypanosomal infection in cattle immunized against contagious bovine pleuropneumonia, *Parasite Immunol.,* 4, 273, 1982.

147. **Greenwood, B. M.,** Immunosuppression in malaria and trypanosomiasis, in *Parasites in the Immunized Host: Mechanisms of Survival,* Porter, R. and Knight, J., Eds., Ciba Foundation Symp. 25 (New Series), Associated Scientific Publishers, Amsterdam, 1974, 137.

148. **Calderon, R. A. and Thomas, D. B.,** *In vivo* cyclic change in B lymphocyte susceptibility to T-cell control, *Nature (London),* 285, 662, 1980.

149. **Clarke, I. A., Virelizier, J.-L., Carswell, E. A., and Wood, P. R.,** Possible importance of macrophage-derived mediators in acute malaria, *Infect. Immun.,* 32, 1058, 1981.

150. **Marshall-Clarke, S. and Playfair, J.H. L.,** B cells: subpopulations, tolerance, autoimmunity and infection, *Immun. Rev.,* 43, 109, 1979.

151. **Askonas, B. A.,** unpublished observations.

152. **Beer, S.,** to be published.

153. **Bancroft, G. J. and Vessey, A. E.,** to be published.

154. **Bancroft, G. J.,** unpublished results.

155. **Corsini, A. C.,** unpublished results.

156. **Selkirk, M. E., Ogilvie, B. M., and Platts-Mills, T. A.,** Activation of human peripheral blood lymphocytes by a trypanosome-derived mitogen, *Clin. Exp. Immunol.,* 45, 615, 1981.

Chapter 6

IMMUNE RESPONSES OF CATTLE TO AFRICAN TRYPANOSOMES

W. Ivan Morrison, Max Murray, and George W. O. Akol

TABLE OF CONTENTS

I. INTRODUCTION

Tsetse flies harboring trypanosomes pathogenic for domestic animals are found over 37% of the African continent. Despite attempts to control animal trypanosomiasis by strategic use of trypanocidal drugs and by application of insecticides to kill the tsetse, the disease remains as the most important constraint to livestock production in infested areas. The main trypanosome species involved, *Trypanosoma congolense*, *T. vivax*, and *T. brucei*, are extremely ubiquitous. This is due in part to the widespread presence of suitable insect vectors. Thus, cyclical development of trypanosomes can occur in a number of different species of tsetse, each of which is adapted to different climatic conditions and vegetation.[1] Furthermore, the trypanosomes are capable of infecting not only most domestic animal species but also many species of wildlife.[2,3] The latter usually do not suffer from severe clinical disease but become carriers and, thus, constitute an important reservoir of infection.

The success of the trypanosome as a pathogen is to a large extent due to its ability to undergo antigenic variation, thus enabling it to evade host immune responses and establish persistent infections.[4-6] Added to the complexity of multiple variable antigen types (VATs) expressed during a single infection, there is also an unknown number of different strains or serodemes of each trypanosome species, each strain being capable of elaborating a different repertoire of VATs.[7] However, despite the apparent advantages which the trypanosome holds over its mammalian hosts in certain animals, notably wild Bovidae, a stable relationship is achieved whereby a low level of infection is established with minimal deleterious effects on the host.[3] This would indicate that such animals may have evolved responses which are effective at limiting the level of parasitosis. By contrast, cattle, most of which have not been under the selective pressure of trypanosome challenge, develop higher levels of parasitosis and suffer a severe clinical disease often resulting in death.[8] However, certain animals, particularly those belonging to the trypanotolerant breeds, manage to survive and recover from the infection.[7]

The purpose of this article is to review the current state of knowledge on the responses of cattle to infection with the African trypanosomes, with particular reference to specific antitrypanosome immune responses. It is not our intention to present a comprehensive historical analysis of the subject as this has been covered adequately in a previous review.[9] Rather, we wish to present relevant recent findings and ideas on the subject. Although emphasis is placed on studies in cattle, investigations in other animals which corroborate or extend the findings in cattle are also considered.

II. DISEASES PRODUCED IN CATTLE BY TRYPANOSOME INFECTIONS

Before embarking on a discussion of immune responses, it is worth considering briefly the disease syndromes produced by trypanosome infections in cattle. Because of the complexity of the situation in the field where animals are usually exposed over prolonged periods to challenge with a number of different serodemes of each of the trypanosome species, it is extremely difficult to obtain a clear picture of the clinical progression of a particular infection. Such information can more readily be obtained from the study of single experimental infections.

Based on observations of both field and experimental infections we consider that there are three main types of disease syndrome in cattle associated with trypanosome infections.

A. Anemia and Wasting or Poor Growth

The first of these and by far the most common manifestation of trypanosome infections is characterized by progressive anemia with persistent fluctuating parasitemia.[8,10] All of the three common trypanosome species can produce this disease syndrome.

Usually there is a progressive decrease in the packed red blood cell volume (PCV) to levels around 20% over the first 4 to 6 weeks of the infection. At this stage, the PCV may continue to decrease until death of the animal occurs. In other instances the PCV stabilizes and is maintained at a low level for a variable period of time. Some of these animals may eventually die. In others, after a variable length of time, parasitemia gradually disappears, the PCV rises, and the animals recover. Thus, anemia as measured by the PCV is a reliable marker for the severity of the disease.

In general, the degree of anemia correlates with the level and duration of the parasitemia which, in turn, are dependent on the species and particular serodeme of trypanosome involved. We have observed marked variation in virulence among the different serodemes of *T. congolense* which we have studied. Thus, some serodemes produce fluctuating parasitemia for about 6 to 8 weeks followed by gradually diminishing levels of parasitemia and recovery of the majority of cattle. At the other extreme, certain serodemes result in more sustained parasitemia which may persist for 6 to 8 months. The majority of these cattle die at varying times during the infection but a few animals manage to survive to the stage when parasitemia starts to diminish, and thereafter their hematological values slowly return to normal.

B. Hemorrhagic Disease

Infection with certain isolates of *T. vivax* can produce an acute hemorrhagic syndrome usually resulting in death 2 to 4 weeks after infection.[11,12] This is characterized by fever, sustained high levels of parasitemia, and often blood-stained diarrhea. At necropsy, there are diffuse petechial or ecchymotic hemorrhages on the visceral surfaces and usually massive hemorrhage into the alimentary tract. The hemorrhagic nature of the disease is thought to be due to defective clotting as a consequence of thrombocytopenia.[13]

C. Meningoencephalitis

In addition to causing anemia, certain serodemes of *T. brucei* also give rise to a disease characterized by clinical abnormalities of the central nervous system (CNS).[14,15] This syndrome may occur either during the period of patent parasitemia or at a later stage following the disappearance of parasites from the blood. In both instances trypanosomes are present in the cerebrospinal fluid and the nervous symptoms are attributable to a diffuse meningoencephalitis similar to that found in cases of human trypanosomiasis. A similar disease may also develop in cattle infected with *T. brucei* at varying periods after treatment with the trypanocidal drug Berenil (Hoechst, West Germany).[15] This appears to be associated with the persistence of trypanosomes in the CNS after treatment. The disease can be induced more readily with certain serodemes of *T. brucei* than with others and only a percentage of animals infected with any one of these serodemes develop the disease. Indeed, in the studies which we carried out,[15] all of the *T. brucei* serodemes involved had been isolated from areas of endemic human trypanosomiasis. This is of particular interest since the closely related human pathogen *T. rhodesiense* is infective for cattle and has been shown to produce a very similar CNS disease syndrome in cattle.[16] The question, therefore, arises whether some of these putative *T. brucei* populations are in reality *T. rhodesiense*. We have obtained some support for this idea in our studies;[15] we found in one animal, which developed CNS disease, a population of trypanosomes which was resistant to lysis by human serum, in the blood incubation infectivity test (BIIT), despite the fact that the population (GUTat 3.1) used to infect the animal was sensitive to human serum.

III. GENERAL CONSIDERATION OF BOVINE IMMUNE RESPONSES TO TRYPANOSOMES

From the foregoing outline of the diseases produced by trypanosome infections in cattle, it is apparent that in many cattle infected with a single trypanosome serodeme are able to exert sufficient control over the infection to enable them to eliminate the parasite and recover. However, these animals often undergo a phase of illness during which there is marked loss of productivity, and there is little doubt that under field conditions where they would be required to forage for themselves and would be exposed to much harsher environmental conditions many more animals would succumb to the infections. Nevertheless, the ability of cattle to recover from infection indicates that the mechanisms by which they control the infection can be relatively effective. This is in contrast to the situation in laboratory animals in which experimental trypanosome infections very often have a lethal outcome.[17] Further-more, there is evidence that within the cattle population as a whole there are certain indigenous African breeds which have a greater capacity to control the level and duration of parasitemia and, thus, survive the infection.[3] These cattle, the best example of which is the N'Dama breed, are confined mainly to West and Central Africa and it is considered that they have achieved their more resistant status as a result of natural selection in trypanosomiasis endemic areas. The term trypanotolerance is used to describe this innate characteristic.

There is a large body of evidence that immunity to trypanosome challenge is mediated by antibody responses against the variable surface glycoprotein (VSG).[9] However, because of antigenic variation, complete immunity can only be achieved against the VATs which form a major component of the population of trypanosomes used for immunization. It is also believed that once trypanosome infections become established antibody responses are important in controlling the infections. However, from recent findings it appears likely that other host responses may influence the growth of the parasite. For this reason we will discuss separately responses mediating protective immunity and those which modulate established infections.

IV. ACQUISITION OF PROTECTIVE IMMUNITY

A. Immunity to Bloodstream Trypanosomes

1. Induction of Immunity to Bloodstream Forms

Over the years numerous studies have demonstrated that protective immunity can be induced in cattle against specific populations of bloodstream trypanosomes. The most com-monly used methods for induction of immunity have been establishment of infection followed by treatment with trypanocidal drugs and inoculation of irradiated noninfective trypanosomes.

In several early studies with trypanocidal drugs in the field it was claimed that animals which had been treated were immune or partially immune to reinfection.[18-21] Subsequent experimental studies demonstrated that cattle could be rendered immune to homologous challenge by a brief period of infection followed by trypanocidal treatment. In 1968, Cunningham[22] reported that three of four cattle which had been infected from a *T. brucei* stabilate and treated with Berenil were fully immune when challenged with the same stabilate 2 to 3 months after treatment. In a similar experiment with *T. congolense,* Wilson[23] infected five cattle with stabilated organisms on two occasions at an interval of 11 weeks. On each occasion the animals were treated with Berenil 3 weeks after infection. When challenged with stabilate after a further 11 weeks, all five cattle were immune, although on subsequent challenge within the next few months three of the five animals became infected. In a study carried out by Wellde and colleagues,[24] nine cattle which were treated with Berenil at varying periods of 5 to 28 weeks after infection were challenged at intervals of 28 to 128 weeks after treatment; all animals became infected although in most instances there was a prolonged prepatent period and five of the nine cattle self-cured the ensuing infection. By contrast, in the same study five cattle which had self-cured a primary infection with *T. congolense* after periods of 30 to 61 weeks of infection were fully immune when challenged with the same stock of *T. congolense* 25 to 54 weeks after parasitemia had disappeared.

Initial studies with irradiated trypanosomes in cattle indicated that very large numbers of organisms were required to induce immunity. Thus, Duxbury et al.[25] were not successful in immunizing cattle against *T. congolense* by giving four to seven weekly doses of irradiated trypanosomes ranging from 10^8 to 10^9 organisms. The animals were challenged with 10^4 or 10^5 trypanosomes and the only effect was an increase of about 3 days in prepatent period. A similar result was obtained with *T. brucei* in a small experiment involving three cattle.[26] However, in further studies with *T. rhodesiense* the same group of workers were able to induce complete immunity in five cattle given six weekly i.v. inoculations of irradiated trypanosomes totaling from 3.5 to 6×10^{10} and challenged 1 week later.[27] The same animals were still completely immune when challenged again 8 months later.

At face value, these results would indicate that trypanosomes are not particularly immunogenic and that complete immunity against challenge with the homologous trypanosome populations is not readily achieved. However, a major flaw in all of these studies is the fact that they utilized uncharacterized stocks of trypanosomes. We have conducted a series of experiments in which we have examined the immunogenicity of either irradiated trypanosomes or purified VSG from a well-defined clone of *T. brucei* (ILT at 1.3).[28] By using hyperimmune serum to the purified ILT at 1.3 VSG in a neutralization assay, the population of trypanosomes used in these studies was shown to be antigenically homogeneous to a level of 10^4 organisms. It was found that a single inoculum of as few as 10^7 irradiated trypanosomes administered intravenously into cattle conferred complete protection against challenge with 10^3 trypanosomes 14 days later. Furthermore, in animals which received 10^6 irradiated organisms, there was a delay in the onset of parasitemia after challenge as compared to controls. Confirmation that such immunity was mediated by antibodies to the VSG was obtained by immunizing cattle with purified VSG. Although 200 μg of VSG, when administered on its own, failed to immunize, the same amount of antigen when incorporated in several different adjuvants resulted in immunity against challenge with 10^4 trypanosomes.[28,29]

2. The Role of Antibody

It is generally assumed, by extrapolation from results obtained in laboratory animals, that the immunity induced in cattle is mediated by antibody. In mice, immunity can be transferred passively with serum from immunized animals.[30-33] Adoptive transfer of spleen cells from immunized mice has also been shown to confer immunity.[33-35] Similar immunity can be attained by transfer of a B cell-enriched fraction of spleen cells but not with a T cell-enriched fraction.[33,35] Furthermore, congenitally athymic nude mice can readily be immunized with irradiated trypanosomes or by infection and treatment,[36] although it has been shown that nude mice infected with *T. congolense* generate a population of Thy 1[+] lymphocytes in their spleens.[37] On the other hand, mice rendered B cell-deficient by treatment from birth with anti-μ serum were highly susceptible to infection and could not be immunized with irradiated organisms.[38]

In cattle there are major difficulties in carrying out passive or adoptive transfer experiments. However, we have found a strong correlation between protection and the levels of neutralizing antibody.[28,29] As few as 10^6 irradiated trypanosomes inoculated intravenously into cattle elicited detectable neutralizing antibody and the levels of antibody increased with higher doses of trypanosomes. Of interest was the finding that inoculation of trypanosomes either subcutaneously or intradermally resulted in significantly lower levels of antibody than obtained by the intravenous route.

By comparison with intact trypanosomes, purified VSG was much less immunogenic, although the immunity could be potentiated by the use of adjuvants. Based on the size of the VSG molecule and the surface area of the trypanosome, Cross[39] estimated that 10^9 trypanosomes contained about 750 μg of VSG. The dose of 200 μg used in our studies to immunize cattle would, therefore, be equivalent to about 2.5×10^8 trypanosomes. This produced a scarcely detectable antibody response and no protection.

Table 1
THE IMMUNE RESPONSE OF PAIRS OF CATTLE TO DIFFERENT DOSES OF IRRADIATED *T. BRUCEI* OR PURIFIED VSG WITH AND WITHOUT ADJUVANT

	VSG equivalent[b] (μg)	Antibody titers[c]		Protection against homologous challenge
		Farr assay	Neutralization	
Immunization with irradiated trypanosomes[a]				
10^9	750	1.78	10^4	Yes
10^8	75	0.75	10^2	Yes
10^7	7.5	0.95	10^2	Yes
Immunization with VSG	200	0.39	—	No
	200 in adjuvant[d]	1.89	10^1	Yes

[a] Trypanosomes were subjected to 60,000 rads of γ-irradiation and inoculated intravenously.

[b] Calculation of the equivalent amounts of VSG in different numbers of intact trypanosomes was based on bindings of Cross.[39]

[c] The titers of antibody in the Farr assay are expressed as $\log^{10}$ antigen binding capacity (ABC). Titers for preinoculation sera were <0.2. The titers of neutralizing antibodies are expressed as the reciprocal of the highest dilution of serum which gave complete neutralization.

[d] Purified VSG was emulsified in an equal volume of incomplete Freund's adjuvant and inoculated intramuscularly.

By preabsorbing sera with either viable bloodstream trypanosomes or uncoated procyclic forms prior to testing for antibody in the solid phase radioimmunoassay, it was possible to obtain information on the specificity of the antibody elicited by the different immunization procedures.[28] The results suggested that most of the antibody induced by irradiated trypanosomes was directed against VSG determinants on the surface of live trypanosomes. We did not detect any significant antibody response to uncoated trypanosomes nor did the uncoated organisms remove any of the antibody activity to whole ILT at 1.3 trypanosomes. The antibody induced by immunization with VSG in adjuvant was found to differ in specificity from that produced by intact trypanosomes. Thus, a substantial proportion of the antibody elicited by VSG was directed against determinants on the molecule which are not accessible on live trypanosomes and, therefore, are probably not important in protective immunity. A comparison of the neutralizing activity of the different sera with levels of antibody detected in the Farr assay (utilizing purified VSG) also provided evidence to support this suggestion. Although similar titers of antibody to VSG were detected in sera from animals given VSG in adjuvant and those which received 10^9 irradiated trypanosomes, the former only exhibited neutralizing activity for trypanosomes to a dilution of 10^{-1}, whereas the latter neutralized to a dilution of 10^{-4} (Table 1).

The level, specificity, and class of the antibody elicited by irradiated trypanosomes were found to be very similar to those of the antibody produced during infection with *T. brucei*.[28] In both instances, the antibody consisted of a mixture of IgM and IgG and was specific mainly for determinants on the surface of live trypanosomes. There was also no detectable response to uncoated trypanosomes during the first 14 days of infection, although more prolonged infection was found to result in detectable antibody to uncoated forms.[40] These findings indicate that immunological recognition of the VSG occurs mainly at the level of the intact trypanosome rather than the released soluble VSG. Evidence for this has also been obtained in mice.[41]

The detection of both IgM and IgG classes of antibody agrees with observations by Luckins in cattle infected with *T. congolense*[42] and by Musoke et al.[43] in cattle infected with *T. brucei*. In both of these studies evidence was presented that IgM antibody was much more effective than IgG at neutralizing trypanosome infectivity, although Musoke et al.[43] found that in animals which exhibited second peak of antibody to the infecting VAT, the IgG was as effective as IgM at neutralizing infectivity. Based on these observations, Musoke et al.[43] concluded that during the initial antibody response the IgG antibody was of low avidity.

The mechanism by which VSG-specific antibody eliminates the parasite in vivo in cattle has not been studied. It is well established that anti-VSG antibody can operate against the trypanosome in vitro either by inducing complement-mediated lysis[44] or by interaction with macrophages to effect phagocytosis.[45] In specifically immunized mice inoculated with radio-labeled trypanosomes, it was found that the organisms were rapidly cleared from the circulation and taken up by the mononuclear phagocytic system.[46] Furthermore, in passively immunized mice depleted of C3 by treatment with cobra venom factor, there was marked impairment of clearance of trypanosomes from the circulation.[46] By contrast, Shirazi et al.[47] found that mice depleted of C3 during the first 3 weeks of infection with *T. brucei* showed little difference in parasitemia as compared to nondepleted mice, suggesting that C3 was not required for elimination of the parasite.

Because of the problem of antigenic variation, efforts have been made to identify common antigenic determinants on different VSG molecules which might be used to induce cross-protective immunity. Barbet and McGuire[48] were able to show that antisera raised against purified VSG recognized a determinant on the molecule which was common between all VSGs studied, including those from different serodemes and different trypanosome species. However, this determinant was not exposed on the surface of viable trypanosomes and, therefore, was not accessible to an immune response. More recent studies have shown that some VATs from different serodemes of the *Trypanozoon* subspecies possess cross-reacting determinants which are exposed on the surface of live trypanosomes and are cross-protective.[49,50] These variable antigens, which are referred to as iso-VATs, are not identical, since they have different isoelectric points. It is not known to what extent iso-VATs occur in *T. congolense* or *T. vivax*. In cattle experimentally infected with *T. congolense* or *T. brucei*, secondary peaks of antibody to the infecting VAT have been detected several weeks or months after infection.[5,51] It was not clear whether these responses were induced by recurrence of the infecting VAT or by an iso-VAT within the same serodeme. Support for the latter comes from the recent finding by Barbet et al.[52] that two VATs from the same serodeme of *T. brucei* share some but not all surface-exposed epitopes.

Although non-VSG common trypanosome antigens are known to induce antibody responses in trypanosome-infected cattle,[53] they are thought not to play a role in immunity. However, Shapiro and Murray,[54] using radioimmune precipitation techniques, demonstrated an association between the capacity of cattle to control *T. brucei* infections and their responses to three common protein antigens. Thus, the majority of animals which recovered from the infection produced detectable antibody to at least one of these three molecules, whereas most of the animals which died showed no response. While the significance of this observation remains to be determined, it may be that the detection of antibody to these molecules merely reflects the superior immune responsiveness of cattle undergoing recovery.

3. The Role of Cell-Mediated Immune Responses

Because of the strong evidence that immunity to trypanosome infection is mediated by antibody, little effort has been made to investigate cell-mediated immune responses to the trypanosome. Mansfield and Kreier,[55] working in rabbits infected with *T. congolense*, failed to demonstrate delayed-type hypersensitivity (DTH) reactions following inoculation of ul- trasonicated trypanosome antigen. On the other hand, Tizard and Soltys[56] described DTH responses in rabbits infected with *T. rhodesiense* for periods greater than 30 days, using as antigen sonicated dead trypanosomes which had been killed by leaving in suspension for several days at 4°C. In mice, Finerty[57] described the induction of DTH responses, as evaluated by delayed foot pad swelling, to freeze-thawed antigen prepared from *T. rhodesiense* in animals primed with formalin-fixed trypanosomes. Gasbarre et al.,[58] also working in mice, demonstrated in vitro T cell proliferative responses to live *T. brucei* with lymph node cells from mice immunized with viable trypanosomes emulsified in Freund's complete adjuvant (FCA). In this study, live trypanosomes were required both for priming and in the in vitro proliferative assay.

Emery et al.[59] investigated the development of DTH responses in cattle subjected to various infection and immunization procedures with *T. congolense*. They demonstrated that cattle which had been infected with *T. congolense* and treated with Berenil developed characteristic DTH skin reactions when inoculated intradermally with ultrasonicated *T. congolense* antigen. Moreover, a marked proliferative response was obtained in vitro when peripheral blood leukocytes (PBL) from these animals were cultured in the presence of the ultrasonicated antigen. PBL from cattle immunized with formolized *T. congolense* in FCA exhibited a similar proliferative response in vitro to trypanosome antigen. However, no response was detected in cattle undergoing an active infection with *T. congolense*. In a later study which was carried out to compare the capacity of different adjuvants to potentiate immune responses in cattle to *T. brucei* VSG, it was shown that PBL from cattle immunized with VSG in certain adjuvants exhibited a poliferative response in vitro to sonicated *T. brucei* antigen.[29] This response, which was considered to be characteristic of a DTH reaction, was shown to be specific for the VSG used for immunization. The induction of this DTH response did not occur in animals immunized with VSG alone and was dependent on the particular adjuvant used. Thus, FCA and muramyl dipeptide were particularly potent at stimulating the response, whereas other adjuvants such as *Bordetella pertussis* and saponin induced virtually no response. This was of particular interest because saponin was very effective at boosting antibody responses and inducing protective immunity, indicating that the induction of DTH responses was not requied for protective immunity.

B. Immunity to Metacyclic Trypanosomes

1. The Local Skin Reaction

The first interaction between the trypanosome and its host occurs in the skin following the successful feed of an infected tsetse fly. The metacyclic trypanosomes extruded by the fly establish themselves at this level and proliferate for several days prior to dissemination to the bloodstream.[60,61] Thus, in the first 10 days of infection, trypanosomes can be seen in increasing numbers within collagen bundles, lying in the inflammatory edema which sep- arates and disrupts the collagen fibers, and within dilated lymphatics in the papillary dermis and hypodermis. Thereafter, the numbers decline rapidly.

The presence of proliferating trypanosomes in the skin induces a striking skin reaction, commonly called a chancre (Figure 1). This reaction develops within a few days of a susceptible animal being bitten and reaches maximum dimensions during the second week before declining to nondetectable levels during the third week. The chancre reaction is specific for the trypanosome. No comparable response occurs to bites of uninfected tsetse flies, although animals repeatedly bitten develop distinct skin reactions.[62] However, these lesions are smaller and occur much earlier (i.e., 24 to 72 hr) than the chancre. The size and severity of the chancre depends on the number of trypanosomes which become established[63,64] and the species of trypanosome involved. In cattle, *T. congolense* and *T. brucei* induce local skin reactions which can measure up to 10 cm in diameter; they are red, edematous, hot, and very painful. The reaction produced by *T. vivax* is much smaller, measuring only 2 to

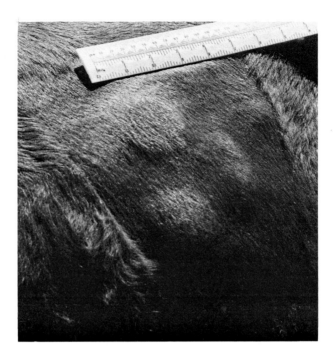

FIGURE 1. Chancre reactions on the flank of a 9-month-old Friesian 10 days after being bitten by tsetse flies infected with *T. congolense*.

3 cm at its maximum, and with some strains of *T. vivax* no detectable reaction develops, although the cattle subsequently become infected. In addition to cattle,[60,61,65-69] chancres have been reported in goats,[70,71] sheep,[68,72] wildlife,[73] and in man.[74] Chancres can also be produced in cattle by inoculation of bloodstream forms of *T. brucei* or *T. vivax*.[69] However, bloodstream forms of *T. congolense* do not induce a reaction[65,69] although they will readily infect cattle when inoculated intradermally. The findings that certain *T. vivax* isolates do not give chancres[75] and that infection with *T. congolense* can be initiated by intravenous inoculation of metacyclics[76] indicate that the local skin reaction is not a prerequisite for establishment of infection with metacyclic trypanosomes. Furthermore, laboratory animals such as mice, rats, and guinea pigs do not develop a chancre but become infected following tsetse challenge.[77] This would appear to be related to skin thickness, as in these species the tsetse probes its proboscis into the subcutaneous tissue.

In cattle, the development of the chancre is accompanied by marked enlargement of the lymph nodes draining the lesion, precedes the onset of parasitemia and fever and, therefore, predicts imminent parasitemia.[61] The composition of the cells within the chancre suggests that the reaction consists of two components, an initial inflammatory reaction followed by an immune response. The early lesion is characterized by severe congestion, exudation of fluid, and marked cellular extravasation. At this time, the cells invoved are mainly neutrophils and small and medium lymphocytes. The degree of neutrophil infiltration varies with the severity of the reaction and is more prominent in reactions produced by *T. brucei* and *T. congolense* than those induced by *T. vivax*. As the reaction reaches its peak, neutrophils disappear and cellular infiltration increases and is dominated by immunological cell types. Lymphocytes are the main cell type present and include numerous proliferating large lymphocytes (Figure 2) and plasma cells. The number of plasma cells increases progressively during the third week as the reaction subsides.

The dynamics of this cellular reaction in cattle are also reflected in the responses in efferent lymph from lymph nodes draining the chancre.[78] By surgical insertion of indwelling cannulae

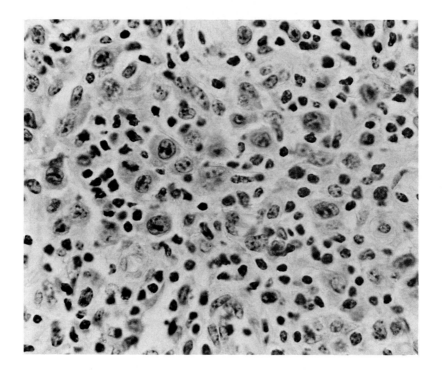

FIGURE 2.   Marked infiltration of large lymphocytes into the papillary dermis of an 18-day chancre reaction. (H & E; magnification × 400.)

into lymphatics, it was possible to monitor continuously the response of drainage lymph nodes in cattle infected with cyclically transmitted *T. congolense*. Trypanosomes were first detected in the lymph as early as 6 to 7 days after infection which was 3 to 5 days before their appearance in the bloodstream. Shortly thereafter there was a marked increase in lymph flow, total cell output, and output of blast cells. The response paralleled the development of the skin reaction and a its peak was associated with an increase in blast cells from normal levels of 1 to 20%, at which time 6% of the cells in the lymph were plasma cells. Similar results have been obtained in goats infected with *T. congolense*, *T. brucei*, or *T. vivax*, although the time intervals between infection and detection of trypanosomes in blood and in lymph and the appearance of the chancre were shorter than in cattle.[78]

The cellular responses in the skin and drainage lymph nodes of cattle infected with *T. congolense* are accompanied by the appearance in the serum, between 14 and 16 days, of antibodies which neutralize the metacyclic trypanosomes.[76] In addition, we have found in cattle cyclically infected with *T. congolense* that leukocytes from peripheral blood or lymph exhibit a marked proliferative response when cultured in vitro with ultrasonicated trypanosome antigen prepared from the first bloodstream population.[79] Moreover, this response, which appears to be T cell mediated, is demonstrable prior to development of the chancre, between 3 and 7 days after infection, but is no longer detectable once the chancre has developed. Thus, there appears to be very rapid sensitization of T cells to trypanosome antigen(s).

While the establishment of infection with metacyclic trypanosomes is not dependent either on inoculation into the skin or on the development of a chancre, it is probable that the skin provides a favorable environment for the growth of metacyclic trypanosomes. Components of skin such as dermal collagen have been found to be important ingredients for in vitro cultivation of metacyclic trypanosomes.[80] Since the skin is also the site of initial interaction between the trypanosome and cells of the immune system, the reaction that develops therein probably plays an important role in induction of immune responses which exert control over the infection. However, whether all of the immunological and inflammatory components of the chancre are to the benefit of the host or whether some of the responses may result in stimulation of trypanosome growth is not yet known.

2. Induction of Immunity to Cyclical Challenge

Cattle primed by infection using tsetse (cyclical) infected with cloned derivates of *T. congolense* and treated with Berenil after 3 or 4 weeks were found to be immune to cyclical challenge from 3 weeks to 6 months later.[62,76] In these animals, localized skin reactions and parasitemia did not develop. On the other hand, cattle primed in the same way but subjected to cyclical challenge with heterologous clones were completely susceptible to infection as demonstrated by the development of chancres followed by parasitemia. Immunity to homologous challenge was achieved irrespective of the bloodstream VATs used to infect the tsetse employed for challenge. These results confirmed the findings of Nantulya et al.,[81] in mice, although in their study mice had to be primed on two occasions with tsetse infected with *T. congolense*. Similar results have been obtained with *T. congolense* in rabbits[82] and in goats.[69] Furthermore, in studies with *T. brucei*, Emery et al.[69] demonstrated that goats were immune to cyclical challenge, providing parasites from the same serodeme were used.

Immunity to cyclical challenge has also been achieved in cattle with uncloned stocks of *T. congolense* providing the same stock was used for challenge, even when the stock was known to consist of more than one serodeme.[62] The use of metacyclic trypanosomes grown in tissue culture for immunization has also been examined. Cattle inoculated intradermally with cultured *T. congolense* metacyclics developed chancres, and when treated 3 weeks later with Berenil were subsquently found to be immune to tsetse challenge with the same serodeme.[83] These results indicated that organisms cultured in vitro are biologically and antigenically similar to metacyclics which develop in the tsetse fly.

In studies with *T. congolense* in cattle, it appeared that protective immunity was effected against the metacyclic population at the level of the skin, as no detectable skin reaction, indicative of trypanosome proliferation, developed at the site of challenge.[62] Similarly, results with *T. brucei* in goats indicated that protection occurred at the level of the skin or at least in the regional lymph node, in that following homologous cyclical challenge immune goats did not develop any chancres nor could trypanosomes be found in the efferent lymph from lymph nodes draining the bite size.[69]

The view that protection is operative against the metacyclic population of *T. congolense* was supported by the findings that the metacyclics were completely neutralized by lymph and serum.[76] Furthermore, the timing of appearance of antibody which completely neutralized the metacyclics (days 14 to 16) coincided with the time at which cattle achieved complete protection to homologous challenge. Thus, while cattle infected with cyclically transmitted *T. congolese* and treated with Berenil on day 15 were completely immune, animals treated on day 5 or on days 10 to 12 were still susceptible, although those treated on days 10 to 12 sometimes showed a delay in chancre development and onset of parasitemia. These results suggest that the chancre must go through its full cycle of development in order for protective immunity to be achieved, since it usually reaches peak reactivity by days 10 to 13 and has started to regress by day 15. However, there was evidence that cattle treated with Berenil on day 5 or days 10 to 12 had been sensitized to the trypanosome, as on challenge a marked necrotizing reaction developed within the chancres. This consisted of a severe necrotizing vasculitis and thrombosis accompanied by infiltration wih large numbers of neutrophils, changes indicative of an Arthus reaction.

The results of experiments on immunization indicate that the antigenic composition of the metacyclic population is constant and characteristic for any one particular serodeme of *T. congolense* and is distinct from that produced by unrelated serodemes. Similar conclusions have been made on the basis of serological studies. Using immunofluorescence and neutralization tests, evidence has been obtained that the antigenic composition of the metacyclic population of *T. congolense* and *T. brucei* is constant for any one serodeme,[84,85] although subsequent studies have shown both for *T. congolense*[86] and *T. brucei*[87-89] that this population consists of an as yet undefined number of VATs. Since, in the case of *T. congolense,* the tsetse extrudes only very small numbers of metacyclics, the time required for development of protective immunity might reflect the time taken for all of the constituent VATs in the metacyclic population to expand to immunogenic levels. Thus, cattle which showed evidence of partial immunity following treatment with Berenil on days 10 to 12 after cyclical infection, probably had generated adequate antibody responses to some but not all of the metacyclic VATs. Whether all of the expansion of the metacyclic VATs occurs in the skin, so that immunological priming takes place predominantly in the skin and drainage lymph node, or whether there is also significant growth of some or all of these populations in the blood is not clear, although it is known that in mice metacyclic VATs do appear in the blood.[87-90] The relative roles of IgM and IgG antibodies in protection against cyclical challenge in vivo is also not known.

To date the results obtained by cyclical infection followed by cyclical challenge with *T. vivax* are in complete contrast to *T. congolense* and *T. brucei*. Initial studies have shown that goats treated after tsetse-transmitted infection of *T. vivax* are susceptible to homologous as well as heterologous cyclical challenge,[91] despite in some cases being cyclically primed several times.[92] These results indicate either that *T. vivax* does not revert to a constant metacyclic VAT composition or that there is rapid antigenic variation in the metacyclic population with insufficient expansion of metacyclic VATs to induce protective antibody responses.

Recent studies by Nantulya and colleagues[93,94] have shown that infection of cattle with bloodstream forms of *T. congolense, T. brucei,* and *T. vivax,* results in the production of antibodies to metacyclic trypanosomes of the respective serodemes. Infections with bloodstream forms of each trypanosome species in cattle were allowed to progress until the animals became negative for parasitemia and were recovering from the disease. When the animals were then subjected to homologous cyclical challenge they were found to be immune. At least for *T. congolense* and *T. brucei*,[93] serum antibodies to all metacyclic VATs had developed within 2 months of infection, as judged by immunofluorescence and neutralization assays. These results indicated that bloodstream VATs had been expressed which were identical or cross-reactive with metacyclic VATs. This has also been observed in rabbits infected with *T. brucei*.[87]

With the information which is now available on immunity to cyclical infection with the African trypanosomes, it should be possible to determine whether conventional immunization of livestock against the disease is a feasible proposition. Immunity to homologous challenge, of several months duration, can be achieved in cattle by cyclical infection followed by chemotherapy. However, the principal limitation in practical application of such a procedure is the number of different serodemes which occur in any given endemic area. As antisera to different metacyclic populations become available, it will be possible to analyze field isolates in order to determine the number of serodemes present in a location. This problem can also be tackled by using the chancre as a marker for infection. Thus, an animal immunized against one or more characterized serodemes can be cyclically challenged with several different isolates to determine, on the basis of chancre development, which of the challenge populations differ from those used for immunization.

V. RESPONSES OF THE HOST WHICH CONTROL OR MODULATE AN ESTABLISHED INFECTION

It has been known for many years that in animals undergoing chronic trypanosome infections each wave of parasitemia is followed by the appearance of antibodies specific for the major VATs of that parasite population. Thus, it has been assumed that the degree of control of parasitemia is dependent on the replication rate of the parasite and the rapidity with which the host can mount an antibody response. However, this is probably an over-simplification of the situation. Recent studies with *T. brucei* indicate that induction of an antibody response is not merely dependent on the number of trypanosomes with which the host is confronted but also on the differentiative status of the trypanosome population. Furthermore, the inherent immune responsiveness of the host may alter during the course of infection due to the effects of the disease. Evidence is also emerging that responses other than specific antibody may be activated during trypanosome infections which influence the growth rate of the parasite.

A. Antibody Responses and Parasite Differentiation

During each parasitemic wave of a relapsing infection with *T. brucei* the composition of the parasite population changes from being predominantly slender forms during the rising phase to contain progressively larger numbers of stumpy forms.[95] These stumpy forms are senescent nondividing organisms which have a limited lifespan. A relationship between the rate of morphological differentiation and virulence was demonstrated by Barry et al.[96] who showed that the capacity to differentiate was unrelated to VAT; they observed that populations of *T. brucei* which produced rapidly fulminating infections in mice maintained predominantly slender-form morphology (monomorphic), whereas parasites of the same VAT which produced chronic infections differentiated to stumpy forms (pleomorphic). Black and colleagues[41,97] have presented evidence that slender and stumpy forms of *T. brucei* differ in their capacity to induce VAT-specific antibody responses. It was found that slender-form parasites did not release free VSG into the plasma of their infected hosts, whereas VSG was released by stumpy forms. However, this released VSG did not react with monoclonal antibodies which recognize VSG on the surface of intact trypanosomes but did react with monoclonal antibodies which recognize the native VSG molecule. These observations, together with the finding that the anti-VSG antibody response in infected mice was directed mainly against determinants displayed on the surface of intact trypanosomes, suggested that intact trypanosomes or fragments of degenerating trypanosomes are more important than free VSG in the induction of the antibody response. Black and colleagues[97] went on to show that a monomorphic population of *T. brucei* failed to induce any antibody response in mice, as evaluated both by the absence of any specific antibody in the serum and the inability to demonstrate antibody-producing cells in the spleens of infected mice by cell fusion techniques. By contrast, antibody production could readily be demonstrated in mice infected with pleomorphic populations of *T. brucei*. That this difference was not due to an inherent difference in the antigenicity of the two morphological types was demonstrated by the finding that antibody responses could readily be induced with irradiated noninfective monomorphic organisms. These results suggested that differentiation to senescent stumpy-form parasites was required in order to induce a specific antibody response.[97] Thus, differentiation can influence the kinetics of infection in two ways: first, by slowing the growth rate of the population as a result of the development of nondividing forms and, second, by stimulating VSG-specific antibody responses.

In more recent studies, it has been shown that the host exerts an important influence on the degree of differentiation exhibited by a given population of *T. brucei*. Thus, Black et al.[98] found that two populations of *T. brucei* which were pleomorphic and monomorphic, respectively, in mice were equally pleomorphic when inoculated into cattle. When these parasites were recloned back into mice they reverted to the original phenotypes. From these observations it was apparent that differences in the rate of parasite differentiation might play a central role in determining the susceptibility to infection of different host species and individuals within a species. Parasite differentiation was, therefore, compared in C3H/He and C57BL/6 mice which differ in their susceptibility to infection with *T. brucei*.[99] It was found that the lower level of parasitemia displayed by the less susceptible C57BL/6 was associated with more rapid parasite differentiation and a superior antibody response as compared to the C3H/He. However, the rate of differentiation was similar in both strains of mice when they were subjected to γ-irradiation (650 rads). This result along with the observations that the initial infectivity of the parasites and the kinetics of parasite growth and differentiation over the first few days of infection were similar in both strains of mice, suggested that the difference which emerged in the rate of differentiation was the result of a process which was activated after infection of the mice and was at least partially dependent on the presence of a radiosensitive cell.[99] Evidence was presented that this process was not mediated by antibody, nor was it due to selective clearance of slender-form parasites by antibody.

Despite the finding that the C57BL/6 mice mounted a superior antibody response to the trypanosome than the C3H/He, the two strains of mice did not differ intrinsically in their capacity to respond to the trypanosome, as evaluated by antibody responses to fixed doses of irradiated trypanosomes.[95] Differences in the antibody responses during infection could, therefore, have been due to the observed differences in differentiation rate. However, there was also evidence that the C3H/He mice were suppressed for antibody responses.[99] Thus, the relative roles of differentiation and immunosuppression in determining susceptibility to infection were unclear.

It has been suggested by Black et al.[98] that the mammalian host exerts its influence on parasite differentiation via soluble mediators, for which the parasite must have a receptor. Since it was found that plasma from cattle, which supported differentiation of *T. brucei*, when inoculated into mice had no effect on the course of infection with a monomorphic population of *T. brucei*, Black et al.[98] proposed that the mediator involved provided a signal for growth/multiplication of the parasite and that differentiation occurred in the absence of this signal. Thus, the variation in parasite differentiation observed in different hosts was considered to reflect the levels of the growth-promoting mediator(s). On the basis of the finding that pleomorphic and monomorphic *T. brucei* populations retained their respective phenotypes in coinfected mice, it was proposed that differences exhibited by different parasite populations in the same host were due to a difference in their avidity for the host molecules which promote growth.[98]

To date, studies on parasite differentiation have been confined to *T. brucei* because of the ease with which the different morphological types of this parasite can be identified. However, preliminary evidence based on the numbers of proliferating organisms present during the course of infection suggests that a similar process of differentiation may also occur with *T. vivax*.[100]

That differentiation may have a role in susceptibility of cattle to infection was indicated by the results of a small experiment in which the response of pairs of 1-week-old and yearling calves to infection with *T. brucei* was compared; the 1-week-old calves exhibited higher levels of parasitemia, a slower rate of parasite differentiation, and a more severe anemia than the yearlings.[3] Much more effort is required to define the role of parasite differentiation in the susceptibility of domestic animal species to trypanosomal infections and to dissect the mechanism by which differentiation is regulated. Such an approach offers the possibility of being able to manipulate the process of differentiation in order to control parasite growth and, thus, alleviate the pathogenic effects of the infection.

B. Immunosuppression

During infection with the African trypanosomes there is profound activation of the immune system manifesting as marked lymphoid hyperplasia and hypergammaglobulinemia.[8,101] While part of this response is undoubtedly due to specific responses to the large amounts of trypanosomal antigen which are generated during infections, there is also evidence for activation of responses which are not specific for the trypanosomes. Thus, in infected mice there is an increase in the number of background plaque-forming cells to xenogeneic erythrocytes[102,103] and in infected mice and monkey serum antibodies unrelated antigens have been detected.[97,104]

Associated with this activation of the immune system, some hosts suffer from a severe immunosuppression. Over the past decade a large body of literature has accumulated on this subject. While much of this work has concentrated on trypanosome infections in laboratory animals, there is also evidence for immunosuppression in human[105] and bovine trypanosomiasis,[106-108] although in cattle the suppression has usually been relatively mild. Since the subject of immunosuppression in laboratory animals is dealt with in detail in Chapter 5, we will merely summarize the data and concentrate on studies in cattle, with particular emphasis on aspects which relate directly to control of trypanosome infections.

1. Immunosuppression in Laboratory Animals

The immunosuppression observed in infected laboratory animals can be considered under four headings.

a. Depression of Humoral Responses to Unrelated Antigens

Infections with trypanosomes in mice are associated with a profound suppression in antibody responses, as measured both by serum antibody levels and numbers of splenic plaque-forming cells, to a variety of antigens including both T-dependent and T-independent antigens.[102,103,109] This suppression is usually apparent shortly after initial detection of parasitemia.

b. Depression of Cell-Mediated Immune Responses

The responses in vitro of spleen cells to both T and B cell mitogens and in mixed leukocyte reactions are markedly suppressed in trypanosome-infected mice.[110,111] It is of interest that the degree of suppression of these responses is much greater in spleen cells than in cells from other compartments of the immune system.[112] Even in the advanced stages of infection with *T. congolense* or *T. brucei* there was relatively little suppression of responses of lymph node cells and peripheral blood leukocytes.[112]

Several investigations have found that despite the profound suppression of antibody responses in infected mice, cell-mediated immune responses in vivo, as measured by DTH reactions, remained normal. Thus, unimpaired DTH skin reactions to oxazolone and dinitrofluorobenzene have been observed in mice infected with *T. brucei*.[102,113,114] However, Murray et al.[102] showed that suppression of the response to oxazolone did occur in more chronically infected mice, i.e., infections of 5 to 6 weeks duration. Furthermore, Mansfield and Wallace[115] demonstrated partial suppression of DTH skin reactions to purified protein derivative in rabbits infected for 6 weeks with *T. congolense* and primed 3 weeks previously with FCA. The later onset of the suppression of DTH responses may relect the involvement of lymph nodes rather than spleen in these responses.

c. Altered Susceptibility to Other Diseases

Urquhart et al.[116] examined the influence of *T. brucei* infection on the course of infection with the intestinal helminth *Nippostrongylus brasiliensis* in rats. By contrast to the self-limiting infection produced by *N. brasiliensis* in normal rats, rats infected with *T. brucei* failed to expel the nematode infection. Phillips et al.[117] obtained similar results with *Trichuris muris* in mice infected with *Trypanosoma brucei*. *T. brucei* infections have also been found to increase the susceptibility of mice to infection with louping ill virus.[118] Trypanosome-infected mice were found to support much higher titers of virus than uninfected mice, although there was no difference in the survival of the two groups.

The study of Allt et al.[119] provides an example of how trypanosome infection, by depression of the immune response, can alleviate a disease syndrome. These authors observed that infection of rabbits with *T. brucei* suppressed the development of the autoimmune disease, allergic neuritis. In a later study, however, MacKenzie et al.[120] obtained contradictory results in rats infected with *T. brucei*.

d. Depression of Antitrypanosome Immune Responses

Despite the complete suppression observed in antibody responses to unrelated antigens in mice with chronic trypanosome infections, the animals often retain the ability to respond to the trypanosome, at least over the first few waves of parasitemia. However, Sacks and Askonas[121] found that mice infected with *T. brucei* exhibited depressed antibody responses as compared to uninfected controls, following inoculation of irradiated trypanosomes of a heterologous clone of *T. brucei;* the degree of this depression was related to the virulence of the infecting organisms. Furthermore, by examining the antbody responses of chronically infected mice to organisms derived from each of the first three waves of parasitemia, they found that there was a progressive suppression of both IgM and IgG antibody responses to the parasites, so that by the third parasitemic wave there was no detectable IgG and only low levels of IgM. The possibility that a change in the rate of parasite differentiation might also have contributed to this deterioration in the specific immune response, should also be considered. Nevertheless, in studies to compare the susceptibility of C57BL/6 and C3H/He mice to infection with *T. brucei*, Black et al.[99] also obtained evidence that there was partial suppression of the antibody response to the initial peak of parasitemia in the more susceptible C3H/He mice.

A number of mechanisms have been proposed to explain immunosuppression in trypanosome-infected laboratory animals. These include clonal exhaustion of immunologically reactive cells due to sustained polyclonal activation,[103-116] induction of suppressor cells,[122-124] direct suppressive activity of trypanosome antigens or products,[125,126] and defective macrophage function in uptake and/or processing and presentation of antigens.[127,128] A striking feature of immunosuppression in trypanosome-infected rodents is the rapid return to normal responsiveness following removal of the trypanosome infection by chemotherapy.[102] This argues against depletion of immunologically reactive cells and implicates a direct role for the trypanosome. That trypanosome antigens are involved in inducing the suppression is suggested by the finding that suppression can be induced in mice by inoculation of a trypanosome membrane fraction.[126] Furthermore, recent studies by Grosskinsky and Askonas[129] have provided convincing evidence that the macrophage plays an important role in the suppressive mechanism, although it is still unclear to what extent other cell types are also involved.

2. Immunosuppression in Cattle

The degree of derangement of the immune system during trypanosome infections in cattle is much less marked than in laboratory animals. Thus, cattle continue to produce antibodies to the trypanosome for many months after initial infection,[51] they show less evidence of immunosuppression to unrelated antigens, and although the lymphoid organs show marked hyperplasia there is less disruption of the tissue architecture than in laboratory animals.[130,131] However, hypergammaglobulinemia involving IgM and sometimes IgG is a consistent feature of bovine trypanosomiasis,[131-135] although the presence of heterophil antibodies has not been reported. Indeed, Musoke et al.[43] have claimed that the majority of the increase in IgM and IgG in the serum of cattle 2 weeks after infection with *T. congolense* could be accounted for by antibodies against the trypanosome. This conclusion was based on the finding that 85% of the immunoglobulin could be removed by absorption on trypanosomes collected at 3-day intervals during the first 2 weeks of infection from the same animals. Thus, while it could be argued that the procedure used could have resulted in nonspecific removal of immunoglobulins, the results suggest that polyclonal activation is not a prominent feature of bovine trypanosomiasis. On the other hand, it is well established that most specific antibody responses are accompanied by the appearance of small quantities of antibodies specific for a variety of antigens which are unrelated to the immunizing antigen.[136-138] Furthermore, there is evidence that this ''nonspecific'' component of the response is particularly marked against antigens to which the animal has recently been exposed, suggesting that it involves reactivation of recently primed B cells.[138,139] Thus, during trypanosome infections the nonspecific response might be preferentially directed against trypanosome antigens to which the animal has been exposed during previous waves of parasitemia. This would account for the presence of large amounts of antitrypanosomal antibody in the serum of infected cattle and might also contribute to the long-term persistence of anti-VSG antibodies.[5] The degree of specificity of the immune response for the trypanosome is probably dependent on the host species infected and on the severity of infection; responses with a larger component of nonspecific antibodies might be expected in those animals such as mice in which infection gives rise to high levels of parasitemia and invariably, has a fatal outcome.

Attempts to evaluate the immune competence of trypanosome-infected cattle have concentrated mainly on examining antibody responses to various viral and bacterial antigens. Holmes et al.[140] and Scott et al.[106] reported slight depression of antibody responses to *Clostridium oedematiens* and foot and mouth disease virus vaccines, both in naturally infected cattle and in cattle experimentally infected with *T. congolense*. Sollod and Frank[141] found that in cattle infected with *T. congolense* there was a delay of 4 days in the antibody response to the hapten dinitrophenyl, but that the peak titers of antibody were the same as in control cattle; in the same study, infected cattle were found to have normal responses to parainfluenza 3 virus and to an *Escherichia coli* bacteriophage. Significant suppression of the antibody response to louping ill virus was reported by Whitelaw et al.[107] in cattle experimentally infected with *T. congolense* or *T. vivax*, but not in cattle infected with *T. brucei*. Rurangirwa and colleagues,[142-144] working with cattle experimentally infected with *T. congolense* or *T. vivax*, found slight suppression of antibody responses to *Leptospira biflexa*, *Brucella abortus* (S-19), and *Mycoplasma mycoides* antigens but found no evidence of suppression of antibody responses to rinderpest vaccine. In a later study, Rurangirwa et al.[108] observed profound suppression of the antibody response to *B. abortus* (S-19) in cattle infected with *T. congolense*.

A number of studies in which the responses to mitogens of leukocytes from infected cattle were examined failed to demonstrate any evidence of suppression. Initial experiments reported by Sollod and Frank[141] and Masake et al.[145] examined PBL from cattle infected with *T. congolense*. Furthermore, Masake and Morrison[131] found that leukocytes from peripheral blood, lymph nodes, and spleen of cattle infected with *T. vivax* exhibited normal responses to several mitogens. We have also examined the responses in mixed leukocyte reaction of cells from peripheral blood, lymph nodes, and spleens of cattle infected with *T. congolense* and could find no evidence of suppression, even in cattle infected for up to 5 1/2 months.[146]

The cellular responses of bone marrow have also been examined in trypanosome-infected cattle. Evidence of a significant decrease in mobilization of neutrophils from the bone marrow was found in cattle during the first 14 weeks of infection with *T. congolense*.[147] Furthermore, serum from cattle infected with *T. congolense* or *T. vivax* was found to inhibit formation of granulocyte/monocyte colonies in bone marrow cells cultured in methyl cellulose.[148] No inhibition of erythroid colony formation was found. The authors suggested that the inhibitory effect may be due to the release of trypanosome lytic products into the serum.[148]

From these studies of both antibody and cell-mediated immune responses in cattle, the evidence for a significant immunosuppression which may be of functional importance must be questioned. The suppression of peak antibody titers might be explained by a general increase in immunoglobulin catabolism and turnover rate as has been demonstrated by Nielsen et al.[149] Only in the study by Rurangirwa with *B. abortus* was there pronounced suppression of an antibody response.[105] Furthermore, recent experiments reported by Sharpe et al.[150] failed to demonstrate a significant deficiency in immunity to live foot and mouth virus challenge in cattle immunized with foot and mouth vaccine during infection with *T. congolense*. On the other hand, Ilemobade et al.[150a] obtained evidence of partial impairment of immunity to challenge with live *M. mycoides* in two of four cattle vaccinated against the organism and infected with *T. congolense* or *T. vivax*. The inconsistent demonstration of immunosuppression in trypanosome-infected cattle may be related to the fact that all of the studies have concentrated on the first 6 weeks of infection. It is possible that infections of longer duration or with organisms of greater virulence are more likely to result in functionally significant immunosuppression.

The possible role of immunosuppression in influencing antibody responses to the trypanosome has recently been investigated in a study by Nantulya et al.[151] The antibody responses of cattle were examined following simultaneous or sequential challenge with two clones of *T. brucei*. It was found that the responses to one of the clones were partially depressed in animals inoculated with both clones either simultaneously or 2 days apart, but there was no depression of responses in animals inoculated at 4- and 6-day intervals with the two clones. However, it was found that the clone, which gave a normal antibody response, reached 10- to 20-fold higher levels of parasitemia than the second clone in coinfected cattle, although it was not clear whether this difference in parasitemia also occurred in cattle infected with the two clones separately. Thus, while these authors suggested that antigenic competition contributed to the depression in antibody response to one of the clones, they also indicated that a major factor involved could have been the number of trypanosomes of each clone to which the animals were exposed.

We have examined the response of cattle infected for 3 1/2 months with *T. congolense* to fixed numbers of irradiated organisms of a clone of *T. brucei* inoculated either intravenously or subcutaneously.[152] Three of five infected cattle inoculated intravenously and two of five infected cattle inoculated subcutaneously with irradiated *T. brucei* showed marked suppression in antibody responses as measured by the Farr assay with purified VSG (Figure 3). The individual animals which showed suppressed antibody responses were those which had experienced the most severe trypanosome infections and were most anemic at the time of antigenic challenge. However, when these animals were given a second inoculum of the same irradiated *T. brucei* 5 weeks later both control and infected cattle exhibited a vigorous secondary response.

As already discussed, Emery et al.[59] were able to demonstrate an in vitro proliferative response of PBL to ultrasonicated trypanosomal antigen in cattle which had been cured of trypanosome infection by chemotherapy, but found no response in infected cattle. These results suggested that although infected cattle were sensitized to trypanosome antigen(s), the proliferative response was suppressed during infection. Recent studies in our laboratory have shown that in cattle cyclically infected with *T. congolense,* PBL collected between 3 and 7 days after infection (i.e., prior to development of a chancre) exhibit a strong proliferative response to ultrasonicated trypanosome antigen, but that this response then disappears, only to reemerge if the animal is treated.[79] Preliminary results indicate that this is a T cell response. The possibility that such a response is required for development of the chancre reaction is suggested by the results of studies in rabbits and goats in which it has been found that if animals are cyclically challenged within 12 to 20 days with two unrelated serodemes of *T. congolense*, then the second challenge does not provoke a chancre reaction and induces little or no antibody response.[153,154] However, it is unclear whether these findings reflect suppression of the responses required to mediate the chancre and induce antibody or whether there is inhibition of multiplication of the infecting trypanosome population. The latter possibility is suggested by experiments which have demonstrated interference in establishment of su-

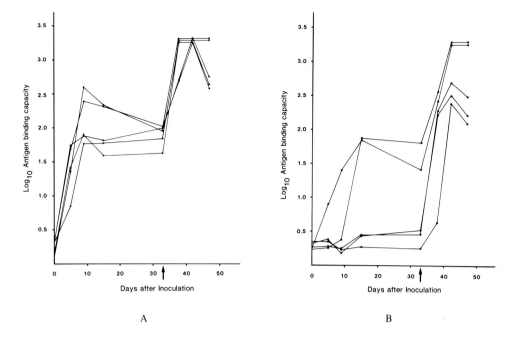

FIGURE 3. Antibody responses in control cattle (A) and cattle infected with *T. congolense* (B) following inoculation with irradiated noninfective *T. brucei*. Cattle were infected by inoculation with 10^7 bloodstream forms of *T. congolense* stock IL-552. After 3 1/2 months of infection the infected cattle, along with controls, were inoculated intravenously with 10^9 irradiated (60,000 rads) *T. brucei* ILTat 1.3. After a further 33 days the animals received a second identical inoculum of irradiated *T. brucei* (arrow). Antibody was measured in a Farr assay using ^{125}I-labeled purified ILTat 1.3 VSG.

perinfections with *T. congolense* in cattle[155] (see next section). Nevertheless, the results to date suggest that there is a suppression of T cell responses to the trypanosome in cattle following the first week of infection. Although there is no evidence that such a response is required for protective immunity, its possible role in exerting positive or negative regulation of trypanosome growth awaits evaluation.

C. Interference in Establishment of Superinfections

We have found, in cattle challenged sequentially with two unrelated serodemes of *T. congolense*, that an already established infection may interfere with the establishment of a second infection.[155] This interference phenomenon was observed in cattle initially infected with bloodstream forms of *T. congolense* and challenged 5 to 6 weeks later either cyclically or with bloodstream forms of the second serodeme. The interference effect did not result from specific immunity and required the presence of an active infection, since treatment of infected animals with Berenil prior to rechallenge resulted in them being fully susceptible to the second infection. In the case of animals subjected to cyclical challenge, although there was no significant increase in parasitemia and most animals did not develop chancre reactions, all produced neutralizing antibodies to the metacyclic population. By contrast, cattle that received the second challenge by bloodstream forms showed only a slight trace of antibody to the infecting trypanosome population. These results suggested that there was inhibition of growth of the superimposed trypanosome population, although following cyclical challenge there must have been sufficient expansion of the metacyclic population to induce an antibody response. Whether the absence of chancres in cyclically challenged animals reflected a suppression of the responses which give rise to the chancre or a reduction of the numbers of trypanosomes growing in the skin to levels which were insufficient to induce a chancre was not clear.

In an experiment carried out by Akol and Murray[62] it was found that infected cattle cyclically challenged 95 days later with an unrelated serodeme of *T. congolense* developed chancres and showed a marked increase in parasitemia. The failure to demonstrate an interference effect in this experiment may have been due to the longer duration of the initial infection and the very low parasitemia which these animals exhibited at the time of challenge.

Recent studies by Luckins and colleagues[82,153] have shown that when rabbits cyclically infected with *T. congolense* were cyclically challenged 14 to 21 days later with an unrelated stock of the same parasite, they failed to develop chancre reactions and did not produce antibody to the initial bloodstream population of parasites. Similarly, we have found that in goats cyclically challenged with two unrelated cloned populations of *T. congolense* at an interval of 12 days, there was minimal chancre development to the second challenge and little evidence of an immune response to the metacyclic trypanosomes.[154] In both of these studies, if animals were challenged within the first week after infection, there was no interference in chancre formation or production of antibodies to the second infection. At present it is not known if these results are due to a suppression of immune responses to the second infection or inhibition of growth of the second trypanosome population to an extent that it does not induce a significant immune response.

Since the interference effect cannot readily be accounted for by specific antibody responses and as it appears to require an active infection, we would suggest that other responses are activated during infection in cattle which can modulate trypanosome growth by mechanisms analogous to those proposed by Black et al.[98] Such responses might result either in production of substances which can inhibit trypanosome growth or suppression of production of substances required to promote trypanosome growth. The ability of the already established infection to maintain growth might be explained by selection of bloodstream populations which have a higher or lower avidity for these putative stimulatory or inhibitory substances, respectively.

In endemic areas of bovine trypanosomiasis where animals come under challenge with numerous trypanosomal serodemes, the interference phenomenon may serve to limit the number of serodemes expressed within the bloodstream of infected animals. Furthermore, our results suggest that in certain circumstances immunity may develop against metacyclic trypanosomes without significant establishment of the infection within the bloodstream. Although at present we do not know if interference is operative between serodemes of different trypanosome species, such an effect might contribute to the tendency for infection with the different species in cattle to appear sequentially following initial exposure to natural tsetse challenge.[156]

VI. ACQUIRED RESISTANCE IN THE FIELD

There is evidence that cattle maintained in a particular field location may acquire a degree of resistance to trypanosome challenge. This has been observed with trypanotolerant N'Dama cattle in West Africa[157-160] and with *Bos indicus* breeds in East Africa[18,19,21,161] (reviewed by Murray et al.[3]). In the latter studies, animals were maintained by strategic use of chemotherapy and evidence of acquired resistance was based on a reduction in the frequency of required treatments.

These observations probably result from the acquisition of immunity to the metacyclics of at least some of the serodemes present in the local area. Since it is known that immunity to homologous cyclical challenge is acquired just after initial detection of parasitemia, then, even in animals in the field which are treated on detection of infection, immunity should have developed to the serodemes which have given rise to parasitemia. The degree of resistance which such animals acquire will probably depend on how many of the local serodemes establish infection in the periods between chemotherapy. In animals such as the

N'Dama which usually do not receive chemotherapy, there is the opportunity to acquire immunity not only to the metacyclic populations but also to many bloodstream VATs. Cross-immunity between serodemes will only occur in the case of iso-VATs. The extent to which this contributes to acquired resistance in the field is questionable, as iso-VATs have not yet been described for *T. congolense* or *T. vivax* and they would be required to occur at a relatively high frequency to give significant immunity between serodemes. Perhaps of greater significance would be the occurrence of iso-VATs between metacyclic populations of different serodemes. Preliminary evidence presented by Esser et al.[90] working with *T. rhodesiense* suggests that this may be the case. The detection of antimetacyclic antibodies in cattle experimentally infected with bloodstream trypanosomes[93] may also be of considerable significance in the acquisition of immunity under field conditions. Thus, in animals such as the N'Dama which do not receive chemotherapy, the occurrence of bloodstream VATs which cross-react with metacyclic VATs may serve to boost responses to the metacyclic population and perhaps result in stronger immunity of longer duration. Furthermore, responses to these bloodstream populations will ensure development of immunity to metacyclic challenge, even in animals infected by mechanical transmission from biting flies. This may be particularly important with *T. vivax*, since mechanical transmission of infection with this parasite is thought to be relatively common.

Another factor which may be important in the acquisition of immunity in the field is the age at which animals are first exposed to infection. It is a widely held view that if calves suckling their mothers are subjected to early exposure to local strains of trypanosomes, they will acquire a degree of resistance to challenge, provided they are not moved to another location.[162] This might be partially explained by a protective effect of maternal colostrum, although critical evidence for this is lacking. However, studies in mice have shown that protection can be transferred from mother to offspring with colostrum.[3] There is also some evidence, at least with *T. congolense*, that young calves are innately less susceptible to trypanosome infection than adults.[3,24,163] This increased resistance, together with maternally derived protective antibodies, may decrease the severity of infections in young calves but allow some establishment of infection sufficient to induce protective immune responses.

At present, there is no convincing evidence that either the common antigenic determinant on the VSG or other common trypanosome antigens contribute to acquired immunity. This is, perhaps, not surprising since such determinants are not exposed on the surface of trypanosomes and, therefore, are not accessible to antibody. However, their possible role in inducing other antibody-independent responses which limit trypanosome growth should not be discounted. That such responses occur in infected cattle is suggested by the finding of interference in establishment of superinfections with unrelated serodemes.[155] While these responses are unlikely to have a direct role in acquisition of protective immunity, as they appear to require the presence of active infection, they may enable survival of the host by limiting the number of different trypanosome serodemes which can grow in the animal at any given time.

VII. CONCLUDING REMARKS

Many of the observations made in laboratory animals infected with the African trypanosome do not necessarily apply to trypanosomiasis in cattle. While infections in mice are invariably fatal and are characterized by progressively increasing levels of parasitemia, infections in cattle are often self-limiting and, after attaining peak levels during the first few weeks of infection, the parasitemia gradually diminished over a period of weeks or months. Thus, fatalities are usually not associated with overwhelming parasitemia but are due to the pathogenic consequences of the infection, the most important of which is anemia. Nevertheless, the severity of the anemia is related to the level and duration of parasitemia. The greater degree of control of parasitemia in cattle probably also accounts for the findings that disruption of lymphoid architecture, production of nonspecific antibodies, and immuno-suppression are much less pronounced than in infected laboratory animals.

Trypanosome infections in cattle provoke a number of different immune responses. Following the bite of an infected tsetse fly, the first evidence of a response by the immune system is the detection in peripheral blood after 3 to 4 days of infection of T cells which are sensitized to trypanosome antigens. This is followed by the development of intense cellular reactions in the skin commencing 5 to 8 days after infection and reaching maximum intensity during the second week of infection. Antibodies which neutralize the metacyclic trypanosomes appear in the serum just after the peak of the local skin reaction and at the time of initial detection of parasitemia. Thereafter, antibodies are produced to the VATs of each successive wave of parasitemia. As the infection progresses, antibodies are also produced against common trypanosome antigens.

The time of appearance of neutralizing antibodies for the metacyclics coincides with the time at which animals acquire protective immunity against cyclical challenge. This immunity is specific for the infecting serodeme, reflecting a difference in the VAT composition of metacyclics of different serodemes. Thus, while immunity can readily be induced to individual serodemes by cyclical infection followed by chemotherapy, the practicability of such an approach awaits further information on the number of serodemes which are likely to be present in a particular field location.

Although there is convincing evidence that VAT-specific antibodies are important in mediating protective immunity and in eliminating each successive wave of parasitemia during an infection, evidence is now emerging that other responses may also be important in regulating parasitic growth. It is apparent that the rate at which the parasite differentiates to senescent nondividing forms may be an important factor in influencng control of parasitemia, since these senescent forms are required to induce an antibody response. In addition, there is evidence that the rate of differentiation is influenced by a process which is activated during infection and that the degree to which it is activated differs in mouse strains of different susceptibility. Moreover, certain parasite populations which show little differentiation in mice readily differentiate in cattle. There is also evidence in infected cattle that responses are activated which markedly inhibit the establishment and growth of a superimposed infection. How these responses in cattle are induced and whether they act by regulating parasite differentiation is not known. However, a dissection of the mechanisms underlying these regulatory processes may provide the key to understanding the basis of differences in host susceptibility to trypanosome infections. Furthermore, this approach offers new possibilities of being able to manipulate host responses in order to control parasite growth and alleviate the pathogenic effects of the infection.

REFERENCES

1. **Ford, J.,** The geographical distribution of *Glossina,* in *The African Trypanosomiases,* Mulligan, H. W., Ed., Allen and Unwin, London, 1970, 274.
2. **MacLennan, K. J. R.,** The epizootiology of African trypanosomiasis in livestock in West Africa, in *The African Trypanosomiases,* Mulligan, H. W., Ed., Allen and Unwin, London, 1970, 751.
3. **Murray, M., Morrison, W. I., and Whitelaw, D. D.,** Host susceptibiliy to African trypanosomiasis; trypanotolerance, *Adv. Parasitol.,* 21, 1, 1982.
4. **Gray, A. R.,** Antigenic variation in a strain of *Trypanosoma brucei* transmitted by *Glossina morsitans* and *G. palpalis, J. Gen. Microbiol.,* 41, 195, 1965.

5. **Wilson, A. J. and Cunningham, M. P.,** Immunological aspects of bovine tryapnosomiasis. I. Immune response of cattle to infection with *Trypanosoma congolense* and the antigenic variation of the infecting organisms, *Exp. Parasitol.*, 32, 165, 1972.

6. **Vickerman, K.,** Antigenic variation in trypanosomes, *Nature (London)*, 273, 613, 1978.

7. **WHO,** Proposals for the nomenclature of salivarian trypanosomes and for the maintenance of reference collections, *Bull. WHO*, 56, 467, 1978.

8. **Morrison, W. I., Murray, M., and McIntyre, W. I. M.,** Bovine trypanosomiasis, in *Diseases of Cattle in the Tropics,* Ristic, M. and McIntyre, W. I. M., Eds., Martins Nijhoff, The Hague, 1981, 469.

9. **Murray, M. and Urquhart, G. M.,** Immunoprophylaxis against African trypanosomiasis, in *Immunity to Blood Parasites of Animals and Man,* Vol. 93, Miller, L. H., Pino, J. A., and McKelvey, J. J., Eds., Plenum Press, New York, 1977, 209.

10. **Murray, M.,** Anaemia of bovine African trypanosomiasis: an overview, in *Pathogenicity of Trypanosomes,* No. 132e, Losos, G. and Chouinard, A., Eds., International Development Research Centre, Ottawa, 1979, 121.

11. **Hudson, J. R.,** Acute and subacute trypanosomiasis in cattle caused by *T. vivax, J. Comp. Pathol.*, 54, 108, 1944.

12. **Mwongela, G. N., Kovatch, R. M., and Fazil, M. A.,** Acute *Trypanosoma vivax* infection in dairy cattle in coast province, Kenya, *Trop. Anim. Health Prod.*, 13, 63, 1981.

13. **Davis, C. E.,** Thrombocytopaenia: a uniform complication of African trypanosomiasis, *Acta Trop.*, 39, 123, 1982.

14. **Losos, G. J. and Ikede, B. O.,** Review of the pathology of diseases in domestic and laboratory animals caused by *Trypanosoma congolense, T. vivax, T. brucei, T. rhodesiense* and *T. gambiense, Vet. Pathol.*, 9 (Suppl.), 1, 1972.

15. **Morrison, W. I., Murray, M., Whitelaw, D. D., and Sayer, P. D.,** Pathology of infection with *Trypanosoma brucei:* disease syndromes in dogs and cattle resulting from severe tissue damage, in *From Parasitic Infection to Parasitic Disease,* Vol. 7, Gigase, P. L. and Van Marck, E. A. E., Eds., Contr. Microbiol. Immunol., S. Karger, Basel, 1983, 103.

16. **Wellde, B. T., Kovatch, R. M., Hockmeyer, W. T., Owiti, S., Masaba, S. C., and Arp Siongok, T.,** *Trypanosoma brucei rhodesiense:* experimental infections in cattle, in *Recent Developments in Medical Research in Eastern Africa,* Njogu, A. R., Tukei, P. M., and Roberts, J. M. D., Eds., Kenya Medical Research Institute and Kenya Trypanosomiasis Research Institute, Nairobi, 1980, 187.

17. **Murray M. and Morrison, W. I.,** Parasitaemia and host susceptibility, in *Pathogenicity of Trypanosomes,* No. 132e, Losos, G. and Chouinard, A., Eds., International Development Research Centre, Ottawa, 1979, 71.

18. **Bevan, L. E. W.,** Notes on immunity in trypanosomiasis, *Trans. R. Soc. Med. Hyg.*, 30, 199, 1936.

19. **Whiteside, E. F.,** Interactions between drugs, trypanosomes and cattle in the field, in *Drugs Parasites and Hosts,* Goodwin, L. G. and Nimmo-Smith, R. H., Eds., Churchill Livingstone, London, 1962, 116.

20. **Wilson, A. J., Le Roux, J. G., Paris, J., Davidson, C. R., and Gray, A. R.,** Observations on a herd of beef cattle maintained in a tsetse area. I. Assessment of chemotherapy as a method for control of trypanosomiasis, *Trop. Anim. Health Prod.*, 7, 187, 1975.

21. **Wilson, A. J., Paris, J., Luckins, A. G., Dar, F. K., and Gray, A. R.,** Observations on a herd of beef cattle maintained in a tsetse area. II. Assessment of the development of immunity in association with trypanocidal drug treatment, *Trop. Anim. Health Prod.*, 8, 1, 1976.

22. **Cunningham, M. P.,** Vaccination of cattle against trypanosomes by infection and treatment, in *Isotopes and Radiation in Parasitology,* International Atomic Energy Agency, Vienna, 1968, 88.

23. **Wilson, A. J.,** Immunological aspects of bovine trypanosomiasis. III. Patterns in the development of immunity, *Trop. Anim. Health Prod.*, 3, 14, 1971.

24. **Wellde, B. T., Hockmeyer, W. T., Kovatch, R. M., Bhogal, M. S., and Diggs, C. L.,** *Trypanosoma congolense:* natural and acquired resistance in the bovine, *Exp. Parasitol.*, 52, 219, 1981.

25. **Duxbury, R. E., Anderson, J. S., Wellde, B. T., Sadun, E. H., and Muriithi, I. E.,** *Trypanosoma congolense:* immunisation of mice, dogs and cattle with gamma-irradiated parasites, *Exp. Parasitol.*, 32, 527, 1972.

26. **Duxbury, R. E., Sadun, E. H., Anderson, J. S., Wellde, B. T., Muriithi, I. E., and Warui, G. M.,** Immunisation of rodents, dogs, cattle and monkeys against African trypanosomiasis by the use of irradiated trypanosomes, in *Isotopes and Radiation in Parasitology,* Vol. 3, International Atomic Energy Agency, Vienna, Austria, 1973, 179.

27. **Wellde, B. T., Duxbury, R. E., Sadun, E. H., Langbehn, H. R., Lotzsch, R., Deindl, G., and Warui, G.,** Experimental infections with African trypanosomes. IV. Immunization of cattle with gamma-irradiated *Trypanosoma rhodesiense, Exp. Parasitol.*, 34, 62, 1973.

28. **Morrison, W. I., Black, S. J., Paris, J., Hinson, C. A., and Wells, P. W.,** Protective immunity and specificity of antibody responses elicited in cattle with irradiated *Trypanosoma brucei, Parasite Immunol.*, 4, 395, 1982.

29. **Wells, P. W., Emery, D. L., Hinson, C. A., Morrison, W. L., and Murray, M.,** Immunisation of cattle with variant specific surface antigen of *Trypanosoma brucei:* the influence of different adjuvants, *Infect. Immun.,* 36, 1, 1982.
30. **Dodin, A. and Fromentin, H.,** Mise en évidence d'un antigène vaccinant dans le plasma de souris expérimentalement infectées par *Trypanosoma gambiense* et par *Trypanosoma congolense, Bull. Soc. Pathol. Exot.,* 55, 123, 1962.
31. **Watkins, J. F.,** Observations on antigenic variation in a strain of *Trypanosoma brucei* growing in mice, *J. Hyg.,* 62, 69, 1964.
32. **Seed, J. R.,** The characterization of antigens isolated from *Trypanosoma rhodesiense, J. Protozool.,* 10, 380, 1963.
33. **Campbell, G. H. and Phillips, S. M.,** Adoptive transfer of variant-specific resistance to *Trypanosoma rhodesiense* with B lymphocytes and serum, *Infect. Immun.,* 14, 1144, 1976.
34. **Luckins, A. G.,** Adoptive immunity in experimental trypanosomiasis, *Trans. R. Soc. Trop. Med. Hyg.,* 66, 346, 1972.
35. **Takayanagi, T. and Nakatake, Y.,** *Trypanosoma gambiense:* enhancement of agglutinin and protection in subpopulations by immune spleen cells, *Exp. Parasitol.,* 38, 233, 1975.
36. **Campbell, G. H., Esser, K. M., and Phillips, S. M.,** *Trypanosoma rhodesiense* infection in congenitally athymic (nude) mice, *Infect. Immun.,* 20, 714, 1978.
37. **Morrison, W. I., Roelants, G. E., Mayor-Withey, K. S., and Murray, M.,** Susceptibility of inbred strains of mice to *Trypanosoma congolense:* correlation with changes in spleen lymphocyte populations, *Clin. Exp. Immunol.,* 32, 25, 1978.
38. **Campbell, G. H., Esser, K. M., and Weinbaum, F. I.,** *Trypanosoma rhodesiense* infection in B-cell-deficient mice, *Infect. Immun.,* 18, 434, 1977.
39. **Cross, G. A. M.,** Identification, purification and properties of clone-specific glycoprotein antigens constituting the surface coat of *Trypanosoma brucei, Parasitology,* 71, 393, 1975.
40. **Murray, M.,** unpublished data, 1982.
41. **Black, S. J., Hewett, R. S., and Sendashonga, C. N.,** *Trypanosoma brucei* variable surface antigen is released by degenerating parasites but not by actively dividing parasites, *Parasite Immunol.,* 4, 233, 1982.
42. **Luckins, A. G.,** The immune response of zebu cattle to infection with *Trypanosoma congolense* and *T. vivax, Ann. Trop. Med. Parasitol.,* 70, 133, 1976.
43. **Musoke, A. J., Nantulya, V. M., Barbet, A. F., Kironde, F., and McGuire, T. C.,** Bovine immune response to African trypanosomes: specific antibodies to variable surface glycoproteins of *Trypanosoma brucei, Parasite Immunol.,* 3, 97, 1981.
44. **Lourie, E. M. and O'Conner, R. J.,** Trypanolysis *in vitro* by mouse immune serum, *Ann. Trop. Med. Parasitol.,* 30, 365, 1936.
45. **Takayanagi, T., Nakatake, Y., and Enriquez, G. L.,** *Trypanosoma gambiense:* phagocytosis *in vitro, Exp. Parasitol.,* 36, 106, 1974.
46. **MacAskill, J. A., Holmes, P. H., Whitelaw, D. D., McConnell, I., Jennings, F. W., and Urquhart, G. M.,** Immunological clearance of ^{75}Se-labelled *Trypanosoma brucei* in mice. II. Mechanisms in immune animals, *Immunology,* 40, 629, 1980.
47. **Shirazi, M. F., Holman, M., Hudson, K. M., Klaus, G. G. B., and Terry, R. J.,** Complement (C3) levels and the effect of C3 depletion in infections of *Trypanosoma brucei* in mice, *Parasite Immunol.,* 2, 155, 1980.
48. **Barbet, A. F. and McGuire, T. C.,** Crossreacting determinants in variant specific surface antigens of African trypanosomes, *Proc. Natl. Acad. Sci. U.S.A.,* 75, 1989, 1978.
49. **Van Meirvenne, N., Magnus, E., and Vervoort, T.,** Comparison of variable antigenic types produced by trypanosome strains of the subgenus *Trypanozoon, Ann. Soc. Belge Med. Trop.,* 57, 409, 1977.
50. **Vervoort, T., Barbet, A. F., Musoke, A. J., Magnus, E., Mpimbaza, G., and Van Meirvenne, N.,** Isotypic surface glycoproteins of trypanosomes, *Immunology,* 44, 223, 1981.
51. **Nantulya, V. M., Musoke, A. J., Barbet, A. F., and Roelants, G. E.,** Evidence for reappearance of *Trypanosoma brucei* variable antigen types in relapse populations, *J. Parasitol.,* 65, 673, 1979.
52. **Barbet, A. F., Davis, W. C., and McGuire, T. C.,** Cross-neutralization of two different trypanosome populations derived from a single organism, *Nature (London),* 300, 453, 1982.
53. **Wilson, A. J. and Cunningham, M. P.,** Immunological aspects of bovine trypanosomiasis. IV. Patterns in the production of common antibodies, *Trop. Anim. Health Prod.,* 3, 133, 1971.
54. **Shapiro, S. Z. and Murray, M.,** African trypanosome antigens recognised during the course of infection in N'Dama and Zebu cattle, *Infect. Immun.,* 35, 410, 1982.
55. **Mansfield, J. M. and Kreier, J. P.,** Tests for antibody — and cell-mediated hypersensitivity to trypanosome antigens in rabbits infected with *Trypanosoma congolense, Infect. Immun.,* 6, 62, 1972.
56. **Tizard, I. R. and Soltys, M. A.,** Cell-mediated hypersensitivity in rabbits infected with *Trypanosoma brucei* and *Trypanosoma rhodesiense, Infect. Immun.,* 4, 674, 1971.

57. **Finerty, J. F., Krehl, E. P., and McKelvin, R. L.,** Delayed-type hypersensitivity in mice immunized with *Trypanosoma rhodesiense* antigens, *Infect. Immun.,* 20, 464, 1978.
58. **Gasbarre, L. C., Hug, K., and Louis, J. A.,** Murine T lymphocyte specificity for African trypanosomes. I. Induction of a T lymphocyte-dependent proliferative response to *Trypanosoma brucei, Clin. Exp. Immunol.,* 41, 97, 1980.
59. **Emery, D. L., Wells, P. W., and Tenywa, T.,** *Trypanosoma congolense:* specific transformation *in vitro* of leukocytes from infected or immunised cattle, *Exp. Parasitol.,* 50, 358, 1980.
60. **Luckins, A. G. and Gray, A. R.,** An extravascular site of development of *Trypanosoma congolense, Nature (London),* 272, 613, 1978.
61. **Akol, G. W. O. and Murray, M.,** Early events following challenge of cattle with tsetse infected with *Trypanosoma congolense:* development of the local skin reaction, *Vet. Rec.,* 110, 295, 1982.
62. **Akol, G. W. O. and Murray, M.,** *Trypanosoma congolense:* susceptibility of cattle to cyclical challenge, *Exp. Parasitol.,* in press.
63. **Hirumi, H., Hirumi, K., Gray, M. A., Moloo, S. K., Akol, G. W. O., and Murray, M.,** *In vitro* cultivation of animal infective forms of *Trypanosoma congolense* and local skin reactions induced by the cultured trypanosomes in cattle, in *The Proc. Int. Scientific Council for Trypanosomiasis Research and Control,* 17th Meeting, Arusha, Tanzania, 1981, in press.
64. **Luckins A. G., Rae, P., and Gray, M. A.,** Development of local skin reactions in rabbits infected with metacyclic forms of *Trypanosoma congolense* cultured *in vitro, Ann. Trop. Med. Parasitol.,* 75, 998, 1981.
65. **Bolton, M. A.,** The local reaction in cattle at the site of infection with *Trypanosoma congolense,* in a report to the government of Southern Rhodesia on Investigation into the Immunological Response of Cattle and Laboratory Animals to Trypanosomiasis, No. 2064, Food and Agriculture Organization, Rome, 1965, 26.
66. **Roberts, C. J., Gray, M. A., and Gray, A. R.,** Local skin reactions in cattle at the site of infection with *Trypanosoma congolense* by *Glossina moristans* and *G. tachinoides, Trans. R. Soc. Trop. Med. Hyg.,* 63, 620, 1969.
67. **Gray, A. R. and Luckins, A. G.,** The initial stage of infection with cyclically transmitted *Trypanosoma congolense* in rabbits, calves and sheep, *J. Comp. Pathol.,* 90, 499, 1980.
68. **Gray, A. R. and Luckins, A. G.,** Features of epidemiological importance in the development of cyclically transmitted stock of *Trypanosoma congolense* in vertebrate hosts, *Insect. Sci. Appl.,* 1, 69, 1980.
69. **Emery, D. L., Akol, G. W. O., Murray, M., Morrison, W. I., and Moloo, S. K.,** The chancre: early events in the pathogenesis of African trypanosomiasis in domestic livestock, in *The Host-Invader Interplay,* Van den Bossche, H., Ed., Elsevier/North-Holland, Amsterdam, 1980, 345.
70. **Emery, D. L. and Moloo, S. K.,** The sequential cellular changes in the local skin reaction produced in goats by *Glossina morsitans morsitans* infected with *Trypanosoma (Trypanozoon) brucei, Acta Trop.,* 37, 137, 1980.
71. **Emery, D. L. and Moloo, S. K.,** The dynamics of the cellular reactions elicited in the skin of goats by *Glossina morsitans morsitans* infected with *Trypanosoma (Nannomonas) congolense* or *T. (Duttonella) vivax, Acta Trop.,* 38, 15, 1981.
72. **Uilenberg, G., Maillot, L., and Giret, M.,** Etudes immunologiques sur les trypanosomes. II. Observations nouvelles sur le type antigenique de base d'une souche de *Trypanosoma congolense, Rev. Elev. Med. Vet. Pays Trop.,* 26, 27, 1973.
73. **Murray, M., Grootenhuis, J. G., Akol, G. W. O., Emergy, D. L., Shapiro, S. Z., Moloo, S. K., Dar, F., Bovell, D. L., and Paris, J.,** Potential application of research on African trypanosomiasis in wildlife and preliminary studies on animals exposed to tsetse infected with *Trypanosoma congolense,* in *Wildlife Diseases Research and Economic Development,* No. 147, Karstad, L., Nestel, B., and Graham, W., Eds., International Development Research Centre, Ottawa, 1981, 40.
74. **Fairbairn, H. and Godfrey, D. G.,** The local reaction in man at the site of infection with *Trypanosoma rhodesiense, Ann. Trop. Med. Parasitol.,* 51, 464, 1957.
75. **Dwinger, R.,** unpublished data, 1983.
76. **Akol, G. W. O. and Murray, M.,** Induction of protective immunity in cattle by cyclical infection with cloned isolates of *Trypanosoma congolense,* in preparation.
77. **Willett, K.C. and Gordon, R. M.,** Studies on the deposition migration and development in the blood forms of trypanosomes belonging to the *Trypanosoma brucei* group. II, *Ann. Trop. Med. Parasitol.,* 51, 471, 1957.
78. **Akol, G. W. O. and Emery, D. L.,** unpublished data, 1983.
79. **Akol, G. W. O.,** unpublished data, 1983.
80. **Gray, M. A., Cunningham, I., Gardiner, P. R., Taylor, A. M., and Luckins, A. G.,** Cultivation of infective forms of *Trypanosoma congolense* from trypanosomes in the proboscis of *Glossina morsitans, Parasitology,* 82, 81, 1981.

81. **Nantulya, V. M., Doyle, J. J., and Jenni, L.,** Studies on *Trypanosoma (Nannomonas) congolense.* IV. Experimental immunisation of mice against tsetse fly challenge, *Parasitology,* 80, 133, 1980.

82. **Luckins, A. G., Rae, P. F., and Gray, A. R.,** Infection, immunity and the development of local skin reactions in rabbits infected with cyclically-transmitted stocks of *Trypanosoma congolense, Ann. Trop. Med. Parasitol.,* in press.

83. **Akol, G. W. O. and Hirumi, H.,** unpublished data, 1983.

84. **Jenni, L.,** Comparisons of antigenic types of *Trypanosoma (T) brucei* strains transmitted by *Glossina m. morsitans, Acta Trop.,* 34, 35, 1977.

85. **Nantulya, V. M., Doyle, J. J., and Jenni, L.,** Studies on *Trypanosoma (Nannomonas) congolense.* II. Antigenic variation in three cyclically transmitted stocks, *Parasitology,* 80, 123, 1980.

86. **Nantulya, V. M. and Musoke, A. J.,** unpublished data, 1983.

87. **Le Ray, D., Barry, J. D., and Vickerman, K.,** Antigenic heterogeneity of metacyclic forms of *Trypanosoma brucei, Nature (London),* 273, 300, 1978.

88. **Hajduk, S. and Vickerman, K.,** Antigenic differentiation of *Trypanosoma brucei:* studies on metacyclic and first parasitaemia populations, *Trans. R. Soc. Trop. Med. Hyg.,* 75, 145, 1981.

89. **Nantulya, V. M., Musoke, A. J., Moloo, S. K., and Ngaira, J. M.,** Analysis of the variable antigen composition of *Trypanosoma brucei* metacyclic trypanosomes using monoclonal antibodies, *Acta Trop.,* 40, 19, 1983.

90. **Esser, K. M., Schoenbechler, M. J., and Gingrich, J. B.,** *Trypanosoma rhodesiense* blood forms express all antigen specificities relevant to protection against metacyclic (insect form) challenge, *J. Immunol.,* 129, 1715, 1982.

91. **De Gee, A. L. W., Shah, S. D., and Doyle, J. J.,** An attempt to immunise against *Trypanosoma vivax* by cyclical infection followed by treatment, in Host-Parasite Relationships in *Trypanosoma (Duttonella) vivax* with Special Reference to the Influence of Antigenic Variation, Ph.D. thesis, University of Utrecht, The Netherlands, 1980, 113.

92. **Emery, D. L., Moloo, S. K., and Murray, M.,** unpublished data, 1983.

93. **Nantulya, V. M., Musoke, A. J., Rurangirwa, F. R., and Moloo, S. K.,** Resistance of cattle to cyclical challenge with *Trypanosoma brucei* or *T. congolense* following self-cure from syringe-passaged infections, submitted.

94. **Musoke, A. J. and Nantulya, V. M.,** unpublished data, 1983.

95. **Ashcroft, M. T.,** The polymorphism of *Trypanosoma brucei* and *T. rhodesiense,* its relationship to relapses and remissions of infections in white rats, and the effect of cortisone, *Ann. Trop. Med. Parasitol.,* 51, 301, 1957.

96. **Barry, J. D., Le Ray, D., and Herbert, W. J.,** Infectivity and virulence of *Trypanosoma (Trypanozoon) brucei* for mice: dissociation of virulence and VAT in relation to pleomorphism, *J. Comp. Pathol.,* 89, 465, 1979.

97. **Sedashonga, C. and Black, S. J.,** Humoral responses against *Trypanosoma brucei* variable surface antigen are induced by degenerating parasites, *Parasite Immunol.,* 4, 245, 1982.

98. **Black, S. J., Jack, R. M., and Morrison, W. I.,** Host: parasite interactions which influence the virulence of *Trypanosoma (Trypanozoon) brucei brucei* organisms, *Acta Trop.,* in press.

99. **Black, S. J., Sendashonga, C. N., Lalor, P. A., Whitelaw, D. D., Jack, R. M., Morrison, W. I., and Murray, M.,** Regulation of the growth and differentiation of *Trypanosoma (Trypanozoon) brucei brucei* in resistant (C57BL/6) and susceptible (C3H/He) mice, *Parasite Immunol.,* in press.

100. **Shapiro, S. Z.,** unpublished data, 1983.

101. **Vickerman, K. and Barry, J. D.,** African trypanosomiasis, in *Immunology of Parasitic Infections,* Cohen, S. and Warren, K. S., Eds. Blackwell Scientific, Oxford, 1982, 204.

102. **Murray, P. K., Jennings, F. W., Murray, M., and Urquhart, G. M.,** The nature of immunosuppression in *Trypanosoma brucei* infections in mice. II. The role of the T and B lymphocytes, *Immunology,* 27, 825, 1974.

103. **Hudson, K. M., Byner, C., Freeman, J., and Terry, R. J.,** Immunodepression, high IgM levels and evasion of the immune response in murine trypanosomiasis, *Nature (London),* 264, 256, 1976.

104. **Houba, V., Brown, K. N., and Allison, A. C.,** Heterophile antibodies, M-antiglobulins and immunoglobulins in experimental trypanosomiasis, *Clin. Exp. Immunol.,* 4, 113, 1969.

105. **Greenwood, B. M., Whittle, H. C., and Molyneux, D. H.,** Immunosuppression in Gambian trypanosomiasis, *Trans. R. Soc. Trop. Med. Hyg.,* 67, 846, 1973.

106. **Scott, J. M., Pegram, R. G., Holmes, P. H., Pay, T. W. F., Knight, P. A., Jennings, F. W., and Urquhart, G. M.,** Immunosuppression in bovine trypanosomiasis: field studies using foot-and-mouth disease vaccine and clostridial vaccine, *Trop. Anim. Health Prod.,* 9, 159, 1977.

107. **Whitelaw, D. D., Scott, J. M., Reid, H. W., Holmes, P. H., Jennings, F. W., and Urquhart, G. M.,** Immunosuppression in bovine trypanosomiasis: studies with louping ill vaccine, *Res. Vet. Sci.,* 26, 102, 1979.

108. **Rurangirwa, F. R., Musoke, A. J., Nantulya, V. N., and Tabel, H.,** Immune response of *Trypanosoma congolense* infected cattle to *Brucella abortus* vaccine, *Parasite Immunol.,* in press.

109. **Goodwin, L. G., Green, D. G., Guy, M. W., and Voller, A.,** Immunosuppression during trypanosomiasis, *Br. J. Exp. Pathol.,* 53, 40, 1972.

110. **Corsini, A. C., Clayton, C., Askonas, B. A., and Ogilvie, B. M.,** Suppressor cells and loss of B-cell potential in mice infected with *Trypanosoma brucei, Clin. Exp. Immunol.,* 29, 122, 1977.

111. **Pearson, T. W., Roelants, G. E., Lundin, L. B., and Mayor-Withey, K. S.,** Immune depression in trypanosome-infected mice. I. Depressed T lymphocyte responses, *Eur. J. Immunol.,* 8, 723, 1978.

112. **Kar, S. K., Roelants, G. E., Mayor-Withey, K. S., and Pearson, T. W.,** Immunodepression in trypanosome-infected mice. VI. Comparison of immune responses of different lymphoid organs, *Eur. J. Immunol.,* 11, 100, 1981.

113. **Freeman, J., Hudson, K. M., Longstaffe, J. A., and Terry, R. J.,** Immunodepression in trypanosome infections, *Parasitology,* 67, xxiii, 1973.

114. **Askonas, B. A., Corsini, A. C., Clayton, C. E., and Ogilvie, B. M.,** Functional depletion of T- and B-memory cells and other lymphoid cell subpopulations during trypanosomiasis, *Parasitology,* 36, 313, 1979.

115. **Mansfield, J. M. and Wallace, J. H.,** Suppression of cell-mediated immunity in experimental African trypanosomiasis, *Infect. Immun.,* 10, 335, 1974.

116. **Urquhart, G. M., Murray, M., Murray, P. K., Jennings, F. W., and Bate, E.,** Immunosuppression in *Trypanosoma brucei* infections in rats and mice, *Trans. R. Soc. Trop. Med. Hyg.,* 67, 528, 1973.

117. **Phillips, R. S., Selby, G. R., and Wakelin, D.,** The effect of *Plasmodium berghei* and *Trypanosoma brucei* infections on the immune expulsion of the nematode *Trichuris muris* from mice, *Int. J. Parasitol.,* 4, 409, 1974.

118. **Reid, H. W., Buxton, D., Finlayson, J., and Holmes, P. H.,** Effect of chronic *Trypanosoma brucei* infection on the course of louping ill virus infection in mice, *Infect. Immun.,* 23, 192, 1979.

119. **Allt, G., Evans, E. M. E., Evans, D. H. L., and Targett, G. A. T.,** Effect of infection with trypanosomes on the development of experimental allergic neuritis in rabbits, *Nature (London),* 233, 197, 1971.

120. **MacKenzie, A. R., Sibley, P. R., and White, B. P.,** Differential suppression of experimental allergic diseases in rats infected with trypanosomes, *Parasite Immunol.,* 1, 49, 1979.

121. **Sacks, D. L. and Askonas, B. A.,** Trypanosome-induced suppression of anti-parasite responses during experimental African trypanosomiasis, *Eur. J. Immunol.,* 10, 971, 1980.

122. **Jayawardena, A. N. and Waksman, B. H.,** Suppressor cells in experimental trypanosomiasis, *Nature (London),* 265, 539, 1977.

123. **Pearson, T. W., Roelants, G. E., Pinder, M., Lundin, L. B., and Mayor-Withey, K. S.,** Immune depression in trypanosome-infected mice. III. Suppressor cells, *Eur. J. Immunol.,* 9, 200, 1979.

124. **Wellhausen, S. R. and Mansfield, J. M.,** Lymphocyte function in experimental African trypanosomiasis. II. Splenic suppressor cell activity, *J. Immunol.,* 122, 818, 1979.

125. **Assoku, R. K. G., Hazlett, C. A., and Tizard, I.,** Immunosuppression in experimental African trypanosomiasis: polyclonal B-cell activation and mitogenicity of trypanosome-derived saturated fatty acids, *Int. Arch. Allergy Appl. Immunol.,* 9, 298, 1979.

126. **Clayton, C. E., Sacks, D. L., Ogilvie, B. M., and Askonas, B. A.,** Membrane fractions of trypanosomes mimic the immunosuppressive and mitogenic effects of living parasites on the host, *Parasite Immunol.,* 1, 241, 1979.

127. **Mansfield, J. M. and Bagasra, O.,** Lymphocyte function in experimental African trypanosomiasis. I. B cell responses to helper T cell-independent and -dependent antigens, *J. Immunol.,* 120, 759, 1978.

128. **Bagasra, O., Schell, R. F., and Le Frock, J. L.,** Evidence for depletion of Ia + macrophages and associated immunosuppression in African trypanosomiasis, *Infect. Immun.,* 32, 188, 1981.

129. **Grosskinsky, C. M. and Askonas, B. A.,** Macrophages as primary targets and mediators of immune dysfunction in African trypanosomiasis, *Infect. Immun.,* 33, 149, 1981.

130. **Morrison, W. I., and Murray, M.,** Lymphoid changes in African trypanosomiasis, in *Pathogenicity of Trypanosomes,* No. 13e, Losos, G. and Chouinard, A., Eds., International Development Research Centre, Ottawa, 1979, 154.

131. **Masake, R. A. and Morrison, W. I.,** Evaluation of the functional and structural changes in the lymphoid organs of Boran cattle infected with *Trypanosoma vivax, Am. J. Vet. Res.,* 42, 1738, 1981.

132. **Clarkson, M. J., Penhale, W. J., and McKenna, R. B.,** Progressive serum protein changes in experimental infections in calves with *Trypanosoma vivax, J. Comp. Pathol.,* 85, 397, 1975.

133. **Luckins, A. G. and Mehlitz, D.,** Observations on serum immunoglobulin levels in cattle infected with *Trypanosoma brucei, T. vivax* and *T. congolense, Ann. Trop. Med. Parasitol.,* 70, 479, 1976.

134. **Kobayashi, A. and Tizard, I. R.,** The response to *Trypanosoma congolense* infection in calves: determination of immunoglobulins IgG₁, IgG₂, IgM and C3 levels and the complement-fixing antibody titres during the course of infection, *Tropenmed. Parasitol.,* 27, 411, 1976.

135. **Nielsen, K., Sheppard, J., Holmes, W., and Tizard, I.,** Experimental bovine trypanosomiasis: changes in serum immunoglobulins, complement and complement components in infected animals, *Immunology,* 35, 817, 1978.

136. **Loor, F.,** On the existence of heterospecific antibodies in sera from rabbits immunised against tobacco mosaic virus determinants, *Immunology,* 21, 557, 1971.

137. **Miller, H. R. P., Ternynck, T., and Avrameas, S.,** Synthesis of antibody and immunoglobulins without detectable antibody formation in cells responding to horseradish peroxidase, *J. Immunol.,* 114, 626, 1975.

138. **Poskitt, D. C., Frost, H., Cahil, R. N. P., and Trnka, Z.,** The appearance of non-specific antibody-forming cells in the efferent lymph draining antigen-stimulated single lymph nodes, *Immunology,* 33, 81, 1977.

139. **Julius, M. H.,** Cellular interactions involved in T-dependent B-cell activation, *Immunol. Today,* 3, 295, 1982.

140. **Holmes, P. H., Mammo, E., Thomson, A., Knight, P. A., Lucken, R., Murray, P. K., Murray, M., Jennings, F. W., and Urquhart, G. M.,** Immunosuppression in bovine trypanosomiasis, *Vet. Rec.,* 95, 86, 1974.

141. **Sollod, A. E. and Frank, G. H.,** Bovine trypanosomiasis: effect on the immune response of the infected host, *Am. J. Vet. Res.,* 40, 658, 1979.

142. **Rurangirwa, F. R., Tabel, H., Losos, G., Masiga, W. N., and Mwambu, P.,** Immunosuppressive effect of *Trypanosoma congolense* and *Trypanosoma vivax* on the secondary immune response of cattle to *Mycoplasma mycoides subsp. mycoides,* *Res. Vet. Sci.,* 25, 395, 1978.

143. **Rurangirwa, F. R., Tabel, H., Losos, G. J., and Tizard, I. R.,** Suppression of antibody response to *Leptospira biflexa* and *Brucella abortus* and recovery from immunosuppression after Berenil treatment, *Infect. Immun.,* 26, 822, 1979.

144. **Rurangirwa, F. R., Mushi, E. Z., Tabel, H., Tizard, I. R., and Losos, G. J.,** The effect of *Trypanosoma congolense* and *T. vivax* infections on the antibody response of cattle to live rinderpest virus vaccine, *Res. Vet. Sci.,* 28, 264, 1980.

145. **Masake, R. A., Pearson, T. W., Wells, P., and Roelants, G. E.,** The *in vitro* response to antigens of leucocytes from cattle infected with *Trypanosoma congolense,* *Clin. Exp. Immunol.,* 43, 583, 1981.

146. **Roelants, G. E. and Morrison, W. I.,** unpublished data, 1983.

147. **Valli, V. E. O., Forsberg, C. M., and Lumsden, J. H.,** The pathogenesis of *Trypanosoma congolense* infection in calves. III. Neutropenia and myeloid response, *Vet. Pathol.,* 16, 96, 1979.

148. **Kaaya, G. P., Valli, V. E. O., Maxie, M. G., and Losos, G. J.,** Inhibition of bovine bone marrow granulocyte/macrophage colony formation *in vitro* by serum collected from cattle infected with *Trypanosoma vivax* or *Trypanosoma congolense,* *Tropenmed. Parasitol.,* 30, 230, 1979.

149. **Nielsen, K., Sheppard, J., Holmes, W., and Tizard, I.,** Experimental bovine trypanosomiasis: changes in the catabolism of serum immunoglobulins and complement components in infected cattle, *Immunology,* 35, 811, 1978.

150. **Sharpe, R. T., Langley, A. M., Mowat, G. N., MacAskill, J. A., and Holmes, P. H.,** Immunosuppression in bovine trypanosomiasis: respose of cattle infected with *Trypanosoma congolense* to foot-and-mouth disease vaccination and subsequent live virus challenge, *Res. Vet. Sci.,* 32, 289, 1982.

150a. **Ilemobade, A. A., Adegboye, D. S., Onaviran, O., and Chima, J. C.,** Immunodepressive effects of trypanosomal infection of cattle immunized against contagious bovine pleuropneumonia, *Parasite Immunol.,* 4, 273, 1982.

151. **Nantulya, V. N., Musoke, A. J., Rurangirwa, F. R., Barbet, A. F., Ngaira, J. M., and Kitende, J. M.,** Immune depression in African trypanosomiasis: the role of antigenic competition, *Clin. Exp. Immunol.,* 47, 234, 1982.

152. **Morrison, W. I.,** unpublished data, 1983.

153. **Luckins, A. G. and Gray, A. R.,** Interference with anti-trypanosome immune responses in rabbits infected with cyclically-transmitted *Trypanosoma congolense,* *Parasite Immunol.,* in press.

154. **Murray, M., Moloo, S. K., and Dwinger, R.,** unpublished data, 1983.

155. **Morrison, W. I., Wells, P. W., Moloo, S. K., Paris, J., and Murray, M.,** Interference in the establishment of superinfections with *Trypanosoma congolense* in cattle, *J. Parasitol.,* 68, 755, 1982.

156. **Wilson, A. J., Paris, J., and Davidson, C. R.,** A study of the development of infections by different trypanosome species in cattle treated regularly with diminazene aceturate, in *Proc. Int. Scientific Council for Trypanosomiasis Research and Control,* No. 109, Dakar, Senegal, OAU/STRC, 1975, 90.

157. **Chandler, R. L.,** Studies on the tolerance of N'Dama cattle to trypanosomiasis, *J. Comp. Pathol.,* 68, 253, 1958.

158. **Desowitz, R. S.,** Studies on immunity and host parasite relationships. I. The immunological response of resistant and susceptible breeds of cattle to trypanosomal challenge, *Ann. Trop. Med. Parasitol.,* 53, 293, 1959.

159. **Toure, S. M., Gueye, A., Seye, M., Ba, M. A., and Mane, A.,** A comparison between the pathology of a natural trypanosome infection in Zebu and N'Dama cattle, *Rev. Elev. Med. Vet. Pays Trop.,* 31, 293, 1978.

160. **Saror, D. I., Ilemobade, A. A., and Nuru, S.,** The haematology of N'Dama and Zebu cattle experimentally infected with *Trypanosoma vivax,* in *Int. Scientific Council for Trypanosomiasis Research and Control,* No. 111, Yaounde, Cameroon, OAU/STRC, 1981, 287.

161. **Bourn, D. and Scott, M.,** The successful use of work oxen in agricultural development of tsetse infested land in Ethiopia, *Trop. Anim. Health Prod.,* 10, 191, 1978.

162. **Desowitz, R. S.,** African trypanosomes, in *Immunity to Parasitic Animals,* Vol. 2, Jackson, G. J., Herman, R., and Singer, I., Eds., Appleton-Century-Crofts, New York, 1970, 551.

163. **Fiennes, R. N. T. W.,** Pathogenesis and pathology of animal trypanosomiasis, in *The African Trypanosomiases,* Mulligan, H. W., Ed., Allen and Unwin, London, 1970, 729.

Chapter 7

COMPLEMENT IN TRYPANOSOMIASIS

Klaus H. Nielsen

TABLE OF CONTENTS

I. INTRODUCTION

The complement system is an important component of the overall defense mechanism against foreign antigens. Thus, complement is responsible for the nonspecific destruction through lysis of invading cells, specificity being imparted in most instances by natural or acquired antibody. In addition, activation of complement sets in motion a number of associated functions, such as phagocytosis, immune adherence, kinin and anaphylatoxin production, and immunoconglutination. These functions have a single goal: the elimination of antigen. Therefore, their impairment may have grave consequences for the host.

Activation of complement in the trypanosome-infected host is a well-described phenomenon (recently reviewed in References 1 to 3). There are basically two separate areas to be considered with respect to complement in the host-parasite relationship. These are the ability of the host defense mechanisms including complement to eliminate the parasite, and the influence of the parasite on the host defenses to avoid elimination. Some of the possible interactions are presented in Figure 1, along with some of the consequences of host complement activation by trypanosomes.

II. HOST ELIMINATION OF TRYPANOSOMES

A. Antibody Mediated

Using mice infected with *Trypanosoma brucei*, Stevens and Moulton[4] demonstrated that peritoneal macrophages phagocytosed and digested the parasites in vivo and in vitro. Interestingly, attachment and digestion appeared to be associated with the flagellum. Normal mouse peritoneal macrophages lacked these abilities, even when supplied with antibody and complement. Similar experiments with deer mice suggested an early production of opsonic antibody which was not apparent in late infection. Their results indicated that antibody and complement were important mediators of macrophage ingestion of *T. brucei*, but that this defense mechanism was largely ineffective as a result of antigenic variation and Ferrante et al.,[6] using *T. lewisi*-infected rats, concluded that while phagocytosis and hepatic clearance were important in removing parasites from circulation, these activities were unrelated to complement-fixing antibody and complement. In a previous paper, Ferrante and Jenkin[7] showed that dividing and adult forms of *T. lewisi* shared common antigens but that adult forms of the parasite were covered with noncomplement fixing, nonopsonic host antibody. Thus, contrary to earlier findings by D'Alesandro[8] who showed antigenic differences between early and late infection stage parasites, Ferrante and Jenkin[7] suggest that antigenic variation does not occur but rather that parasite antigenic determinants are occluded. These data are partly in disagreement with those of Nogueira et al.[9] who showed C3 receptor-dependent ingestion by macrophages of *T. cruzi*-infected mice.

More recently, MacAskill et al.[10] demonstrated that radioactively labeled *T. brucei* were cleared in mice by hepatic phagocytosis dependent on antibody and C3. Interestingly, no evidence to suggest involvement of activated macrophages was found. Again, these findings do not support those of Murray et al.,[11] Corsini et al.,[12] or Stevens and Moulton.[4] That macrophages play an important role is clear from the above discussion and from the contributions of Lumsden and Herbert[13] and Goodwin.[14] Similarly, antibody-dependent cellular cytotoxicity has been demonstrated to participate in protection against *T. cruzi* epimastigote forms[15-18] and trypomastigote forms.[19,20]

However, while the exact mechanisms of cellular elimination of trypanosomes cannot be resolved at present, there is mounting evidence that antibody and complement are important in clearance of the parasite either by lysis or as an immune complex.[21] Several contributions have clearly established the presence of parasite-antibody complexes both in circulation,[22] as cryoprecipitates,[23] and in tissues.[24-26] Although some variations were noted (depending

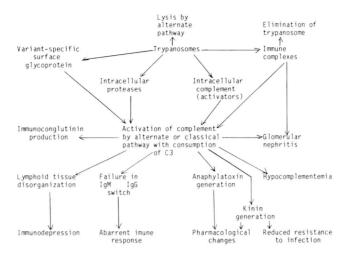

FIGURE 1. Consequences of activation of complement by trypanosomes.
(Adapted from Tizard, I., Nielsen, K. H., Seed, J. R., and Hall, J. R.,
Microbiol. Rev., 42, 661, 1978.)

on the species and strain of trypanosomes studied), complement appeared to play an important role. The role of complement has been further emphasized with regards to trypanolytic antibody. Flemmings and Diggs[27] showed that antibody-mediated cytotoxicity to *T. rhodesiense* was dependent upon an alternate pathway of complement activation. This was demonstrated by the lack of effect on lysis of EGTA and abolition of lysis by cobra venom factor (CoF)-treated or C4-deficient sera. Similar findings were reported by Jarvinen and Dalmasso.[28] These investigators showed that *T. lewisi* infection in rats resulted in activation of the classical complement pathway and to a lesser extent an alternate pathway. The importance of complement in trypanolysis was further emphasized by Balber et al.[29] and Powell and Kuhn.[30] The former investigators demonstrated the absolute complement requirement for lysis of antibody-treated *T. brucei* and *T. congolense* and that parasites surviving this treatment could eliminate or inactivate surface immune complexes, that the variant-specific glycoprotein was involved, and that survival led to antigenic variation. Powell and Kuhn[30] investigated production of trypanolytic antibody in mouse strains with differing susceptibility to *T. cruzi*. Interestingly, no apparent difference in cytolytic antibody responses of highly susceptible and resistant mice was noted. These data are in agreement with those of Kierszenbaum and Howard[31] who showed that lower antibody production to *T. cruzi* in genetically low responder mice caused increased susceptibility that could be remedied by passive transfer of antibody.

B. Nonantibody Mediated

It would appear that antibody, complement, and cells of the immune system play an important but not all-inclusive role in clearance of parasites from the host. While the exact mechanism(s) remains elusive, a second and nonspecific elimination mechanism dependent on serum factors also exists. Anziano et al.[32] demonstrated that epimastigote forms of *T. cruzi* had surface receptors for C3 and C4. This finding was supported by Nogueira et al.[33] who reported the reaction of these forms of *T. cruzi* with complement caused antibody-independent lysis, presumably through some mechanism that bound or inactivated complement components. These findings confirmed the work of Budzko et al.[34] and Kierszenbaum et al.[35] who demonstrated lysis of bloodstream forms of serum *T. cruzi* by fresh chicken serum, but not sera from man and guinea pig. In fact, in the latter communication, it was observed that chicken serum could (1) be from immunosuppressed birds and (2) act independently of calcium, thereby suggesting the activation of complement by an alternate pathway. Warren[36] had failed in similar experiments, and based on the evidence of Budzko et al.,[34] Kierszenbaum,[37] and Krettli et al.,[22] the cause of lysis may be activation of human complement through both pathways by antibody bound to membranes of *T. cruzi* isolated from blood of infected mice. In contrast, Cunningham et al.[38] reported interaction of complement from several mammalian species with *T. cruzi* in the absence of antibody. All of the above results have been disputed by Kipnis et al.[39] who demonstrated that for *T. cruzi* from irradiated mice (i.e., without antibody), to activate an alternate pathway of complement (human) pretreatment of the parasite with trypsin or sialidase was essential.

T. cyclops was lysed by normal human serum by an alternate pathway of complement activation in the absence of antibody. This may be a result of *T. cyclops* expressing surface complement activators which, unlike *T. brucei*, makes it susceptible to lysis by the alternate pathway of complement activation.[40] However, Rifkin[41] has shown lysis of *T. brucei* by normal human serum, in the absence of factors essential to the classical or alternate complement pathways, by a single nonimmunoglobulin serum protein of a high molecular weight (500,000 daltons).

Although similar in its mechanism to antibody-mediated trypanolysis, nonantibody-mediated destruction of parasites remains a controversial topic. It would seem unreasonable that trypanosomes should not be phagocytosed in the classical fashion via opsonization by antibody and complement. It would also be unreasonable to suggest that trypanosomes cannot be lysed by antibody-activated complement by either pathway or both. However, while controversy will always arise where absence of antibody is indicated in direct activation of complement, such mechanisms exist as shown in the literature, the classical example being zymosan activation of complement.[24] The truth in the final analysis will probably turn out to be a combination of all the above mechanisms acting in concert to eliminate the parasite from the infected host.

III. EFFECT OF TRYPANOSOMES ON HOST COMPLEMENT

A. Immune Complex Lesions

Rhesus monkeys infected experimentally with *T. rhodesiense* were shown to have glomerular deposits of C3, properdin, and IgM, but not IgG and IgA by immunofluorescence.[24] The deposits were granular and provoked a proliferative glomerulonephritis. The sera from such monkeys were hypocomplementemic suggesting that immune complex deposition may play an active role in activation of complement. Similar findings have been reported by Lindsley et al.[25] in *T. rhodesiense*-infected rats with the additional demonstration of anti-nucleic acid (DNA and RNA) antibodies in serum and activation of complement by the classical and alternate pathways. Lindsley et al.[43] also demonstrated the presence of immune complexes in rabbits infected with *T. rhodesiense*. In contrast to the findings in monkeys, these immune complexes were found to contain IgM and IgG and usually C3.

In human cases of sleeping sickness a high level of serum immune complexes and/or cryoglobulins has frequently been found.[23,44] Tissue damage by immune complexes, however, has not been established in man except for, perhaps, disseminated intravascular coagulation.[45] In a recent study, Lambert et al.[46] found large amounts of immune complexes in serum and cerebrospinal fluid in patients with *T. brucei gambiense* infection. These authors observed a negative correlation between serum C3 values and immune complex levels as measured by a C1q binding assay. However, they did suggest that the circulating immune complexes were an expression of polyclonal B cell activation as shown by a positive correlation between immune complex levels, and IgM levels or rheumatoid factor-like anti-immunoglobulin antibodies. Rheumatoid factor-like IgM has also been described in rats infected with *T. lewisi*.[47] The IgG antibody response to *T. lewisi* was amplified by this rheumatoid factor-like IgM, thereby providing protection. Autoantibodies have been described in other animal species infected with trypanosomes. Thus, Mackenzie et al.[48] detected antiliver, anti-Wassermann, and antifibrinogen antibodies in cattle infected with *T. brucei* and/or *T. congolense*. Similar autoantibodies have been described in rabbit and human sera but not in lion and hyena sera.[48]

The immunopathology of trypanosomiasis will be described elsewhere, however, immune complex and autoantibody activation of complement are probably important mechanisms of tissue damage, particularly as they relate to thrombosis,[49] erythrocyte destruction by "innocent bystander" lysis,[50] and damage to small vessels in muscles and brain.[51]

B. Activation of Complement in the Trypanosome-Infected Host

Cobra venom factor injected into mice infected with *T. cruzi* caused a significant increase in parasitemia and mortality when compared to untreated infected mice.[34,37] This finding amply demonstrated that complement was important for in vivo control of parasitemia and it was confirmed by Cunningham et al.[38] This finding, however, was not confirmed by Dalmasso and Jarvinen,[52] studying the infection of mice and guinea pigs with a different strain of *T. cruzi*. Mice genetically deficient in C5 did not have higher parasitemias than normal mice, and measurement of serum C3 revealed no differences in serum levels of the two groups. Similar studies with guinea pigs genetically deficient in C4 and normal guinea pigs gave no indications of differences in the course of infection. These experiments led the authors to suggest a minor, if any, role of at least the classical complement pathway. Other experiments by the same group[28] with *T. lewisi*-infected rats have shown tremendous decreases in serum complement, C3, and C4 levels. The serum C3 levels correlated with parasitemia, returning to normal after elimination of the trypanosomes. Interestingly, C6 levels were not decreased as measured by a hemolytic assay, and the parasitemia in C4-deficient rats were not significantly different from those of normal rats. This was also true in C3 or late complement component-depleted animals. It was concluded that the classical pathway of complement activation resulted from *T. lewisi* infection with consumption of early acting components as well as in low level activation of the alternate pathway. Thus, it was determined that complement does not play a major role in elimination of *T. lewisi* infection in rats. These findings were also the case in mice infected with *T. musculi*.[53]

Cattle experimentally infected with *T. congolense* showed marked and persistent decreases in total hemolytic complement, C1, C1q, and C3.[54] Serum properdin levels correlated with parasitemia and C8 appeared not to be activated, indicating consumption by the classical and an alternate pathway without either sequence reaching the terminal stages. In the same study,[55] a marked increase in the catabolic rate of C1 and C3 was found, possibly contributing to the overall low complement levels. These findings are in agreement with the low C3 levels in *T. congolense*-infected cattle observed by Kobayashi and Tizard[56] and hypocomplementemia of *T. congolense*- and *T. vivax*-infected cattle described by Rurangirwa et al.[57]

Hypocomplementemia has been reported in various species infected with the *T. brucei* group of trypanosomes. For example, Rhesus monkeys infected with *T. rhodesiense* developed substantial hypocomplementemia associated with glomerulonephritis.[24] Some of these animals had low C3 and C4 levels, also. In human cases of trypanosomiasis a persistent low level of total hemolytic complement has been observed.[23,45] In addition, low levels of C4, C4, and factor B have been recorded,[45] indicating activation of both classical and alternate pathways. These findings are substantiated by high immunoconglutinin levels both in man and experimental animals.[49,58-63] The latter report also described hypocomplementemia in mice infected with *T. rhodesiense*.

Other contributions, however, partially contradict the above findings. Normal and T cell-depleted mice chronically infected with *T. brucei* were shown to have elevated C3 levels early in the infection, the levels subsequently returned to normal.[64] These authors did not find significant differences in parasitemia between normal and C3-depleted mice, thus, casting considerable doubt on the role of complement in control of infection. Further doubt has been cast on the effectivity of complement in control of parasitemia by Tizard et al.,[65] who found an inhibition of the immunoconglutinin response to *Brucella abortus* S19 in cattle infected with *T. congolense*. This finding may be explicable in two ways. Profound immunosuppression induced by trypanosomes has been described,[66-71] and since immunoconglutinin is an autoantibody, its production would presumably also be depressed. Alternatively, depletion of some complement components during trypanosome infection may result in diminished availability of immunoconglutinogen. Hypercatabolism of immunoglobulin isotypes may also play a role.[55] An alternate explanation for the lack of immunoconglutinin response reported by Tizard et al.[65] may be that *B. abortus* S19 is independently capable of activating complement (unpublished data) thus leading to confusion with regards to which microorganism is responsible for immunoconglutinogen production.

C. In Vitro Activation of Complement by Trypanosomes

The obvious need to resolve the mechanism(s) by which trypanosomes activate complement is not readily accomplished by studying the in vivo response. Therefore, it became necessary to study the interaction of the parasite with complement in vitro. The effects of complement on viable trypanosomes have been described above (see Section II.B). To avoid repetition, only antigens or fragments of trypanosomes will be considered in this discussion.

The variant-specific surface antigen of *T. brucei* has been shown to activate human complement by the classical pathway.[72] These authors also described a second factor, capable of activating the alternate pathway. Interestingly, the variant antigen preferentially consumed C1, C4, and C3 (only slightly), however, intradermal inoculation of the purified variant antigen into rats suggested anaphylatoxin production. These findings are important in that the variant antigen may be released during trypanosome destruction at each parasitemia wave, thereby causing considerable utilization of complement. Similarly, Nielsen and Sheppard[73] and Nielsen et al.[74] demonstrated that both *T. congolense* and *T. lewisi* released factors upon autolysis that activated bovine (and to a lesser extent human and guinea pig complement) at the C1 level. Attempts to characterize this factor revealed the presence of a second and minor component, probably a protease, that also activated bovine complement.[74] The primary component was found to be a glycolipid based on various chemical procedures and the correlation between complement activation and hexose content was positive.[74,75] The potency of this factor as a complement activator was demonstrated in that 1.0 mg injected intravenously into a rat completely destroyed any hemolytic activity in its serum.[76] A similar material has been isolated from *T. cruzi*.[38,77] This factor was found to be nonproteinacious with a molecular weight of 23,000 daltons and could activate mouse, human, and guinea pig complement in vitro and mouse complement in vivo, rapidly.

T. theileri was demonstrated to activate bovine complement by both the classical and an alternate pathway.[65] This activation was mediated by living or autolyzed trypanosomes. Due to the large numbers necessary to induce this, it is questionable whether this is detrimental to the host.

D. Consequences of Complement Activation In Vivo

Many of the proposed consequences of complement activation in vivo in a trypanosome-infected animal are based on attempts to use our current knowledge of immunology to explain immunological and/or pathological findings. Some of these consequences are outlined in Figure 1.

In experimental animals, complement depletion has been shown to have a disruptive effect on the architecture of lymphoid tissue and processing of antigen.[78-80] Similarly, in trypanosomiasis T-dependent areas of lymphoid tissues are disrupted,[11,51,81] and uncontrolled proliferation of plasma cells has been observed[82] as well as interference with T and B cell cooperation in the immune response.[51,82] Therefore, it might be deduced that complement activation may play a role in lymphoid tissue disorganization and interfere with normal cellular function, leading to and perhaps partly responsible for immunodepression, another widely observed phenomenon in trypanosomiasis.[66-70]

A further consequence of in vivo complement activation may be interference with the switch mechanism regulating isotype production of antibody.[79,83-85] This is particularly evident in the IgM-to-IgG switch of CoF decomplemented animals[83] and greatly reduced IgA and IgE responses have also been shown.[84,86] Complement-depleted animals also have a greatly reduced capacity to respond to thymus-dependent antigens.[84,85] These findings correspond to a number of observations in trypanosomiasis. Thus, elevated IgM levels is a well-established finding in most species studied.[23,54,56,68,69,88-93] This macroglobulinemia is closely associated with decreased IgA and IgE immunoglobulin levels[54] and sometimes with unchanged IgG levels,[54,93] (although frequently IgG levels are also somewhat increased.[56,93-95]) Thus, the changes in IgG levels are inconsistent between animals experimentally depleted of complement and the findings in trypanosome infection.

Biologically active peptides such as kinins may readily be generated from complement activation, particularly through immune complexes, but also perhaps through direct activation by microorganisms. Elevated blood kinins have been described in trypanosome-infected animals.[26,96-104] The induction of kinins and its consequences to them are described in detail elsewhere (see Chapter 3). Biologically active products of complement activation other than kinins may include anaphylatoxins generated as C3 and C5 split products.

Increased susceptibility to secondary infection, frequently the cause of mortality, has been described in animals infected with trypanosomes.[51] Increased susceptibility to tumors has also been demonstrated.[105] This enhanced susceptibility to other invasive agents may largely be a result of the well-described immunodepression phenomenon (referred to above); however, a report by Nielsen et al.[76] clearly showed that rats decomplemented with a complement-activating factor isolated from *T. lewisi* or infected with *T. lewisi* were far more susceptible to *Salmonella typhimurium* infection. These rats died much more rapidly and in greater numbers than rats decomplemented with CoF. Thus, the increased susceptibility may be partly a consequence of complement activation, as C3 is of considerable significance in protecting against infection,[106] but other factors cannot be excluded as contributors to this phenomenon. Cunningham et al.[107] have demonstrated that mice infected with *T. cruzi* and challenged with *Aeromonas hydrophila* were actually less susceptible than control mice, regardless of whether mice strains susceptible or resistant to *T. cruzi* were used. The resistance to *A. hydrophila* waned in the mice genetically susceptible to *T. cruzi*. The level of resistance to *A. hydrophila* was dependent on the infective dose of *T. cruzi* used and could apparently be transferred passively. Thus, an inconsistent picture emerges with regard to the level of susceptibility (or resistance) in the trypanosome-infected host to secondary infection, however, it would seem unreasonable that interference with the complement system in the animal would not compromise it to bacterial infections.

IV. SUMMARY

As is clearly evident from this survey of the literature, the involvement of complement with regard to host protection and host dysfunction is not resolved. The consensus would be that with most species of trypanosomes in most hosts some activation of complement occurs by both pathways, probably by immune complexes and directly by certain parasite antigens. Although largely conjecture, complement activation could be visualized to have numerous detrimental effects on the health of the host. Disruption of lymphoid tissue architecture and deregulation of the antibody isotype switch mechanism can be demonstrated in experimentally decomplemented animals and in trypanosomiasis. Immunopharmacological events, anemia, and increased susceptibility to invasive agents are also features frequently found in the infected host, probably as a direct result of complement activation in the infection. Since complement is an important nonspecific defense mechanism, the requirement for further elucidation of its role in parasitic infections is obvious.

ACKNOWLEDGMENTS

Without the contributions of Dr. E. B. Nielsen, Mrs. R. Williams, and Mrs. L. Sroufe, this paper would not have been written on time. The generous help of Dr. F. Kierzenbaum, Department of Microbiology and Public Health, Michigan State University, East Lansing, Mich., in editing this manuscript is gratefully acknowledged.

REFERENCES

1. **Tizard, I., Nielsen, K. H., Seed, J. R., and Hall, J. R.,** Biologically active products from African trypanosomes, *Microbiol. Rev.,* 42, 661, 1978.
1a. **Fine, D. P.,** *Complement in Infectious Diseases,* CRC Press, Boca Raton, Fla., 1981.
2. **Assoku, R. K. G., Tizard, I. R., and Nielsen, K. H.,** Free fatty acids, complement activation and polyclonal B-cell stimulation as factors in the immunopathogenesis of African trypanosomiasis, *Lancet,* 2, 956, 1977.
3. **Santoro, F., Bernal, J., and Capron, A.,** Complement activation by parasites, *Acta Trop.,* 36, 5, 1979.
4. **Stevens, D. R. and Moulton, J. E.,** Ultrastructural and immunological aspects of the phagocytosis of *Trypanosoma brucei* by mouse peritoneal macrophages, *Infect. Immun.,* 19, 972, 1978.
5. **Ferrante, A. and Jenkin, C. R.,** Evidence implicating the mononuclear phagocytic system of the rat in immunity to infections with *Trypanosoma lewisi, Aust. J. Exp. Biol. Med. Sci.,* 56, 201, 1978.
6. **Ferrante, A., Jenkin, C. R., and Reade, P. C.,** Changes in the activity of the reticulo-endothelial systems of rats during an infection with *Trypanosoma lewisi, Aust. J. Exp. Biol. Med. Sci.,* 56, 47, 1978.
7. **Ferrante, A. and Jenkin, C. R.,** Surface immunoglobulins, a possible mechanism for the persistence of *Trypanosoma lewisi* in the circulation of rats, *Aust. J. Exp. Biol. Med. Sci.,* 55, 275, 1977.
8. **D'Alesandro, P. A.,** Non-pathogenic trypanosomes in rodents, in *Immunity to Parasitic Animals,* Vol. 2, Jackson, G. J. et al., Eds., Appleton-Century-Crofts, New York, 1970, 695.
9. **Nogueira, N., Gordon, S., and Cohn, Z.,** *Trypanosoma cruzi:* modification of macrophage function during infection, *J. Exp. Med.,* 146, 157, 1977.
10. **MacAskill, J. A., Holmes, P. H., Whitelaw, D. D., McConnell, I., Jennings, F. W., and Urquhart, A. M.,** Immunological clearance of ^{75}Se labelled *Trypanosoma brucei* in mice. II. Mechanisms in immune animals, *Immunology,* 40, 629, 1980.
11. **Murray, P. K., Jennings, F. W., Murray, M., and Urquhart, A. M.,** The nature of immune suppression in *Trypanosoma brucei* infection mice. I. The role of the macrophage, *Immunology,* 27, 815, 1974.
12. **Corsini, A. C., Clayton, C., Askonas, B. A., and Ogilvie, B. M.,** Suppressor cells and loss of B-cell potential in mice infected with *Trypanosoma brucei, Clin. Exp. Immunol.,* 29, 122, 1977.
13. **Lumsden, W. H. R. and Herbert, W. J.,** Phagocytosis of trypanosomes by mouse peritoneal macrophages, *Trans. R. Soc. Trop. Med. Hyg.,* 61, 142, 1967.
14. **Goodwin, L. G.,** The pathology of African trypanosomiases, *Trans. R. Soc. Trop. Med. Hyg.,* 64, 797, 1970.
15. **Olabuenaga, S., Cardonin, R., Segura, E., Rieva, N., and DeBracco, M.,** Antibody dependent cytolysis of *Trypanosoma cruzi* by human polymorphonuclear leukocytes, *Cell. Immunol.,* 45, 85, 1979.
16. **Sanderson, C., Lopez, F., and Moreno, M.,** Eosinophils and not lymphoid K cells kill *Trypanosoma cruzi* epimastigotes, *Nature (London),* 268, 340, 1977.
17. **Abrahamson, I. A. and Dias da Silva, W. D.,** Antibody-dependent cell-mediated cytotoxicity against *Trypanosoma cruzi, Parasitology,* 75, 317, 1977.
18. **Sanderson, C. J., Bunn Moreno, M. M., and Lopez, A. M.,** Antibody-dependent cell-mediated cytotoxicity of *Trypanosoma cruzi:* the release of tritium-labeled RNA, DNA and protein, *Parasitology,* 76, 299, 1978.

19. **Kierzenbaum, F. and Hayes, M. M.,** Mechanism of resistance against experimental *Trypanosoma cruzi* infection. Requirements for cellular destruction of circulating forms of *T. cruzi* in human and murine *in vitro* systems, *Immunology*, 40, 61, 1980.

20. **Kierszenbaum, F.,** Antibody-dependent killing of bloodstream forms of *Trypanosoma cruzi* by human peripheral lymphocytes, *Am. J. Trop. Med. Hyg.*, 28, 965, 1979.

21. **Lumsden, W. H. R., Herbert, W. J., and McNeillage, E. I. C.,** *Techniques with Trypanosomes*, Churchill Livingston, Edinburgh, 1973.

22. **Krettli, A. W., Weisz-Carrington, P., and Nussenzweig, R. S.,** Membrane-bound antibodies to bloodstream *Trypanosoma cruzi* in mice; strain differences in susceptibility to complement-mediated lysis, *Clin. Exp. Immunol.*, 37, 416, 1979.

23. **Greenwood, B. M. and Whittle, H. G.,** Complement activation in patients with Gambian sleeping sickness, *Clin. Exp. Immunol.*, 24, 133, 1976.

24. **Nagle, R. B., Ward, P. A., Lindsey, H. B., Sandun, E. H., Johnson, A. J., Berkawe, K. E., and Hildebrandt, P. K.,** Experimental infections with African trypanosomes. VI. Glomerulonephritis involving the alternate pathway of complement activation, *Am. J. Trop. Med. Hyg.*, 23, 15, 1974.

25. **Lindsley, H. B., Nagle, R. B., and Stechschulte, P. J.,** Proliferative glomerulonephritis, hypocomplementemia and nucleic acid antibodies in rats infected with *Trypanosoma lewisi*, *Aust. J. Exp. Biol. Med. Sci.*, 56, 201, 1978.

26. **Boreham, P. F. L. and Kimber, C. D.,** Immune complexes in trypanosomiasis of the rabbit, *Trans. R. Soc. Trop. Med. Hyg.*, 64, 168, 1970.

27. **Flemmings, B. and Diggs, C.,** Antibody-dependent cytotoxicity against *Trypanosoma rhodesiense* mediated through an alternative complement pathway, *Infect. Immun.*, 19, 928, 1978.

28. **Jarvinen, J. A. and Dalmasso, A. P.,** Complement in experimental *Trypanosoma lewisi* infections of rats, *Infect. Immun.*, 14, 894, 1976.

29. **Balber, A. E., Bangs, J. D., Janes, S. M., and Praia, R. L.,** Inactivation or elimination of potentially trypanolytic, complement-activating immune complexes by pathogenic trypanosomes, *Infect. Immun.*, 24, 617, 1979.

30. **Powell, M. R. and Kuhn, R. E.,** Measurement of cytolytic antibody in experimental Chagas' disease using a terminal radio labelling procedure, *J. Parasitol.*, 16, 399, 1980.

31. **Kierszenbaum, F. and Howard, J. G.,** Mechanisms of resistance against experimental *Trypanosoma cruzi* infection: the importance of antibodies and antibody forming capacity in the Biozzi high and low responder mice, *J. Immunol.*, 116, 1208, 1976.

32. **Anziano, D., Dalmasso, A., Lelchuck, R., and Vasquez, C.,** Role of complement in immune lysis of *Trypanosoma cruzi*, *Infect. Immun.*, 6, 860, 1972.

33. **Nogueira, N., Branca, C., and Cohn, Z.,** Studies on the selective lysis and purification of *Trypanosoma cruzi*, *J. Exp. Med.*, 142, 224, 1975.

34. **Budzko, D. B., Pizzimenti, M. C., and Kierszenbaum, F.,** Effects of complement depletion in experimental Chagas' disease: immune lysis of virulent blood forms of *Trypanosoma cruzi*, *Infect. Immun.*, 11, 86, 1975.

35. **Kierszenbaum, F., Ivanyi, J., and Budzko, D. B.,** Mechanisms of natural resistance to trypanosomal infection. Role of complement in avian resistance to *Trypanosoma cruzi* infection, *Immunology*, 30, 1, 1976.

36. **Warren, L. A.,** Biochemical studies on chicken macrophages infected in vitro with *Trypanosoma cruzi*, *Exp. Parasitol.*, 7, 82, 1958.

37. **Kierszenbaum, F.,** Cross-reactivity of lytic antibodies against blood forms of *Trypanosoma cruzi*, *J. Parasitol.*, 62, 134, 1976.

38. **Cunningham, D. S., Craig, W. H., and Kuhn, R. E.,** Reduction of complement levels in mice infected with *Trypanosoma cruzi*, *J. Parasitol.*, 64, 1044, 1978.

39. **Kipnis, T. L., David, J. R., Alper, C. A., Sher, A., and de Silva, W. D.,** Enzymatic treatment transforms trypostigotes of *Trypanosoma cruzi* into activates of alternative complement pathway and potentiates their uptake by macrophages, *Proc. Natl. Acad. Sci. U.S.A.*, 78, 602, 1981.

40. **Kierszenbaum, F. and Weinman, D.,** Antibody-independent activation of the alternative complement pathway in human serum by parasitic cells, *Immunology*, 32, 245, 1977.

41. **Rifkin, M. R.,** *Trypanosoma brucei*: some properties of the cytotoxic reaction induced by normal human serum, *Exp. Parasitol.*, 46, 189, 1978.

42. **Pillemer, L., Blum, L., Lepous, I. H., Ross, O. A., Todd, E. W., and Wardlaw, A. C.,** The properdin system and immunity. I. Demonstration and isolation of a new serum protein, properdin, and its role in immune phenomena, *Science*, 120, 279, 1954.

43. **Lindsley, H. B., Janecek, L. L., Gilman-Sacks, A. M., and Hassanein, K. M.,** Detection and composition of immune complexes in experimental African trypanosomiasis, *Infect. Immun.*, 33, 407, 1981.

44. **Greenwood, B. M. and Whittle, H. C.,** The pathogenesis of sleeping sickness, *Trans. R. Soc. Trop. Med. Hyg.,* 74, 716, 1980.

45. **Basson, W., Page, M. L., and Myburgh, D. P.,** Human trypanosomiasis in Southern Africa, *S. Afr. Med. J.,* 51, 453, 1977.

46. **Lambert, P. H., Berney, M., and Kazyumba, G.,** Immune complexes in serum and in cerebrospinal fluid in African trypanosomiasis. Correlation with polyclonal B cell activation and with intracerebral immunoglobulin synthesis, *J. Clin. Invest.,* 67, 77, 1981.

47. **Clarkson, A. B. and Mellow, G. H.,** Rheumatoid factor-like immunoglobulin M protects previously uninfected rat pups and dams from *Trypanosoma lewisi, Science,* 214, 186, 1981.

48. **Mackenzie, A. R., Boreham, P. F. L., and Facer, C. A.,** Autoantibodies in African trypanosomiasis, *Trans. R. Soc. Trop. Med. Hyg.,* 67, 268, 1973.

49. **Rickman, W. J. and Cox, H. W.,** Immunologic reactions associated with anemia thrombocytopenia and coagulopathy in experimental African trypanosomiasis, *J. Parasitol.,* 66, 28, 1980.

50. **Banks, K. L.,** Injury induced by *Trypanosoma congolense* adhesion to cell membranes, *J. Parasitol.,* 66, 34, 1980.

51. **Losos, A. J. and Ikede, B. O.,** Pathology of experimental trypanosomiasis in the albino rat, rabbit, goat an.¹ sheep. A preliminary report, *Can. J. Comp. Med.,* 34, 209, 1972.

52. **Dɛ lmasso, A. P. and Jarvinen, J. A.,** Experimental Chagas' disease in complement-deficient mice and guinea pigs, *Infect. Immun.,* 28, 434, 1980.

53. **Jarvinen, J. A. and Dalmasso, A. P.,** *Trypanosoma musculi:* immunologic features of the anemia in infected mice, *Exp. Parasitol.,* 43, 203, 1977.

54. **Nielsen, K., Sheppard, J., Tizard, I. R., and Holmes, W. L.,** Experimental bovine trypanosomiasis: changes in serum immunoglobulin, complement and complement component levels in infected cattle, *Immunology,* 35, 817, 1978a.

55. **Nielsen, K., Sheppard, J., Holmes, W., and Tizard, I.,** Experimental bovine trypanosomiasis: changes in the catabolism of serum immunoglobulins and complement components in infected cattle, *Immunology,* 35, 811, 1978b.

56. **Kobayashi, A. and Tizard, I. R.,** The response to *Trypanosoma congolense* infection in calves. Determination of immunoglobulins IgG_1, IgG_2, IgM, and C_3 levels and the complement fixing antibody titers during the course of infection, *Tropenmed. Parasitol.,* 27, 411, 1976.

57. **Rurangirwa, F. R.,Table, H., Losos, A., and Tizard, I. R.,** Hemolytic complement and serum C_3 levels in Zebu cattle infected with *Trypanosoma congolense* and *Trypanosoma vivax* and the effect of trypanocidal treatment, *Infect. Immun.,* 27, 832, 1980.

58. **Ingram, D. G. and Soltys, M. A.,** Immunity in trypanosomiasis. IV. Immuno-conglutinin in animals infected with *Trypanosoma brucei, Parasitology,* 50, 231, 1960.

59. **Lachmann, P. J. and Watson, M. J. C.,** Conglutinin and immunoconglutinins, *Adv. Immunol.,* 6, 497, 1967.

60. **Kobayashi, A., Tizard, I. R., and Wood, P. T. K.,** Studies on the anemia in experimental African trypanosomiasis. II. The pathogenesis of the anemia in calves infected with *Trypanosoma congolense, Am. J. Trop. Med. Hyg.,* 25, 401, 1976.

61. **Pantrizel, R., Duret, J., Tribouley, J., and Ripert, C.,** Application of the conglutination reaction to the serologic diagnosis of trypanosomiasis, *Bull. Soc. Pathol. Exotique,* 55, 391, 1962.

62. **Thoongsuwan, S., Cox, H. W., and Patrick, R. A.,** Immunoconglutinin associated with nonspecific acquired resistance in malaria, babesiosis, and other anemia-inducing infections, *J. Parasitol.,* 64, 1050, 1978.

63. **Rickman, W. J., Cox, H. W., and Thoongsuwan, S.,** Interactions of immunoconglutinin and immune complexes in cold autohemagglutination associated with African trypanosomiasis, *J. Parasitol.,* 67, 159, 1981.

64. **Shirazi, M. R., Holman, M., Hudson, K. M., Klaus, C. C. B., and Terry, R. J.,** Complement (C3) levels and the effect of C3 depletion in infections of *Trypanosoma brucei* in mice, *Parasite Immunol.,* 2, 155, 1980.

65. **Tizard, I. R., Mittal, K. R., and Nielsen, K.,** Depressed immunoconglutinin responses in calves experimentally infected with *Trypanosoma congolense, Res. Vet. Sci.,* 28, 203, 1980.

66. **Goodwin, L. G., Green, D. A., Guy, M. W., and Voller, A.,** Immunosuppression during trypanosomiasis, *Br. J. Exp. Pathol.,* 53, 40, 1972.

67. **Urquhart, G. M., Murray, M., Murray, P. K., Jennings, F. W., and Barte, E.,** Iummunosuppression in *T. brucei* infections in rabbits and mice, *Trans. R. Soc. Trop. Med. Hyg.,* 67, 528, 1973.

68. **Hudson, K. M., Byner, C., Freeman, J., and Terry, R. J.,** Immunodepression, high IgM levels and evasion of the immune response in murine trypanosomiasis, *Nature (London),* 264, 256, 1976.

69. **Baltz, T., Baltz, D., Giroud, C., and Pautrizel, R.,** Immune depression and macroglobulinemia in experimental subchromic trypanosomiasis, *Infect. Immun.,* 32, 979, 1981.

70. **Albright, J. W. and Albright, J. F.,** Trypanosome-mediated suppression of murine humoral immunity independent of typical suppressor cells, *J. Immunol.,* 124, 2481, 1980.

71. **St. Charles, M. C., Frank, D., and Tanner, C. E.,** The depressed response of spleen cells from rats infected by *Trypanosoma lewisi* in producing a secondary response *in vitro* to sheep erythrocytes and the ability of soluble products of the trypanosome to induce this depression, *Immunology,* 43, 441, 1981.

72. **Musoke, A. J. and Barbet, A. F.,** Activation of complement by variant-specific surface antigen of *Trypanosoma brucei, Nature (London),* 270, 438, 1977.

73. **Nielsen, K. H. and Sheppard, J.,** Activation of complement by trypanosomes, *Experientia,* 33, 769, 1977.

74. **Nielsen, K. H., Sheppard, J., Tizard, I. R., and Holmes, W. L.,** *Trypanosoma brucei:* characterization of complement activating components, *Exp. Parasitol.,* 43, 153, 1977.

75. **Nielsen, K., Sheppard, J., Tizard, I., and Holmes, W.,** Complement activating factors of *Trypanosoma lewisi:* some physiochemical characteristics of the active components, *Can. J. Comp. Med.,* 42, 74, 1978.

76. **Nielsen, K., Sheppard, J., Tizard, I. R., and Holmes, W.,** Increased susceptibility of *Trypanosoma lewisi* infected or decomplemented rats to *Salmonella typhimurium, Experientia,* 34, 118, 1978.

77. **Cunningham, D. S., Hazen, T. C., and Kuhn, R. E.,** Partial characterization of a *Trypanosoma cruzi* released decomplementing factor, *J. Parasitol.,* 67, 475, 1981.

78. **Papamichail, M., Gutierrez, C., Embling, P., Johnson, P., Holborrow, E. J., and Pepys, M. B.,** Complement dependence of localization of aggregated IgA in germinal centers, *Scand. J. Immunol.,* 4, 343, 1975.

79. **Pepys, M. B., Mirjah, D. D., Dash, A. C., and Wansbrough-Jones, M. H.,** Immunosuppression by cobra venom factor: distribution, antigen-induced blast transformation and trapping of lymphocytes during *in vivo* complement depletion, *Cell. Immunol.,* 21, 327, 1976.

80. **White, R. G., Henderson, D. C., Eslami, M. B., and Nielsen, K. H.,** Localization of a protein antigen in the chicken spleen. Effect of various manipulative procedures on the morphogenesis of the germinal centre, *Immunology,* 28, 1, 1975.

81. **Murray, M.,** The pathology of *Trypanosoma brucei* infection in the rat, *Res. Vet. Sci.,* 16, 77, 1974.

82. **Terry, R. J., Freeman, J., Hudson, K. M., and Longstaffe, J. A.,** Immunoglobulin M production and immunosuppression in trypanosomiasis-linking hypothesis, *Trans. R. Soc. Trop. Med. Hyg.,* 67, 263, 1973.

83. **Nielsen, K. and White, R. G.,** Effect of host decomplementation on homeostasis of antibody production in fowl, *Nature (London),* 250, 234, 1974.

84. **Pepys, M. B.,** Role of complement in induction of the allergic response, *Nature (London),* 237, 157, 1972.

85. **Pepys, M. B.,** Role of complement in induction of antibody production *in vivo.* Effect of cobra factor and other C3 reactive agents and thymus-dependent and thymus-independent antibody responses, *J. Exp. Med.,* 140, 126, 1974.

86. **Pepys, M. B., Brighton, W. D., Hewitt, B. E., Bryant, D. E. W., and Pepys, J.,** Complement and the induction of IgE antibody formation, *Clin. Exp. Immunol.,* 27, 397, 1977.

87. **Houba, V., Brown, K. N., and Allison, A. C.,** Heterophilic antibodies: M-antiglobulins and immunoglobulins in experimental trypanosomiasis, *Clin. Exp. Immunol.,* 4, 113, 1969.

88. **Freeman, T., Smithers, S. R., Targett, G. A. T., and Walker, P. J.,** Specificity of immunoglobulin G in Rhesus monkeys infected with *Schistosoma mansoni, Plasmodium knowlesi* and *Trypanosoma brucei, J. Infect. Dis.,* 121, 401, 1970.

89. **Hudson, K. H., Freeman, J. C., Byner, C., and Terry, R. J.,** Immunodepression in experimental African trypanosomiasis, *Trans. R. Soc. Trop. Med. Hyg.,* 69, 273, 1975.

90. **Luckins, A. G.,** Studies on bovine trypanosomiasis. Serum immunoglobulin levels in Zebu cattle exposed to natural infection in East Africa, *Br. Vet. J.,* 128, 523, 1972.

91. **Luckins, A. G.,** Immunoglobulin response in Zebu cattle infected with *Trypanosoma congolense* and *Trypanosoma vivax, Trans. R. Soc. Trop. Med. Hyg.,* 68, 148, 1974.

92. **Luckins, A. G. and Mehlitz, D.,** Observation on serum immunoglobulin levels in cattle infected with *Trypanosoma brucei, Trypanosoma vivax* and *Trypanosoma congolense, Ann. Trop. Med. Parasitol.,* 70, 479, 1976.

93. **Clarkson, M. J., Penhale, W. J., Edwards, G., and Farrell, P. F.,** Serum protein changes in cattle infected with *Trypanosoma vivax, Trans. R. Soc. Trop. Med. Hyg.,* 69, 2, 1975.

94. **Clarkson, M. J. and Penhale, W. J.,** Serum protein changes in trypanosomiasis in cattle, *Trans. R. Soc. Trop. Med. Hyg.,* 67, 273, 1973.

95. **Seed, J. R., Cornille, R. L., Risby, E. L., and Gam, A. A.,** The presence of agglutinating antibody in the IgM immunoglobulin fraction of rabbit antiserum during experimental African trypanosomiasis, *Parasitology,* 59, 283, 1969.

96. **Boreham, P. F. L.,** Pharmacologically active peptides produced in the tissues of the host during chronic trypanosome infections, *Nature (London),* 212, 190, 1966.

97. **Boreham, P. F. L.,** Immune reactions and kinin formation in chronic trypanosomiasis, *Pharmacol. Chemother.,* 32, 493, 1968.
98. **Boreham, P. F. L.,** *In vitro* studies on the mechanism of kinin formation by trypanosomes, *Br. J. Pharmacol.,* 34, 598, 1968.
99. **Boreham, P. F. L.,** Kinin release and the immune reaction in human trypanosomiasis caused by *Trypanosoma rhodesiense, Trans. R. Soc. Trop. Med. Hyg.,* 64, 394, 1970.
100. **Boreham, P. F. L. and Goodwin, L. G.,** The release of kinins as the result of an antigen-antibody reaction in trypanosomiasis, in *Bradykinin and Related Kinins,* Sicuteri, F. et al., Eds., Plenum Press, New York, 1970, 534.
101. **Boreham, P. F. L. and Wright, I. G.,** Hypotension in rabbits infected with *Trypanosoma brucei. Br. J. Pharmacol.,* 58, 137, 1976.
102. **Richards, W. H. G.,** Pharmacologically active substances in the blood, tissues and urine of mice infected with *Trypanosoma brucei. Br. J. Pharmacol. Chemother.,* 24, 124, 1965.
103. **Veenendaal, G. H., VanMiert, A. S., Van den Ingh, T. S., Schotman, A. J., and Zwart, D.,** A comparison of the role of kinins and serotonin in endotoxin induced fever and *Trypanosoma vivax* infections in the goat, *Res. Vet. Sci.,* 21, 271, 1976.
104. **Wright, I. G. and Boreham, P. F. L.,** Studies on urinary kallikrein in *Trypanosoma brucei* infections in the rabbit, *Biochem. Pharmacol.,* 24, 417, 1977.
105. **Ackerman, S. B. and Seed, J. R.,** The effects of tryphophol on immune responses and its implications towards trypanosome-induced immunosuppression, *Experientia,* 32, 645, 1976.
106. **Crosson, F. J., Jr., Winkelstein, J. A., and Moxou, E. R.,** Participation of complement in the nonimmune host defense against experimental *Haemophilus influenza* type b septicemia and meningitis, *Infect. Immun.,* 14, 882, 1976.
107. **Cuningham, D., Hazen, T. C., and Kuhn, R. E.,** Increased resistance to Aeromonas hydrophila in mice experimentally infected with *Trypanosoma cruzi, J. Parasitol.,* 67, 468, 1981.

Chapter 8

PATHOLOGY OF CHAGAS' DISEASE

Charles A. Santos-Buch and Alberto M. Acosta

TABLE OF CONTENTS

I. INTRODUCTION

A. General Comments

The pathology of Chagas' disease or American trypanosomiasis presents a complicated and diverse picture in both humans and experimental animals. A few infected individuals may be acutely susceptible and die from overwhelming parasitosis in the initial stages of infection,[1] while many others survive the initial infestation and go on to develop the chronic manifestations of the disease months[2,3] or years later.[1,4] Still others remain clinically asymptomatic throughout their lives and die of causes other than Chagas' disease. In recent years it has become increasingly evident that immune mechanisms significantly contribute to the pathology seen in the chronic cardiac form of Chagas' disease[5-8] and may also be implicated in the lesion of myenteric innervation occasionally seen in the chronic form of the disease.[9] Cross-reacting antigenic determinants shared by *Trypanosoma cruzi*, the etiologic agent of Chagas' disease, and mammalian striated muscle,[10] neurons,[11] and basement membrane components[12] have recently been described and their putative immunopathogenic roles are currently being elucidated. The ability of *T cruzi* to reversibly acquire host cell surface components has also recently been reported.[13] The possible role of this mechanism in the immunopathogenic process is also being studied.

B. General Epidemiology of Chagas' Disease

Chagas' disease represents the most common cause of congestive heart failure and sudden death in the world.[14] It is a major public health problem in Central and South America, where an estimated 12 million people are already infected and an additional 45 million are at risk of infection.[14] Although frequently erroneously referred to as South American trypanosomiasis, Chagas' disease is truly a Panamerican disease. *T. cruzi* is found only in the western hemisphere[15] and its natural vector, the *Hemiptera* insects, belonging to the family Reduviidae, subfamily Triatominae, have an extensive geographic distribution extending roughly from the middle of Argentina and Chile up through the middle U.S.[15] There are more than 100 species of Reduviidae (Figure 1) and the majority may harbor *T. cruzi.*[15] Insects in the genera *Rhodnius, Panstrogylus,* and Triatominae are the most common vectors,

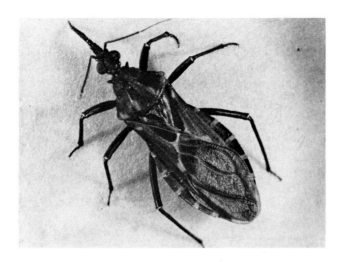

FIGURE 1. *Triatoma infestans*. The laboratory-grown, uninfected insect has introduced its proboscis beneath the epidermis to start its blood meal. (From Santos-Buch, C. A., *Int. Rev. Exp. Pathol.*, 19, 63, 1979. With permission.)

with the proportion of infected insects greater than that of human infection.[16] These aggressive nocturnal insects are popularly known as "kissing bugs" or "assassin bugs" in the southern U.S., as "pitos" or "vinchucas" in Spanish America, and as "barbeiros" in Portuguese Brazil. The most important factor predisposing to human infection is the translation of *T. cruzi*-infected Reduviidae from the sylvatic cycle of the vector to the domestic cycle, namely, the disposition of the vector into human dwellings. Continuity between cycles is known to occur.[17,18] The Reduviidae insects conceal themselves within crevices and cracks in the walls and roofs of poorly constructed dwellings and sally forth at night to feed on the human and domestic animal inhabitants. Badly infected houses have been estimated to contain up to several thousand insects, 70% of which may be infected.[19] In such situations, the incidence of infection of the human inhabitants is close to 100%.[19] Significantly, in areas where insect adaptation to houses has not occurred, only a few isolated cases of Chagas' disease are found even though the infection rate of sylvatic Reduviidae may be high.[20]

Up to 80% of the population in some endemic areas may be infected with *T. cruzi*.[21,22] In the U.S., seroepidemiologic studies estimate that 2 to 4% of the population in certain rural areas of the Southwest are infected.[23] *T. cruzi* has been isolated from sylvatic animals as far north as the state of Maryland,[24] but no human infection has been reported there. Patients suffering from Chagas' disease may also be found in nonendemic areas because of travel to and relocation away from endemic areas.[25]

C. Life Cycle of *T. cruzi*

T. cruzi is a hemoflagellate protozoan that was first described by Chagas in 1909.[26] It exists in three morphologically distinct forms corresponding to the different phases of its life cycle. The infective trypomastigote or bloodstream form exists as a freely swimming, extracellular, nonmultiplying flagellate in the mammalian host (Figure 2a). It is approximately 20 μm long by 2 μm wide and has a characteristic sickle-shaped appearance in thin blood smears. The trypomastigote serves to transfer the infection from cell to cell within the mammalian host. It may be ingested during a blood meal by the vector, the *Reduviida* insect. In the midgut of the insect the ingested trypomastigotes transform into the epimastigote form, which replicates by binary fission (Figure 2b). It is approximately 20 μm long and

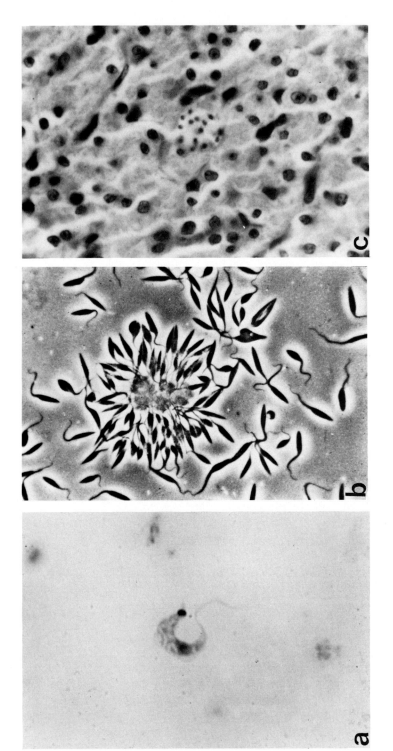

FIGURE 2.   Morphologic forms of *T. cruzi.* (a) Extracellular trypomastigote form in a peripheral blood smear. Note the characteristic sickle-shaped appearance. (Wright stain); (b) individual and clustered epimastigote forms that are found in the digestive tract of the vector and in cell-free laboratory culture. (Wright stain); (c) intracellular amastigote forms in an infected dog. (Hematoxylin and eosin.)

Table 1
TARGET CELL
SYSTEMS OF *T. CRUZI*

In acute symptomatic infection
  Neuroectoderm
    CNS neurons
    Glia
    Parasympathetic ganglia
  Mesoderm
    Macrophages
    Myocardium
    Skeletal muscle
    Smooth muscle

In chronic Chagas' disease
  Neuroectoderm
    Parasympathetic ganglia
  Mesoderm
    Myocardium
    Heart conduction fibers

2 μm wide. Within the hindgut and rectum, epimastigotes transform into infective metacyclic trypomastigotes which are released in the feces of the insect. The deposited trypomastigotes may then enter the body of the victim through the puncture wound of the insect bite. More often, however, since the insects feed at night and attach to the face, the infective feces may get smeared over the face, allowing the trypomastigotes to penetrate the mucous membranes of the mouth, nose, or eyes. Trypomastigotes may also enter the body through cuts or abrasions on the skin, by transplacental transmission,[27,28] by blood transfusion,[29] and by laboratory accidents. There is a local inflammatory reaction at the site of entry, where macrophages and/or local tissue become parasitized. The parasitized cells rupture 4 or 5 days later, releasing trypomastigotes that gain access to the circulation and disseminate through the body. *T. cruzi* is an obligate intracellular protozoan and, thus, does not replicate extracellularly within its mammalian host. Most cells can be parasitized, but there appears to be a tropism for striated muscle, smooth muscle, and neuroectodermal elements (Table 1). Within parasitized cells, trypomastigotes transform into the spherical amastigote or intracellular form (Figure 2c). It is approximately 2 μm in diameter and replicates by binary fission. Unlike other intracellular parasites, the nidi of amastigotes of *T. cruzi* are not known to possess a limiting membrane contributed by the host and are, therefore, not contained in cysts. At the end of 4 to 5 days, amastigotes of heavily parasitized cells elongate their bodies and transform into trypomastigotes, which are released from the ruptured pseudocyst. The released trypomastigotes may then parasitize other cells or be ingested by the vector to continue the life cycle.

II. HISTORICAL BACKGROUND OF CHAGAS' DISEASE

The chronicles of colonization of the New World contain many indirect references to Chagas' disease. As early as 1587, descriptions appear of a disease in Brazil called *Mal de Bicho* or *Bicho*, that was characterized by a distended rectum often filled with worms.[30] These signs may have been due to achalasia of the colon that is sometimes associated with cases of chronic Chagas' disease, particularly in Brazil. In 1590 the first description of the *Reduviida* insect and its nocturnal blood-sucking habits was made by a missionary priest in Tucuman, Argentina,[31] an area endemic for Chagas' disease. In the next 300 years, reports continued of *Bicho*, or *Mal de Culo*, as it was referred to in Spanish America, as well as though its course towards the sea-coast is very imperfectly known : it is even doubtful whether, in passing over the plains, it is not evaporated and lost. We slept in the village of Luxan, which is a small place surrounded by gardens, and forms the most southern cultivated district in the Province of Mendoza ; it is five leagues south of the capital. At night I experienced an attack (for it deserves no less a name) of the *Benchuca*, a species of Reduvius, the great black bug of the Pampas. It is most disgusting to feel soft wingless insects, about an inch long, crawling over one's body. Before sucking they are quite thin, but afterwards they become round and bloated with blood, and in this state are easily crushed. One which I caught at Iquique, (for they are found in Chile and Peru,) was very empty. When placed on a table, and though surrounded by people, if a finger was presented, the bold insect would immediately protrude its sucker, make a charge, and if allowed, draw blood. No pain was caused by the wound. It was curious to watch its body during the act of sucking, as in less than ten minutes it changed from being as flat as a wafer to a globular form. This one feast, for which the benchuca was indebted to one of the officers, kept it fat during four whole months ; but, after the first fortnight, it was quite ready to have another suck.

March 27th.—We rode on to Mendoza. The country was beautifully cultivated, and resembled Chile. This neighbour-

FIGURE 3.   Charles Darwin's description of the nocturnal attack of the Reduviidae, the natural vector of Chagas' disease.[32] The insect was ready to have another blood meal after 14 days ("fortnight"). It has been postulated that Darwin contracted Chagas' disease during an expedition to Argentina.[33]

of the *Reduviida* insect. Interestingly, Charles Darwin encountered the *Reduviia* while visiting an endemic area, Mendoza, Argentina, during his voyage on the H.M.S. Beagle.[32] He accurately describes the nocturnal attack of the aggressive "Benchuca", or *Reduviida* insect (Figure 3). It has been conjectured that the heart failure and edema that plagued Darwin in his later years may be attributed to the pathologic manifestations of chronic Chagas' heart disease.[33]

A. Carlos Justiano Chagas (1879 to 1934)

The insight and investigative ability that Carlos Chagas exhibited at the turn of the 20th century is quite remarkable. In 1907 Chagas went to Minas Gerais, Brazil to direct a malaria control campaign. He noted the large number of Reduviidae insects infesting the poorly constructed rural dwellings. Chagas knew that arthropods were important vectors of human disease and, thus, studied the insects and found trypanosomes in their hindgut.[30] Armed with a vector and a possible agent, he then sought to establish a mammalian host. Allowing the Reduviidae to feed on laboratory animals, he subsequently found trypomastigotes in their blood. Chagas continued his studies and on April 11, 1908 established the first documented case of human *T. cruzi* infection in a 2-year-old girl.[26] The sequence of events of Chagas' studies is noteworthy. Usually a clinical illness is described and then the etiologic agent and vector are sought. Chagas, however, did the reverse, first finding the vector, then the etiologic agent, and finally the disease.[34] Furthermore, the time period in which Chagas accomplished this is also of note. Chagas worked by himself in a rural area using a converted railroad car as his home, office, and laboratory. Within a period of less than 2 years he described many of the salient characteristics of the disease so rightly named after him.[34]

B. Major Contributors to Our Knowledge

Many other investigators also contributed greatly to the understanding of Chagas' disease. Vianna,[35] a colleague of Chagas, made the original histopathologic observations of *T. cruzi* infection and described the intracellular amastigote form of *T. cruzi* in 1911. Brumpt[36] delineated the life cycle of *T. cruzi* by demonstrating that *T. cruzi* is a stercorarian trypanosome which is transmitted in the feces of the Reduviidae. He was also the first to describe xenodiagnosis as a diagnostic method to determine *T. cruzi* parasitemia.[37] Guerreiro and Machado[38] developed the complement fixation test in 1913 that still bears their names for the serologic diagnosis of *T. cruzi* infection. This was the first time a specific serologic test was developed to diagnose a parasitic disease.[39] Villela[40] showed the possibility of congenital transmission of *T. cruzi* infection in experimental animals in 1923. Salvador Mazza was the first to describe Chagas' disease in Argentina in 1934, corroborating its existence and showing that it was not limited to Brazil.[34] Koberle,[41] in Brazil in the 1950s, elucidated the anatomic basis for the development of achalasia of the esophagus and colon associated with chronic Chagas' disease in Brazil.

It is now more evident that the heart is the most important site for pathologic lesions in the chronic form of Chagas' disease.[42] Andrade,[43] in 1956, was the first to describe the apical aneurysm found in cases of congestive cardiomyopathy associated with long-term *T. cruzi* infection. Later, Zilton and Sonia Andrade[44] described the predilected injury to the conduction system and have continued making significant contributions to the study of the cardiac immunopathology found in chronic Chagas' disease.[45] Rosenbaum and Alvarez[46] elaborately studied the associated electrocardiographic abnormalities of Chagas' cardiomyopathy. Mott and Hagstrom[47] compiled an extensive review of the literature associated with Chagas' cardiomyopathy and categorized the lesions associated with the disease. They correlated their own findings with the available data and showed destruction of the cardiac autonomic nervous system in chronic cardiomyopathy. In 1974, Cossio et al.[48,49] showed the presence of antiheart antibodies in patients with the chronic cardiac form of Chagas' disease. The antiheart activity was later attributed to heterophile antibody and no clear relationship to pathogenicity is now linked to chagasic cardiomyopathy.[50] At the same time, Teixeira,[51] in our laboratory, showed the destruction of allogeneic heart cells by *T. cruzi*-sensitized lymphocytes in vitro.

Kierszenbaum[52] showed the complement-mediated immune lysis of virulent forms of *T. cruzi*. De Bracco[53] demonstrated the sequence of complement-dependent phagocytosis and cytotoxicity to *T. cruzi* by human polymorphonuclear leukocytes. Da Silva[54] showed antibody-dependent cell-mediated cytotoxicity to trypomastigote bloodstream forms. Hoff[55] reported that armed macrophages kill *T. cruzi* in vitro. Trischmann et al.[56] reported that natural resistance to *T. cruzi* infection was related to the genotype of specific inbred strains of mice, and the genetics of murine resistance to *T. cruzi* was later worked out in more detail.[57]

Ribeiro dos Santos[58-60] demonstrated the adsorption of *T. cruzi* antigens from ruptured pseudocysts of amastigotes onto normal host tissue and their subsequent destruction by immune elements. He postulated that this mechanism gives rise to the antihost immune responses.[59,60] Sadigursky,[7,10,61] in our laboratory, demonstrated a common immunogen in heart and *T. cruzi* and that this immunogen was related to the calcium regulatory factors of the sarcolemma.

Much has been learned about *T. cruzi* infection and its sequela, Chagas' disease, since its first description in 1909. However, it is apparent that we have merely scraped the surface of the subject matter. A great deal more will be learned about the biology of *T. cruzi* and the pathogenesis of Chagas' disease as investigators continue to unravel this puzzle of nature.

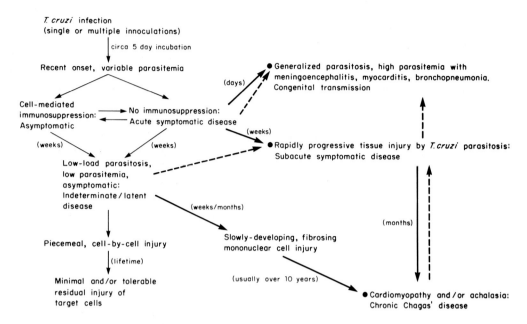

FIGURE 4.   Natural history of *T. cruzi* infection in humans as envisioned by the authors. The thin arrows indicate the usual evolution of the disease. The thick arrows denote the direction of the less frequent pathophysiologic injury produced by *T. cruzi* (estimate: 15 to 20% of those initially inoculated). The broken arrows indicate the effect of corticosteroid treatment without adequate coverage with antitrypanosomal chemotherapy.

III. NATURAL HISTORY OF *T. CRUZI* INFECTION

The natural history of human *T. cruzi* infections has not been worked out; however, salient characteristics are now generally recognized, and inferences drawn from experimental, pathologic, and epidemiologic studies have clarified some of the obscure gaps of our knowledge (Figure 4). It is well to remember that Berenice, who was the first case of Carlos Chagas' study, lived to the seventh decade in spite of demonstrable parasitemias throughout her lifetime.[26,34] Significantly, the girl and her parents did accurately describe face bites by the vector, the *Reduviida,* and there is little doubt that her household was infested by many *T. cruzi*-infected insects.[34] It is ironic that the first human case of Chagas' disease very aptly illustrates the paradox presupposed by *T. cruzi* infections; that is, parasitosis — even of many years' duration — may not produce enough tissue injury to evoke a significant pathophysiologic change. We now classify asymptomatic patients with serologic evidence of *T. cruzi* infection who have no significant pathologic injury as having the indeterminate form of Chagas' disease. It is now believed that human *T. cruzi* infection of many years' duration is a low-load parasitosis which produces a nearly consistent low level of parasitemia.[62] It is estimated that only up to 20% of asymptomatic patients with no significant pathologic changes are at risk of developing extensive cardiac tissue injury later,[1,3,21] and of these only up to 30% of the hearts studied at autopsy show microscopic foci of myofiber parasitosis,[63] and very rarely is there parasitosis of intracardiac ganglioneurons.[47] Experimental work has shown that pathologic changes produced by *T. cruzi* may be the result of the size and frequency of the inocula, of the degree of genetically determined susceptibility to infection of the host, of the innate tissue tropism and the characteristic rate of proliferation of the particular infecting strain of *T. cruzi* (see Hoff in this volume), and of the degree of the immunopathology the infection may evoke. The sum of each of these factors probably also determines the outcome of the infection in humans.

Epidemiologic studies suggest that the majority of patients with positive serology for *T. cruzi* infection do not remember the early phase of the infection, which usually occurs before age 15.[64] A recent study showed that children with demonstrable parasitemias can be divided into two groups, one which exhibits clinical symptoms and the other which does not.[65] Significantly, the patients who lacked the symptomatology of infection were clearly immunosuppressed. Thus, when we speak of acute *T. cruzi* infection, we are referring to a parasitemia of recent onset that requires hospitalization and treatment (Figure 4). In a few patients requiring hospitalization the mortality rate approaches 5 to 10%, and in these subjects the parasitosis is generalized; however, death is more frequently attributed to massive involvement of the brain.[42] If antitrypanosomal treatment is not started early, patients with infection of recent onset develop fixed positive serologic tests for *T. cruzi* antigens later and conversion cannot be effected even with prolonged chemotherapy.[66] The majority of untreated patients with symptomatic acute infection (90 to 95%) progress to the indeterminate form of Chagas' disease in a period of weeks or a few months and become asymptomatic. They remain seropositive throughout their lifetime, even after prolonged chemotherapeutic trials later.[62] The reduction of the parasitosis is related to complement-mediated lysis and to macrophage phagocytosis and destruction as the immune response becomes more effective.[53-55] Untreated patients with the indeterminate form of Chagas' disease have low-grade parasitemias, since some surveys have shown that only 40% have positive xenodiagnostic tests.[62] If xenodiagnosis is repeated at different intervals, the prevalence of positive tests approaches 80 to 90%.[67] Corticosteroid therapy for other reasons (e.g., prednisolone treatment of systemic lupus erythematosis) results in exacerbation of symptomatic parasitosis with high-level parasitemia (Figure 4).

There is insufficient data to document that symptomatic *T. cruzi* parasitemias of recent onset may enter a subacute but progressive phase of tissue injury eventually resulting in a devastating cardiomyopathy of the congestive type (Figure 4). The data from experimentally induced infections and anecdotal reports clearly suggest that this pathogenic mechanism may be operative in some patients.[42] In a typical prototype, the patient with recent onset *T. cruzi* parasitemia would relentlessly continue to develop new and progressive tissue injury in a subacute course, perhaps lasting a matter of months without ever entering the usually long-lasting clinically asymptomatic hiatus of the indeterminate form of the disease (Figure 4). Development of potentially pathogenic immune reactions against parasympathetic neurons and/or myofibers in this rapidly progressive phase may aggravate the disease process, but probably play a minor role to cell parasitosis and subsequent piecemeal cellular necrosis produced by *T. cruzi*. On the other hand, epidemiologic studies have shown that the great majority of patients with *T. cruzi* parasitemia of recent onset evolve into an asymptomatic, indeterminate form of the disease.[64,68] The majority of these patients appear to tolerate *T. cruzi* parasitosis without further clinical developments, and when they come to autopsy for other reasons show minimal focal scars in target organs of no pathophysiologic consequence.[42] Serologic testing for antibodies specific for components of the myocardial cell sarcolemma in asymptomatic *T. cruzi*-infected patients of long duration has shown a low prevalence of antiheart cell immunity (25%).[69] On the other hand, patients with *T. cruzi* infection and progressive congestive cardiomyopathy have nearly two times the prevalence of circulating antisarcolemma antibodies.[69] Experimental data also support the notion that the development of pathoimmunity during the asymptomatic indeterminate phase of the disease ushers an incubation period before the clinical onset of cardiomyopathy[42] (Figure 4). Adoptive transfer of either *T. cruzi*-sensitized or heart sarcolemma-sensitized lymphocytes into normal, syngeneic inbred (Balb/c) mice results in the development of lymphocyte cytotoxicity to syngeneic neonatal myofibers.[70,71] Allogeneic *T. cruzi*-sensitized lymphocytes adhere to parasympathetic ganglia[4] but syngeneic *T. cruzi*-sensitized lymphocytes showed cytotoxicity to Balb/c neuroblastoma cells.[59] The mechanism of development of pathologic immunity has not been strictly verified in humans, although a number of different studies suggest its predominance.[6-8,69] *T. cruzi*-infected asymptomatic patients who appear to tolerate the parasitosis without further tissue injury may escape pathologic immunity by development of immunosuppressive regulatory mechanisms in a normal fashion, whereas those who develop pathoimmunity and cardiomyopathy probably bypass regulatory immunosuppression in a fashion similar to that postulated for other well-studied "autoimmune" diseases.[72]

The appearance of cardiomyopathy with or without achalasia of the hollow viscera (chronic Chagas' disease) marks a devastating event to the *T. cruzi*-infected patient. Pathophysiologic damage becomes clinically apparent slowly at first but is irreversible and progressive[3,4] and spells a terrible prognosis (Figure 4). Fortunately, the rate of conversion from the indeterminate form to the chronic form of Chagas' disease is of the order of 15 to 20% and most patients escape.[1,3,4] The usual mean age of onset of chronic Chagas' disease is in the fourth decade of life, long after the *T. cruzi* inoculation in childhood.

IV. THEORIES OF THE PATHOGENESIS OF CHAGAS' DISEASE

A. Direct Tissue Destruction by *T. cruzi*

Initially, it was thought that the lesions found in the chronic form of Chagas' disease were due to the effects of tissue parasitosis by *T. cruzi*. Parasitosis with subsequent rupture of pseudocysts would lead to inflammatory reactions and subsequent fibrosis. Inasmuch as complete remission of *T. cruzi* infection has not been absolutely verified, individuals can harbor *T. cruzi* throughout their lifetime and, thus, have repeated episodes of tissue infection-rupturing pseudocysts-inflammation-fibrosis. After many years of this continued process, individuals would present with the pathologic manifestations of the chronic form of Chagas' disease. This theory presupposes the continuous presence of *T. cruzi* within the mammalian host and its consistent specific parasitosis of the heart. However, it is very difficult to demonstrate amastigotes of *T. cruzi* in the heart after the initial infestation during the acute form of the disease. Pseudocysts of amastigotes are only incidentally found in the hearts of patients with the indeterminate form of the disease who have died of causes other than Chagas' disease.[42] Andrade and Andrade[68] have shown the presence of amastigotes in only 62 of 208 (30%) hearts from patients who died of Chagas' cardiomyopathy, whereas Suarez et al.[73] have found no amastigotes in 160 chagasic hearts. The significant absence of amastigotes during both the indeterminate and chronic forms of Chagas' disease thus contradicts the basis for the pathogenic role of direct tissue destruction.

B. Destruction of the Autonomic Innervation of the Heart

Achalasia of the esophagus and/or colon occasionally occurs in conjunction with chronic Chagas' heart disease. Almost all reports of such come from Brazil, where the incidence ranges from 2.6%[42] to 20%[74] of autopsied cases of Chagas' cardiomyopathy. No cases have been reported in studies originating in Venezuela[73] or in Panama.[75] The characteristic lesion is a partial or complete destruction of the parasympathetic myenteric plexus innervating the hollow viscera with a reduction in the number of neurons.[42] The pathogenic mechanism leading to this destruction is not known.

Destruction of the ganglion cells of the heart has also been reported, Koberle[41] described the destruction of cardiac parasympathetic ganglia and their subsequent fibrosis in both the presence or absence of inflammatory cells. Mott and Hagstrom[47] reported neuronophagia of the intracardiac ganglia in 10 of 12 autopsied cases of Chagas' cardiomyopathy. Inflammatory infiltrates were present around the nerves in all 12 cases.

The destruction of the parasympathetic ganglia in the target organs of chronic Chagas' disease has led Koberle[74] to propose a neurogenic hypothesis for the pathogenesis of chronic Chagas' disease. He postulates that *T. cruzi* produces a neurotoxin that preferentially affects the parasympathetic ganglion cells within target organs.[76] Once the parasympathetic innervation is destroyed, then the sympathetic innervation will predominate rendering cardiac muscle cells hypersensitive to the actions of catecholamines.[74] This hypersensitivity produces metabolic changes within cells that subsequently would lead to cell lysis and an ensuing inflammatory response. In an effort to prove this hypothesis, Oliveira[77] treated rats with a single injection of a beta-adrenergic agent (isoproterenol: 20 to 340 mg/kg subcutaneously) and produced left ventricular aneurysms in the hearts of these animals.

To date, Koberle's hypothetical *T. cruzi* neurotoxin has eluded experimental isolation. Seneca and Peer[78] claimed to have isolated a *T. cruzi* toxin; however, Andrade and Andrade[42] were unable to produce any toxic effects with material provided by Seneca. Eichbaum[79] and Musacchio and Meyer[80] were unable to show any toxic effects of *T. cruzi* on cultures of nerve cells. Similarly, Ribeiro dos Santos and Hudson[59] observed no specific ^{51}Cr release from tissue cultures of murine neuroblastoma, murine fibrosarcoma, human rhabdomyosarcoma, or human mammary carcinoma that were treated with preparations derived from either amastigotes or epimastigotes of *T. cruzi*. Furthermore, the experimental design of the report attempting to show myocardial damage due to sympathetic hypersensitivity is flawed. The administered dose of isoproterenol used in these experiments is 5000- to 10^5-fold the recommended dosage for use in humans.[81] The pathophysiologic conclusions drawn from such a nonphysiologic system are not justified. Isoproterenol causes a marked reduction in diastolic pressure and may reduce the pressure required for adequate coronary artery perfusion.[82] It also increases myocardial oxygen consumption because of increased cardiac output and ventricular work.[82] This combined effect of decreased blood supply and increased oxygen use creates severe ischemia in the myocardium that may lead to infarction. Since 85% of ventricular aneurysms are caused by ischemic damage of the myocardium,[83] it is reasonable to speculate that the ventricular aneurysms reported by Oliveira are due to ischemic damage induced by the massive dose of isoproterenol used in his study.

If the cardiac damage seen in chronic Chagas' disease was due to a lack of parasympathetic innervation, as Koberle theorizes, then interruption of such input to the heart should produce lesions similar to those seen in chagasic hearts. Campbell and Santos-Buch[84] and Dammin et al.,[85] in separate reports, cut the cardiac branches of the vagus nerve in rabbits and dogs, respectively, thus removing the parasympathetic innervation of the heart. These investigators did not find any cardiac lesions in the experimental animals months[84] or even years[85] after vagectomy. The chronic use of atropine, a parasympathetic blocker, also does not produce any of the cardiac lesions associated with chronic Chagas' disease.[86] If destruction of the parasympathetic innervation of the heart was the cause of Chagas' cardiomyopathy, then denervation should be found in virtually all chagasic hearts. This is certainly not the case. Many chagasic hearts do not exhibit any destruction or replacement fibrosis of the cardiac ganglia. For example, in a meticulous study, Suarez et al.[73] found no neuronophagia, replacement fibrosis, or reduction in the number of cardiac neurons in 24 of 28 chagasic hearts from Venezuela. The presence of neuronal destruction in some chagasic hearts from Brazil is an undisputed fact. The cause of this destruction is not known. However, the data at hand indicate that as a general hypothesis, destruction of the parasympathetic innervation of the heart is not the likely underlying pathogenic mechanism for the lesions seen in chronic Chagas' heart disease.

C. Autoimmune Cardiomyopathy Induced by *T. cruzi*

1. Antiheart Immune Reactions in Human and Experimental Chagas' Disease

One of the fundamental paradoxes of Chagas' disease is the severe destruction of target organs in the absence of either intracellular or extracellular forms of *T. cruzi*. The first histopathologic descriptions of *T. cruzi* infection made by Vianna[35] in 1911 refer to the degeneration of cardiac myofibers in the absence of *T. cruzi*. This has been a consistent finding since its initial report. Andrade and Andrade[68] found inflammatory infiltrates and fibrous replacement in 208 hearts from patients with Chagas' cardiomyopathy and only 30% of these had pseudocysts of amastigotes. Suarez et al.[73] were unable to find any amastigotes in 160 chagasic hearts.

As early as 1930, Magarinos-Torres[87] suggested that the cardiac lesions found in chronic Chagas' disease may be due to an allergic reaction of the host elicited by *T. cruzi* that destroyed normal heart cells. Chagas[88] himself also postulated the existence of such an allergic state in chronic *T. cruzi* infection. In 1958, Tejada-Valenzuela and Castro[89] demonstrated that sera from three patients with chronic Chagas' cardiomyopathy formed precipitin lines with human heart extracts. In 1959 Jaffe et al.[90] and in 1961 Kozma and Drayer[91] showed a high degree of correlation between precipitin antibodies to heart extracts and chronic Chagas' disease. These observations suggested that antiheart autoantibodies could play a role in the pathogenesis of chronic Chagas' disease.

a. Humoral Antiheart Immune Reactions

Antiheart antibodies have been detected in patients with Chagas' disease using immunofluorescence techniques;[48,92-103] however, the validity of these results has been questioned.[50] Cossio et al.[48,92] reported the presence of antibodies in the sera of patients with *T. cruzi* infection that bound to endothelial, vascular, and interstitial (EVI) structures in cardiac and skeletal muscle. The EVI antibody reactivity was apparently of clinical specificity since the sera of 95% of patients with Chagas' cardiomyopathy and 45% of asymptomatic individuals in the indeterminate phase of the disease exhibited positive EVI immunofluorescence staining.[48] Sera from a large number of control individuals from nonendemic areas and sera from patients with other parasitic diseases, with the exception of visceral leishmaniasis, lacked EVI antibody activity.[94] Further studies using immunofluorescence and electron microscopy demonstrated the presence of autologous antibody on myofibers from cardiac and skeletal muscle biopsies of patients with *T. cruzi* infection.[49,96] Variable amounts of tissue damage were coincident with the apparent in vivo deposition of immunoglobulin,[49,96] suggesting a cause and effect relationship. Other reports also demonstrated the presence of EVI antibodies in the sera of patients with Chagas' disease;[93-102] however, the specificity of the EVI reaction was not as high as that reported by Cossio and colleagues. In an effort to establish an experimental model for EVI antibody production, Lenzi et al.[103] immunized rabbits with *T. cruzi* antigens as well as mammalian tissue preparations. Their results showed that immunization with *T. cruzi* antigens or heart antigens elicited EVI antibodies; however, immunization with lung and kidney antigens produced EVI antibodies as well. The lack of tissue antigen specificity for the induction of EVI antibodies indicated that EVI antibodies could interact with antigens present on a variety of different tissues.

Nicholson et al.,[104] in an elegant series of experiments, classified the immunofluorescence staining pattern of various reported antiheart antibodies. The description of a pattern evoked by heterophile antibodies on murine or rat cardiac tissue was indistinguishable from that of the EVI antibody. Heterophile antibodies were also able to react with rat gastric parietal cells, and rat kidney brush border and proximal tubule cells. The reactivity of these antibodies could be abolished by prior incubation with guinea pig red blood cells. Since heterophile antibodies have been described in *T. cruzi* infection,[105,106] Khoury et al.[50] attempted to differentiate between EVI antibody activity and that due to heterophile antibodies. Absorption of EVI positive sera with human blood group A or blood group O red blood cells or with human liver powder did not diminish EVI antibody reactivity on cryostat sections of rat or mouse cardiac or skeletal muscle. However, EVI antibody activity was completely abolished on these substrates after absorption with guinea pig red blood cells, liver, or kidney powders. EVI positive sera were unable to stain human cardiac or skeletal muscle specimens. Furthermore, EVI positive sera reacted with rat gastric parietal cells and rat kidney samples and all EVI activity was abolished by prior absorption with guinea pig red blood cells. These results indicate that EVI antibodies do not have a specific antiheart reactivity, but rather are heterophile in nature.

With these considerations in mind, Khoury et al.[50] attempted to reproduce their previous experiments demonstrating the in vivo deposition of autologous antibodies on cardiac and skeletal muscle biopsies from patients with *T. cruzi* infection and positive EVI serum reactivity. None of the skeletal muscle biopsies tested exhibited any deposition of autologous IgG or C3 on the sarcolemma by immunofluorescence assays. Furthermore, although the sera from all these individuals showed positive heterophile EVI antibody activity on rat and mouse substrates, no staining of autologous skeletal muscle specimens was observed.

Antibodies reacting with Schwann cells have also been described in the sera of EVI antibody-positive, *T. cruzi*-infected individuals.[107] However, subsequent reports have shown that the anti-Schwann cell activity could be abolished by prior absorption of sera with rat liver or kidney powders, or with guinea pig red blood cells.[108] The lack of specificity of these reactions indicated that the anti-Schwann cell activity could be attributed to the presence of heterophile antibodies and not to antibodies directed against specific neuronal components.[108]

The heterophile nature of the EVI antibody activity casts much doubt on their significance in the pathogenesis of Chagas' cardiomyopathy. However, these observations do not preclude the possibility that specific antiheart humoral reactions may contribute to the immunopathogenesis of Chagas' heart disease. For example, Cabral et al.[109] passively transferred parasite-free immune sera from *T. cruzi*-infected rats into normal recipients and observed the development of a chronic myositis and myocarditis in the recipients. Data from our laboratory have shown that treatment of normal rabbit lymphocytes with high titer antisera to subcellular fractions of *T. cruzi* produces a marked lymphocytic adherence and cytolysis of normal allogeneic heart cells in vitro.[51] Further studies are needed to determine the importance of antiheart antibody-mediated reactions in chronic Chagas' disease.

b. Cell-Mediated Antiheart Immune Reactions

Specific cell-mediated antiheart reactions have been reported and confirmed in both humans and experimental animals with *T. cruzi* infections.[5-8] Cossio et al.[5] described the interaction of peripheral blood lymphocytes from 3 of 12 patients with the indeterminate form of Chagas' disease and normal heart. The three patients had positive leukocyte migration inhibition factor (MIF) tests when incubated with heart antigens. Teixeira et al.[6] described the specific lysis of normal human heart cells in vitro by peripheral blood lymphocytes from patients with the acute and chronic forms of Chagas' disease. No specific lysis was demonstrated by lymphocytes from normal volunteers. All chagasic patients in this report exhibited positive MIF tests with both heart and *T. cruzi* antigens, whereas normal controls did not. Reports from our laboratory have shown that lymphocytes obtained from *T. cruzi*-infected rabbits or from rabbits immunized with the microsomal fraction of *T. cruzi* destroy both *T. cruzi* parasitized and normal allogeneic rabbit heart cells in vitro.[51] This cytolysis was specific since no destruction of allogeneic kidney cells was observed.[51] These rabbits had positive MIF tests with both heart and *T. cruzi* antigens. Histopathologic examination of the hearts from infected or immunized animals revealed a myocarditis with myofiber destruction similar to that seen in human chronic Chagas' disease.[110]

One of the difficulties in interpretation of the antiheart cell-mediated reactions just described is the lack of histocompatibility of the target and effector cells. It may be argued that the observed interaction with and destruction of the heart cells exhibited in these experiments is due to allogeneic differences between the interacting cells. In order to establish that there is a specific antiheart cell-mediated cytotoxicity, a syngeneic system must be employed in which the target and effector cells share an identical genetic make-up. Accordingly, we pursued the study of *T. cruzi*-induced antiheart cell-mediated cytotoxicity

Table 2
T. CRUZI-SENSITIZED
LYMPHOCYTE
CYTOTOXICITY OF
NORMAL SYNGENEIC
CARDIAC MYOFIBERS

Days postinfection	Average % specific ^{51}Cr release
15	1.7[a]
45	2.4[a]
90	1.4[a]
120	5.7[a]
150	41.7[b]

[a]   Vs. normal controls, p not significant.
[b]   Vs. normal controls and vs. other groups $p = 0.001$.

using inbred strains of mice with highly defined genetic backgrounds. Young adult male Balb/c mice were infected with a low dose (50 trypomastigotes per mouse) of the myotropic Colombia strain of *T. cruzi*.[111] A similar group of mice was injected with suspension buffer and served as controls. On days 15, 45, 90, 120, and 150 after infection, the animals were sacrificed. Splenic mononuclear cells were isolated[112] and adherent cells were removed.[113] The purified mononuclear cells were incubated with syngeneic (Balb/c) neonatal cardiac myofibers in vitro.[114] Cytotoxicity of cardiac myofibers was measured with the use of a ^{51}Cr release assay.[115] The results are summarized in Table 2. No antiheart lymphocyte cytotoxicity was detectable during the early or intermediate stages of infection. However, during the later phase marked autoreactive lymphocyte cytotoxicity to normal syngeneic cardiac myofibers was evident. No specific cytotoxicity was shown by lymphocytes from control mice. The antiheart immune reaction was correlated with the presence of a widely distributed focal myocarditis with myocardial cell necrosis in the absence of intracellular amastigotes of *T. cruzi*[111] (Figure 5). These data indicate that long-term infection with a low dose of *T. cruzi* elicits the induction of autoimmune antiheart lymphocyte cytotoxicity with a concomitant myocarditis. Furthermore, they indicate that the lymphocyte cytotoxicity previously exhibited in allogeneic systems[6,51] is, at least in part, due to specific antiheart reactions.

In order to conclusively establish that the cardiac damage seen in chronic Chagas' disease is due to antiheart autoimmune cytotoxic reactions, *T. cruzi*-sensitized lymphocytes from the Balb/c mice that had demonstrated antiheart cell lymphocyte cytotoxicity, as described above, were used in adoptive transfer studies.[70] Lymphocytes from the *T. cruzi*-infected mice and also from their matched controls were cultured in the presence of Balb/c cardiac sarcoplasmic reticulum preparations for 5 days. The lymphoblasts were harvested and extensively washed to remove any cardiac sarcoplasmic reticulum present in the medium. Lymphoblasts were then injected into normal young adult male syngeneic recipients. Electrocardiographic tracings were recorded at biweekly intervals. One mouse developed right bundle branch block and atrial fibrillation 4 weeks after transfer. At the end of 6 weeks, the mice were sacrificed and splenic lymphocyte cytotoxicity against normal syngeneic cardiac myofibers was measured as described above.[115] Adoptive transfer recipients of *T. cruzi*-sensitized lymphocytes developed autoreactive lymphocyte cytotoxicity to normal syngeneic cardiac myofibers (Table 3). Recipients of lymphocytes from matched controls did not exhibit these aberrations. None of these mice developed anti-*T. cruzi* serology, indicating that *T. cruzi* parasites were not accidentally carried over from lymphocyte donors. These

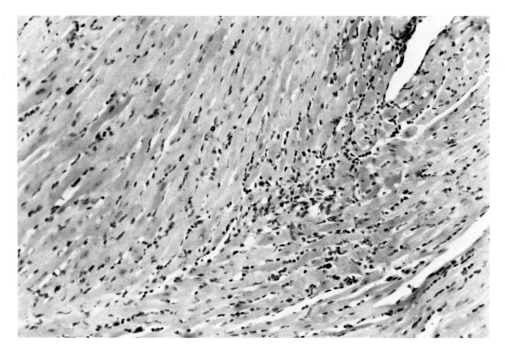

FIGURE 5. Ventricular wall of a Balb/c mouse infected with *T. cruzi* for 150 days that developed lymphocyte cytotoxicity against normal syngeneic cardiac myofibers in vitro. Histologic exam revealed a focal myocarditis with mononuclear cell infiltrates widely distributed throughout the heart in the absence of intracellular forms of *T. cruzi*. (Hematoxylin and eosin.)

Table 3
ADOPTIVE TRANSFER OF LYMPHOCYTE CYTOTOXICITY OF NORMAL SYNGENEIC CARDIAC MYOFIBERS

Syngeneic source of adoptive transfer lymphocytes	Treatment of recipient mice	Average % specific ^{51}Cr release
T. cruzi infected	None	26.4[a]
Matched control	None	1.5
T. cruzi infected	Prednisolone	3.3[b]
Matched control	Prednisolone	2.7

[a] Vs. other groups, $p = 0.001$.
[b] Vs. matched controls, p not significant.

results show that adoptive transfer of *T. cruzi*-sensitized lymphocytes elicits autoimmune antiheart reactions resulting in myocardial cell destruction in vitro.

In further adoptive transfer studies,[70] young adult male syngeneic recipients were treated with 1 mg prednisolone before adoptive transfer of *T. cruzi*-sensitized lymphocytes. These mice received a 1-mg subcutaneous injection of prednisolone per week for the 6-week duration of the experiment. Splenic lymphocytes were isolated and antiheart cytotoxicity measured as described above. The results are summarized in Table 3. The prednisolone-treated mice did not exhibit any antiheart cytoxicity.

The observations that antiheart autoimmune reactions were produced by the adoptive transfer of *T. cruzi*-sensitized lymphocytes and that a viable *T. cruzi* infection was not required give strong support to the hypothesis that the myocardial damage seen in Chagas' disease is at least partly due to antiheart autoimmune reactions elicited by *T. cruzi*. The abrogation of these reactions by glucocorticoid immunosuppressive therapy lends further credence to the theory of an autoimmune-mediated cardiomyopathy in chronic Chagas' disease.

2. Two Theories on the Mechanism of Induction of the Antiheart Autoimmune Response
a. Autoimmunity Produced by Adsorption of T. cruzi Antigens onto Host Cells with Subsequent Release of Self Antigens

The presence of antiheart immune reactions in Chagas' disease has led many investigators to postulate that autoimmune phenomena play a role in the pathogenesis of chronic Chagas' heart disease.[4-10,59,60] Two theories exist as to the mechanism by which the antiheart reactions are elicited.

Ribeiro dos Santos and Hudson,[58] in in vitro studies, have shown that rupturing pseudocysts of amastigotes release *T. cruzi* antigens that adsorb onto neighboring uninfected host cells. Adsorption of *T. cruzi* antigens derived from either epimastigotes or amastigotes rendered cultured human or murine cells vulnerable to immune destruction by rabbit anti-*T. cruzi* serum plus complement; antibody-directed cellular cytotoxicity using rabbit anti-*T. cruzi* serum and normal mouse (Balb/c) splenocytes; or nylon wool nonadherent splenocytes from *T. cruzi*-infected Balb/c mice.[59] Nylon wool nonadherent splenocytes from *T. cruzi*-infected Balb/c mice were also able to destroy normal, uninfected cells 60 days postinfection but not at 15 days postinfection.[59] Immunofluorescence studies using cryostat sections of hearts from C57B1 mice infected with *T. cruzi* for 7 to 10 days show the presence of *T. cruzi* antigens on infected myocardial cells as well as uninfected neighboring cells.[60] Hearts from mice infected for 15 days did not show any fluorescence when treated with anti-*T. cruzi* serum. Monocytes from *T. cruzi*-infected C57B1 mice exhibited a positive MIF test with *T. cruzi* antigen at 10 days postinfection which remained positive throughout the duration of the experiment (90 days).[60] Myocardial and neuronal antigens also yielded positive MIF tests starting at day 20 and remaining so until day 90.[60]

Based on these results, Ribeiro dos Santos and Hudson[59,60] have postulated the following theory for the pathogenesis of chronic Chagas' heart disease. Rupturing pseudocysts of amastigotes in the early phase of infection release *T. cruzi* antigens that are adsorbed onto neighboring uninfected host cells. The parasite-modified host cells are then destroyed by the host anti-*T. cruzi* immune response, thus, releasing self antigens. The released self antigens elicit autoimmune responses that lead to the pathologic lesions found in chronic Chagas' disease.

The basis for the theory of *T. cruzi*-induced autoimmunity proposed by Ribeiro dos Santos and Hudson is that the release of host components after the lysis of *T. cruzi*-modified host cells elicits an autoimmune response. However, there are data that indicate that this series of events is not sufficient to evoke autoimmune reactions. Doherty et al.[116] have shown that infection of inbred mice with lymphocytic choriomeningitis virus produced T-lymphocyte cytotoxicity to virus-infected syngeneic cells but not to normal syngeneic cells. Shearer et al.[117] have reported that the modification of normal murine cells with trinitrophenyl evokes a cytotoxic T-lymphocyte response against trinitrophenyl-modified cells but not against normal cells. Several other reports similarly indicate that cytotoxic T lymphocytes elicited by modified self-antigens will not produce an autoimmune attack of nonmodified syngeneic targets in experimental animals.[118-120] These investigations tend to exclude the possibility that the release of host components after the lysis of *T. cruzi*-modified cells per se will evoke an autoimmune response which will destroy nonmodified syngeneic targets.

Other difficulties lie in Ribeiro dos Santos' and Hudson's theory. Their theory requires a viable *T. cruzi* infection in order to initiate the antigenic modification of host cells. However, data from our laboratory indicate that infection is not prerequisite for the induction of antiheart immune responses or for the production of cardiac lesions characteristic of Chagas' cardiomyopathy. Immunization of rabbits[51] or mice[71] with *T. cruzi* antigens, or passive transfer of *T. cruzi*-sensitized lymphocytes in mice[70] elicits antiheart lymphocyte cytotoxicity and a chronic myocarditis. Furthermore, their theory does not explain the antiheart specificity of the autoimmune reactions seen in Chagas' disease. Since *T. cruzi* has the capacity to infect many different cell types,[42] their theory would predict a widespread autoimmune destruction of many organs due to the adsorption of *T. cruzi* antigens onto different cell types. This phenomenon is not observed in *T. cruzi* infection of long duration.

There is much evidence against the theory of Ribeiro dos Santos and Hudson for the induction of autoimmune responses in Chagas' disease. Their data, however, represent an autoimmune reaction, albeit most probably evoked by a mechanism distinct from that which they proposed. The equivalent lysis of *T. cruzi*-modified and unmodified tumor cells by nylon wool nonadherent splenocytes at 60 days postinfection may be attributed to a type-specific autoreactive immune response. The target tumor cell lines used in these experiments were derived from syngeneic Balb/c striated muscle or from allogeneic murine neuroblastoma.[59] Purified mononuclear cells from the 60-day infected Balb/c mice exhibited positive MIF tests with cardiac muscle and neuronal antigens.[59] The lysis of the unmodified target cells may, therefore, be attributed to auto- or alloreactive immune responses. The mechanism of induction of these reponses, however, is most likely different from that postulated by those authors.

The reports of Ribeiro dos Santos and Hudson showing the adsorption of *T. cruzi* antigens onto neighboring normal host cells and the destruction of *T. cruzi* antigen-modified host cells in vitro may describe a mechanism by which the host's immune response may clear the body of *T. cruzi* and *T. cruzi*-related antigens. The significance of this mechanism in the elicitation of the antiheart autoimmune reaction seen in chronic Chagas' disease has yet to be determined.

b. Autoimmunity Produced by Cross-Reacting Antigens of Host and T. cruzi

The antiheart reactions of immunocompetent cells from *T. cruzi*-infected humans[5,6] and experimental animals[51,111] and the observation that mononuclear cells from these subjects exhibited positive MIF tests with heart antigens led us to propose the hypothesis that *T. cruzi* and striated muscle share a cross-reacting antigen and that the shared *T. cruzi*-striated muscle antigen plays a causative role in the pathogenesis of the cardiac lesions seen in chronic Chagas' cardiomyopathy. The data indicate that *T. cruzi* does, indeed, have an antigenic determinant that is cross-reactive with striated muscle.[9,10,61,121] Reports from our laboratory have shown that the cross-reactive antigen is related to purified preparations of the calcium-sequestering sarcoplasmic reticulum adenosine triphosphatase (SRA).[10,121] Immunofluorescence studies using antisera raised against striated muscle SRA showed specific intracellular staining of *T. cruzi* flagellates.[10] The nucleus and outer membrane did not stain. Similar staining patterns were obtained using antisera raised against *T. cruzi* small membranes. When these antisera were tested against murine myocardium, a specific fine intracellular staining was seen.[10] There was also staining of the cardiac sarcolemma; however, the endpoint titer of the intracellular stain was two twofold dilutions more concentrated than that of the sarcolemma (1:1280 vs. 1:320, respectively).[10] Staining of endothelial, vascular, or interstitial structures characteristic of the heterophile EVI antibodies[50] was not seen. The anti-SRA staining pattern is also distinct from the patterns elicited by other heterophile antibodies on cardiac substrates.[104] Hemagglutination studies using striated muscle SRA- or *T. cruzi* small membrane-sensitized red blood cells and antisera to either striated muscle

SRA or antisera to *T. cruzi* small membranes also showed a specific cross-reactivity.[10] This hemagglutinating activity could be inhibited by microgram quantities of either striated muscle SRA or *T. cruzi* small membranes.[10] Ouchterlony double diffusion studies in gel showed two lines of identity using either striated muscle SRA or *T. cruzi* small membranes as antigen, and antisera against striated muscle SRA and antisera against *T. cruzi* membranes.[10] Enzyme-linked immunosorbent assays (ELISA) also confirmed the cross-reactivity.[122] Furthermore, cell-mediated cross-reactivity was shown using foot pad reactions.[121] In all serologic assays, high titered antisera against muscle tropomyosin, ox red blood cells, sheep red blood cells, or murine kidney extract did not show any reactivity with striated muscle SRA or *T. cruzi* small membranes.[10,122] These results indicate that SRA is not related to ubiquitous blood group, Forssman or heterophile determinants, or to tropomyosin which is part of the muscle contraction/relaxation system.

SRA has a wide phylogenetic distribution. Using highly specific reference antisera to either the small membranes of *T. cruzi* or a tryptic fragment of striated muscle SRA, it was shown that SRA is present in the striated muscle of animals representative of the evolutionary scale ranging from nonhuman primate (monkey) to fish (osteichthyes).[122] Furthermore, nine different strains of *T. cruzi*, including strains isolated from sylvatic animals of North America, also showed cross-reactivity with the reference antisera.[122] These data indicate that SRA is present among all *T. cruzi* strains tested and suggest that the cross-reactive striated muscle determinant may be prevalent among all *T. cruzi* strains of the American continents.

SRA is apparently present in both cardiac and skeletal muscle.[10] Unlike skeletal muscle fibers, the sarcolemma of myocardial cells has calcium transport properties.[123,124] Antisera to either skeletal muscle SRA or to *T. cruzi* small membranes localized antibody on the sarcolemma of cardiac myofibers by immunofluorescence tests.[10] Furthermore, by gel immunoprecipitation, antiserum to heart membrane preparation and antiserum to *T. cruzi* membrane formed two lines of identity with purified SRA.[10] The cardiac sarcolemmal localization of SRA is consistent with the observations that elements of the immune response in chronic Chagas' disease interact with the sarcolemma of cardiac myofibers. In this regard, lymphocytes from individuals with Chagas' disease interact with[5] and destroy[6] normal allogenic heart cells in vitro. Lymphocytes from *T. cruzi*-infected rabbits or rabbits immunized with *T. cruzi* small membranes destroy allogeneic cardiac cell cultures[51] and sera from these animals reacted with the sarcolemma of heart fibers.[110] More importantly, inbred mice infected with *T. cruzi* develop antiheart autoimmune lymphocyte cytotoxicity[111] and the adoptive transfer of *T. cruzi*-sensitized lymphocytes similarly induces antiheart autoimmune lymphocyte cytotoxicity in syngeneic recipients.[70]

A pathogenic role cannot be assigned to the shared *T. cruzi*-striated muscle SRA unless it can be shown that immunization with SRA produces antiheart immune reactions and the development of cardiac lesions similar to those seen in chronic Chagas' disease. With this in mind, young adult male Balb/c mice were immunized with either autologous murine (Balb/c) SRA or heterologous monkey SRA emulsified in Freund's complete adjuvant (FCA).[71] A control group of mice was injected with suspension buffer emulsified in FCA according to the same immunization schedule. Splenic lymphocytes were isolated and antiheart cytotoxicity was determined as described above. Specific antiheart cytotoxicity was exhibited by lymphocytes from mice immunized with monkey SRA (Table 4). Significantly, mice immunized with autologous SRA also developed antiheart lymphocyte cytotoxicity. No cytotoxicity was shown by control mice. These data indicate that SRA can induce a cytotoxic response to normal syngeneic heart cells in vitro. Histopathologic examination of the hearts from these animals demonstrated the presence of cardiac lesions in 70% of heterologous monkey SRA-immunized mice and in 40% of autologous murine SRA-immunized mice.[71] There was an extensive lymphocytic atrial myocarditis attended with cytolysis of myofibers. There were also severe focal lesions with destruction of cardiac myofibers attended by

Table 4
SRA-SENSITIZED LYMPHOCYTE
CYTOTOXICITY OF NORMAL SYNGENEIC
CARDIAC MYOFIBERS

SRA source	Average % specific ^{51}Cr release	Myocarditis
Autologous (Balb/c)	23.2[a,b]	4/10
Heterologous (monkey)	17.2[a]	7/10

[a]   Vs. controls, $p = 0.001$.
[b]   Vs. heterologous, p not significant.

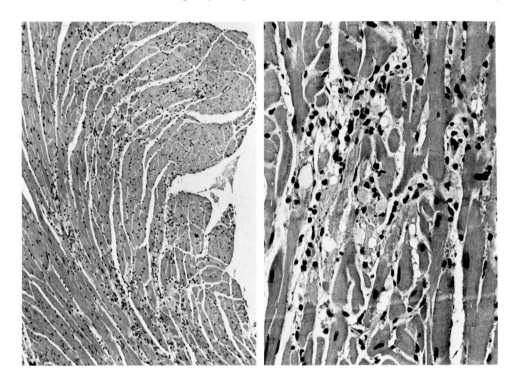

FIGURE 6.   Ventricular wall of a Balb/c mouse immunized with syngeneic (Balb/c) SRA. The mouse developed lymphocyte cytotoxicity against normal syngeneic cardiac myofibers in vitro. (A) Low-power magnification showing several focal areas of myocarditis (Hematoxylin and eosin.); (B) high-power magnification demonstrating destruction of myofibers attended by intermediate-sized lymphocytes. (Hematoxylin and eosin.)

intermediate-sized lymphocytes widely distributed throughout both ventricles (Figure 6). These data showing the elicitation of autoimmune reactions and the subsequent destruction of cardiac myofibers both in vitro and in vivo indicate that SRA is, indeed, immunopathogenic.

There are data that indicate that SRA may be a heteroantigen. Immunization of experimental animals with striated-muscle SRA preparations, particularly those of nonhuman primate, chicken, and turtle, give rise to antiallogenic muscle SRA activity, whereas immunization with rabbit, frog, or fish SRA does not.[122] Immunization with the small membranes from different strains of *T. cruzi* also gives rise to antiallogeneic muscle SRA antibody activity in some, albeit not all immunized animals.[122] Analogously, only a percentage of humans infected with *T. cruzi* go on to develop chronic Chagas' cardiomyopathy.[1] The degree of immunological identity between the SRA heteroantigen present in *T. cruzi* and that present in the host may, thus, modulate the nature of the immune response evoked by the infective organism. An exact identity between the two may result in recognition as self and lack immunogenicity. On the other hand, partial identity between the two may elicit an immune response to the mismatched heteroantigen, resulting in antiheart autoimmune reactions and cardiomyopathy. Further studies are required in order to establish the dynamics of the anti-SRA immune response with the development of cardiomyopathy in *T. cruzi*-infected humans.

V. SUBCLINICAL DISEASE

The diagnosis of acute Chagas' disease is usually assigned to patients who present with a generalized malaise and fever, splenomegaly, edema at the portal of entry, and the presence of *T. cruzi* flagellates in the peripheral blood. It is thought that these patients represent a minority of the cases of recent *T. cruzi* infection, whereas the majority are characterized by a subclinical illness with little or no symptomatology. Many older patients suffering from the chronic cardiac form of the disease do not remember developing any of the signs or symptoms of the acute disease or ever being exposed to the vector. Teixeira et al.,[65] in a provocative report, have shown the presence of an acquired T lymphocyte immunosuppression in a group of patients with recent *T. cruzi* infection and no symptomatology. This is in sharp contrast with a matched set of patients with symptomatic acute Chagas' disease and normal T lymphocyte function. Both groups had equivalent humoral antibody responses. The exact mechanism of the specific T lymphocyte immunosuppression is not known. It is interesting to speculate whether or not those individuals with an initially suppressed T lymphocyte response will go on to develop the chronic autoimmune cardiac manifestations of Chagas' disease due to aberrant T lymphocyte function. On the other hand, it may be that these individuals will be spared and those with normal T lymphocyte function will succumb to the chronic cardiac form because of cell-mediated responses to cross-reacting antigenic determinants present in both *T. cruzi* and the human host. Clearly, longitudinal studies are required to establish the effect of this initial T lymphocyte immunosuppression on the chronic manifestations of Chagas' disease.

VI. ACUTE SYMPTOMATIC CHAGAS' DISEASE

A. Clinical Manifestations

The designation of acute Chagas' disease is reserved for those patients with a recent symptomatic *T. cruzi* infection, the highest incidence of which is found in children under the age of 5 with rare occurrences after the age of 15.[1,64] In 38% of the nonhospitalized cases the symptoms and signs directly relate to those of the developing parasitemia and myocarditis.[1] The disease is manifested by fever, muscular pains, sweats, general malaise, irritability, anorexia, and sometimes vomiting and diarrhea. There is generalized lymphadenopathy and moderate hepatosplenomegaly. Signs related to acute myocarditis, including moderate enlargement of the heart accompanied by electrocardiographic changes such as lengthening of the P-R interval, a low-voltage QRS, sinus tachycardia, and primary alterations of the T waves, are also present.

Edema at the portal of entry with satellite lymphadenopathy are usually present. The eye serves as the portal of entry in approximately 50% of the cases.[68] There is a unilateral bipalpebral edema with reddening of the skin which is referred to as Romana's sign. Frequently, there is also enlargement of the lacrimal gland. These signs persist for approximately 1 month before subsiding. In approximately 25% of cases, the skin serves as the portal of entry.[68] Initially, there is a small painful red spot that enlarges to several centimeters in diameter within a week. This skin lesion, referred to as a *chagoma*, resolves within 30 days and often leaves a pigmented scar.

Most symptoms of acute Chagas' disease resolve within 3 to 4 months. However, residual signs such as an elongated P-R interval, lymphadenopathy and lymphocytosis, fever, and elevated erythrocyte sedimentation rates are transiently recorded for periods of months to years in a few patients.[1] These ''residual'' signs may be due to reinfection since individuals often return to endemic areas where the incidence of *T. cruzi*-infected Reduviidae insects is high.

Circulating antibodies to *T. cruzi* can be detected within 2 to 3 weeks of infection by immunofluorescence, complement fixation, or other serologic techniques. False positive results may be obtained when testing the sera of patients with leishmaniasis because of cross-reacting antigenic determinants present in *T. cruzi* and *Leishmania* species.[125] Sera from patients with mononucleosis, syphilis, or other diseases that induce heterophile antibody production may also yield false positive results. It should be noted that infection with *T. cruzi* can itself induce heterophile antibody production, especially in the acute phase of infection.[105,106] The detection of *T. cruzi* flagellates in the peripheral blood can be accompanied by direct observation of trypanosomes in stained smears of fresh blood or after lysis of red blood cells under a glass coverslip. Other much lengthier indirect techniques exist, such as blood inoculation of media in laboratory culture tubes. At present, the most widely used laboratory method for the detection of *T. cruzi* is xenodiagnosis due to the high biologic amplification of its sensitivity to detect low levels of parasitemia.[62] Uninfected laboratory-grown Reduviidae insects are allowed to feed on the individual who is suspected of having *T. cruzi* infection, and after several weeks the insects are examined for metacyclic trypomastigotes in the hind gut. Cerisola et al.[62] have compared the relative sensitivities of the different detection methods and have reported that xenodiagnosis, although being the most cumbersome of all the methods, is the one with the highest sensitivity for detection of low levels of parasitemia.

The fatality rate for acute Chagas' disease is 5 to 10%.[68] Most fatal cases are due to acute myocarditis with congestive heart failure, meningoencephalitis, and rarely to complications such as bronchopneumonia.[68]

B. Pathology

Histopathologic examination at the portal of entry shows a mononuclear cell infiltrate with amastigotes of *T. cruzi* present in parasitized macrophages.[68] There is also reticulum cell and fibroblast proliferation and interstitial edema. Multinucleated giant cells are occasionally detected. *T. cruzi* has the capacity of infecting many different cell types and, thus, may be found in many different organs. Most frequently pseudocysts of amastigotes are found in cardiac and skeletal muscle, smooth muscle, and glia.[42] There is usually a coincident mononuclear cell infiltrate, with congestion, edema, and often granulomatous areas. Amastigotes are rarely found in the testis, ovary, or thyroid.[42]

The most consistent finding in fatal cases of acute Chagas' disease is a severe myocarditis. The heart is usually slightly dilated, and subepicardial and endocardial petechia may be present.[42] Mononuclear cell infiltrates may involve any and all structures of the heart including myofibers, valvular tissue, neuronal elements, and the conduction system. Amastigotes of *T. cruzi* are quite abundant.

Focal inflammatory lesions may also be found in skeletal muscle. Parasitosis of smooth muscle cells in the esophagus and colon are also observed. Lymphocytic infiltrates around Auerbach's parasympathetic myenteric plexus are occasionally found. In cases of acute Chagas' disease involving the brain, mononuclear cell infiltrates are found in the leptomeninges.[42] There may also be perivascular hemorrhages, neuronophagia, and glial cell proliferation. Rarely is there parasitism of neurons. Infrequently there are reports of necrotic arteriolar lesions of the gastrointestinal tract.[68] There is no evidence of immune deposits in renal glomeruli, nor of the secondary amyloidosis that are sometimes seen in African trypanosomiasis or in visceral leishmaniasis, respectively.

VII. TRANSPLACENTAL TRANSMISSION AND CONGENITAL CHAGAS' DISEASE

A. Clinical Manifestations

The reported incidence of transplacental transmission of *T. cruzi* is low. Approximately 2 to 4% of the live births of *T. cruzi*-infected mothers have congenital Chagas' disease.[95] The mothers are usually in the indeterminate phase of Chagas' disease[126,127] and may have had uninfected babies prior to or after the birth of the infected infant.[95] Most newborns with congenital Chagas' disease are premature and/or small for gestational age with 80% of them weighing less than 2000 g at birth.[127] The clinical manifestations of congenital Chagas' disease are similar to those observed in the acute form of the disease.[27] Hepatosplenomegaly is usually present[27] and anemia with a hematological profile similar to that seen in erythro-blastosis is also encountered.[127] Parasitemia is initially low but increases with time after birth.[27] Saleme et al.[128] demonstrated a correlation between the level of parasitemia and the prognosis of the infant, showing the imminent demise of the child whenever the parasitemic load reached ten or more *T. cruzi* flagellates per milliliter of blood. The mortality rate for congenital cases of Chagas' disease is high. Bittencourt[27] reported that of 90 observed cases of transplacental transmission of *T. cruzi*, 24 infants were stillborn, and of the remaining 66 live births, only 27 survived for more than 24 months. This indicates a mortality rate of 59% for live births and an overall mortality rate of 70% for all cases of congenital Chagas' disease. *T. cruzi* infection also has the capability of inducing abortion.[129,130]

The factors predisposing to congenital transmission of *T. cruzi* are not well understood. Bittencourt[27] and Rassi et al.[131] have reported the births of uninfected infants even though the mothers exhibited *T. cruzi* parasitemias throughout their pregnancies. This indicates that *T. cruzi* parasitemia alone is not sufficient to produce congenital transmission. Some authors believe that the integrity of the trophoblastic layer of the placenta is essential in the prevention of transplacental transmission of *T. cruzi*. Rassi et al.,[131] in a study of human placentas, suggested that the trophoblastic layer constituted a barrier to the penetration of *T. cruzi* by virtue of its phagocytic properties and thickness. Bittencourt et al.[27] indicated that the first step in transplacental passage of *T. cruzi* may be parasitosis of the trophoblast. However, studies conducted in our laboratory in which the reticuloendothelial system of pregnant mice was blocked have shown that transplacental transmission of *T. cruzi* can occur in the presence of an intact trophoblastic layer that does not show any evidence of parasitosis by *T. cruzi*.[28] These experiments suggested that transplacental transmission was effected by blood-born trypomastigotes that penetrated the fetal circulation across the highly permeable yolk sac placenta. Furthermore, these studies showed that congenital transmission was dependent on the strain of *T. cruzi* used for infection and on the immunophagocytic competence of the placenta. Infection of mice with a pathogenic strain of *T. cruzi* following reticuloendothelial system blockade produced transplacental transmission, where infection with the same strain without blockade or infection with a nonpathogenic strain with or without blockade did not.[28] The importance of the infective strain of *T. cruzi* contradicts previous experiments that showed no strain difference in relation to congenital transmission.[132] Similar factors may be involved in congenital Chagas' disease in humans.

B. Pathology

Most of the lesions found in congenital Chagas' disease are related to the parasitosis of tissue by *T. cruzi*. However, amastigotes have not been observed in the necrotizing arteriolitis occasionally seen in the fetus and placenta.[133,134] The heart, skeletal muscle, hollow viscera, brain, and skin are most frequently affected.[27] There is a mononuclear cell infiltrate, some-times accompanied by chronic granulomas composed of lymphocytes, monocytes, and mac-rophages. The most consistent findings in the placentas of cases of congenital Chagas' disease are villous and intervillous inflammatory reactions.[27]

VIII. INDETERMINATE CHAGAS' DISEASE

As previously indicated, the mortality rate for symptomatic acute Chagas' disease is 5 to 10%.[68] The survivors, as well as a large number of individuals with an asymptomatic subclinical disease process, enter into a vaguely defined clinical state: the indeterminate form of Chagas' disease. The undetermined aspect of this form of Chagas' disease lies in whether or not the *T. cruzi*-infected individual will progress to the chronic form of the disease and develop the sequelae of chronic Chagas' cardiomyopathy eventually resulting in death. The factors that contribute to this "decision" are not known. Variability in the pathogenicity of the different infective strains of *T. cruzi*, their geographic distribution, and their epidemiology most probably play a role. Several factors in the mammalian host may also participate, the most important possibly being the variability in genotype susceptibility to the development of the chronic form of the disease.

Individuals in the indeterminate phase of Chagas's disease show no symptoms attributable to *T. cruzi* parasitemia or myocarditis. Routine physical examination including electrocardiograph and chest X-ray reveal no clinical manifestations of *T. cruzi* infection. All carriers have continuously high antibody titers against *T. cruzi*. Inasmuch as the remission of *T. cruzi* infection has never been reported, an individual may harbor the parasite throughout his or her lifetime and parasitemias are thus occasionally detected.[62]

Recent studies using advanced cardiologic diagnostic techniques have demonstrated minor functional and morphologic changes in the hearts of patients with the indeterminate form of Chagas's disease. Decourt et al.,[135] using the HIS bundle electrocardiogram, reported the presence of mild interatrial conduction defects in patients with *T. cruzi* infection and normal standard 12-lead electrocardiographic tracings. Echocardiographic studies by Friedmann et al.[136] demonstrated impaired left ventricular performance, as shown by decreased percent diameter variation, mean circumferential fiber shortening, and ejection fraction in patients with the indeterminate form of Chagas's disease. Histopathologic examination of the hearts from asymptomatic *T. cruzi*-infected patients who died of causes other than Chagas' disease has shown occasional foci of inflammation with fibrosis.[68] Studies of endomyocardial biopsies from patients in the indeterminate phase of the disease have similarly shown inflammatory infiltrates and degenerative changes. Mady et al.[137] have reported minor inflammatory infiltrates in the cardiac biopsies of 12 of 20 patients with the indeterminate form of Chagas's disease. Fibrosis was also found in 3 of the 12 cases. Carrasco et al.[138] have reported the presence of ultrastructural degenerative changes in cardiac biopsies of 8 of 14 patients with the indeterminate form of the disease.

Many investigators believe that the cardiomyopathy seen in chronic Chagas's disease evolves from a slowly progressive, subpatent disease process. Laranja et al.[1] reported the development of permanent electrocardiographic defects in 12 of 75 *T. cruzi*-infected individuals over a 10-year period. The above-mentioned minor functional and morphologic changes in the indeterminate form of Chagas's disease tend to support the hypothesis of a smouldering disease process. However, longitudinal studies are required in order to clearly establish the progression and pathogenesis of Chagas' heart disease.

IX. CHRONIC CHAGAS' DISEASE

A. Clinical Manifestations

An estimated 12 million people are infected with *T. cruzi*.[14] Approximately up to 20% of these individuals go on to develop the chronic form of Chagas' disease.[1,3] The factors predisposing to the development of the chronic form of the disease are not known. The presence of *T. cruzi* parasitemia is very difficult or almost impossible to establish and is not necessary to make a diagnosis of chronic Chagas' disease. The unequivocal history of having developed Romana's sign or a *chagoma* in an endemic area and/or a positive serologic test for *T. cruzi*, in addition to characteristic cardiac or gastrointestinal tract lesions, is sufficient to make the diagnosis.

The highest incidence of chronic Chagas' cardiomyopathy occurs in the third and fourth decades of life.[1,64] Typically, patients enter the hospital complaining of right upper-quadrant pain often complemented by edema of the lower extremities and progressive dyspnea.[68] On physical exam, marked dilatation of the heart with right- and left-sided failure and acites with pedal edema is commonly found. The point of maximal impulse is generally diffuse or of low intensity and is located outside the midclavicular line and may sometimes reach the midaxillary line. Left ventricular heave, a wide and fixed split second sound with P2 equal to A2, and a systolic regurgitation murmur at the mitral area radiating to the axilla and followed by a third heart sound are very often encountered.[68]

Examination of chest X-rays of patients with chronic Chagas' disease reveals moderate to severe cardiomegaly with an increase in size of all cardiac chambers.[139] Severe conduction disturbances are typically present in chronic Chagas' disease. Electrocardiographic studies of patients with Chagas' cardiomyopathy show first-degree atrioventricular block and complete right bundle branch block in approximately 50% of the cases.[1,140] Left anterior hemiblock is also present in about the same incidence and frequently coexists.[1,44,140] Characteristically, incomplete atrioventricular block with P-R intervals of 0.20 sec or more are also found. Ventricular extrasystole is found in 60% of patients with chronic Chagas' disease.[141,142] Studies using stress tests reveal that 37 of 70 patients with Chagas' cardiomyopathy have variable decreases in work capacity and of these, 36 had extrasystolic arrhythmias.[143] Holter-24-hr electrocardiographic monitoring similarly showed extrasystoles and paroxysmal tachycardia as well.[144] Porto,[141] in a study of 503 patients who died of Chagas' heart disease, reported that sudden death occurred in 37% of the cases.

Mendoza et al.,[145] using electro- and vector-cardiographic techniques, reported that 20 of 26 patients with Chagas' cardiomyopathy demonstrated contraction alterations of the left ventricle. M-mode echocardiographic studies showed that 18 of 47 patients with chronic Chagas' disease had hypokinesia of the left posterior ventricular wall.[146] Of the 47 patients, 11 also showed a generalized hypokinesia of the heart.[146] Investigations using two-dimensional echocardiography demonstrated the presence of ventricular aneurysms or apical dyskinesia in 31 of 41 patients with chronic Chagas' cardiomyopathy.[146] Radionucleotide studies similarly showed aberrations in left ventricular function in 22 of 31 patients with Chagas' cardiomyopathy.[147]

Once the onset of heart failure is noted, wide use of cardiotonic drugs, diuretics, or implantation of pacemakers has been ultimately to no avail. Patients with chronic Chagas' cardiomyopathy inexorably deteriorate and die of Chagas' disease within 6 to 13 months of the initial onset of heart insufficiency.

Those patients suffering from the chronic form of Chagas' disease that principally involves the hollow viscera innervated by the parasympathetic nervous system also have a very poor prognosis. In most cases, varied degrees of Chagas' cardiomyopathy occur concurrently.[148] There is an irregular and indiscriminate destruction of ganglion cells of the myenteric plexus ranging from a complete annihilation in severe cases to a variable decrease in cases where no visceral dilatation is noted.[149,150] Although the entire digestive tract can be affected, as can the ureters and biliary tree, the most commonly found forms are different degrees of achalasia of the esophagus and/or colon with distal and proximal dilatation, respectively.[74,148] Impairment of the propagation of the peristaltic wave prerequisite for the propulsion of solid materials through these organs may prove to be a functional explanation of the predisposition for lesions developing here.[148]

The diagnosis of chronic Chagas' myenteric denervation is made by grouping the following: characteristic electrocardiographic changes, a positive serologic test for *T. cruzi*, abnormal manometric motility tests of the esophagus, and abnormal retention of barium enemas after evacuation.[151] A positive mecholyl test may aid in the diagnosis since parasympathe-ticomimetic drugs will induce spontaneous rhythmic activity in patients with chagasic de-nervation of the esophagus but not in nomal subjects.[151]

Patients with Chagas' myenteric denervation without congestive heart failure may develop lower intestinal obstruction or perforate a dilated segment of colon. Death due to pulmonary infections usually induced by aspiration of esophageal contents aggravated by malnutrition, anorexia, and obstipation may occur in such cases. Patients with achalasia of the esophagus or colon and heart failure may succumb to intractable heart disease first, even though involvement of the myenteric nerve plexus may be extensive.

B. Pathology
1. Microscopic Pathology
a. Piecemeal Cell-by-Cell Injury

Some of the variability found in the pathologic presentation of *T. cruzi* infection in humans may be attributed to the tissue tropism of the infective strain. In the laboratory, significantly different tissue tropism is exhibited among *T. cruzi* isolates.[152-154] Cells of mesodermal origin, principally striated muscle and macrophages, are targeted for preferential parasitosis. The "myotropic" and "reticulotropic" nature of certain *T. cruzi* strains has thus been de-scribed.[152,153] Less frequently and rarely described are *T. cruzi* isolates that preferentially parasitize neuroectodermal cells.[42] However, glial cells and neurons of the central and autonomic nervous systems are readily parasitized in experimental infections of mice.[155] In humans with overwhelming parasitosis and parasitemia, almost every cell in the body is infected, but the heart and brain are most severely parasitized. Using tissue culture mono-layers, different *T. cruzi* isolates show characteristic rates of penetration and proliferation and, also, of the exodus of trypomastigotes to the supernate after rupture of pseudocysts (personal observations). The characteristic rates of each isolate parallel the biology of the corresponding course of the infection in susceptible mice.[154,156] Certain cell lines, like the astrocytoma AO-2 cell line, are readily penetrated by some strains of *T. cruzi* (e.g., Colombia and Brazil strains) resulting in enormous cytoplasmic pseudocysts which eventually swarm with packed swimming trypomastigotes. These are unable to rupture the cytoplasmic mem-brane or gain access to the overlay and eventually die (personal observations). Where *T. cruzi* trypomastigote forms rupture the pseudocyst, the host cell immediately begins to attempt the repair of the injured plasma membrane. In tissue culture studies, plasma membrane repair is accomplished with astonishing rapidity by mesodermal cells and epithelial renal cells.[156] Some, however, are unable to recover and are literally blown up and destroyed, probably by osmotic forces and loss of critical intracellular ions. In living cells of experi-mental animals and humans, *T. cruzi* penetration, proliferation and exodus, and plasma membrane repair may obey similar steps. Andrade and Andrade[45] have shown in *T. cruzi*-infected mice that the liquor which suspends the parasites in the intracellular pseudocyst contains amorphous *T. cruzi*-related antigens. *T. cruzi*-related antigens are also found in cytoplasmic vacuoles of adjacent macrophages and, significantly, in the interstitial space adjacent to ruptured parasitized cells.[42,45] The spillage of partially processed *T. cruzi*-related antigens into the extracellular space may explain why focal polymorphonuclear cell exudates are present only where cytoplasmic cell injury has occurred[42] and not where the parasitized cells have morphologically intact plasma membranes. The polymorphonuclear cell exudate may be attributed to complement-mediated chemotaxis by immune complex formation *in situ*. Piecemeal, cell-by-cell necrosis is followed by healing with fibrous replacement.[42]

b. Slowly Developing Mononuclear Cell Injury with Active Fibrosis

In contrast to what is seen in piecemeal necrosis of parasitized cells, a different and possibly more significant tissue injury may occur both in animals and in humans with *T.*

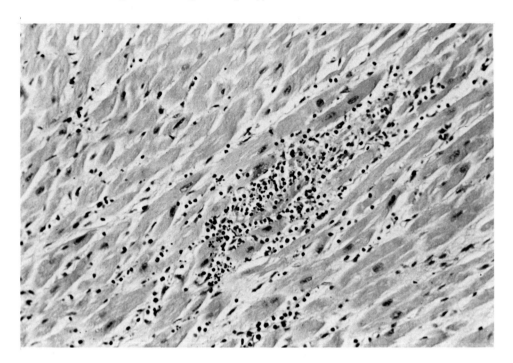

FIGURE 7.   Focal myocarditis in chronic Chagas' disease showing a mononuclear cell infiltrate and myofiber cytolysis. (Hematoxylin and eosin.)

cruzi infection of long duration. In experimental *T. cruzi* infection of long duration, there are seen focal, sometimes confluent, areas of mononuclear exudates always associated with active fibrous replacement of the cellular constituents of target tissues. In experimental situations these fibrous and mononuclear cell lesions make their appearance even when *T. cruzi*-associated piecemeal necrosis is still prevalent, but typically the lesion follows the reduction of polymorphonuclear infiltrates sequentially and bears no relation to ruptured pseudocysts or to parasitized cells.[42] The exudate consists of predominating small and intermediate lymphocytes, some closely applied to the plasma membrane of target cells (Figure 7). Lesser numbers of plasma cells, mast cells, and macrophages are scattered in these lesions. When the target cells are finally replaced by fibrous tissue, a tightly healed scar of relatively acellular collagenous fibers remains (Figure 8). In the human heart, this process may eventually lead to significant loss of working myocardium and diffuse multifocal interstitial fibrous tissue deposition. In Auerbach's parasympathetic plexus of human hollow viscera this process may, in time, lead to significant loss of ganglion cells by neurono-phagocytosis and perineural fibrosis.

The pathogenesis of the lesions produced by the lymphocytic infiltrates of target cell systems in *T. cruzi* infections is not known, but pathoimmunity is strongly suspected to play a major role in its development.[4,121] Teixeira and Santos-Buch showed that allogeneic *T. cruzi*-sensitized lymphocytes selectively adhered to isolated preparations of Auerbach's plexus of rabbit colon, whereas normal, nonsensitized lymphocytes did so only sparingly.[4] A similar phenomenon was observed with tissue culture heart cell monolayers[51] and with freshly cut sections of heart.[5] *T. cruzi* has been shown to possess cross-reacting epitopes of striated-muscle sarcoplasmic reticulum[10] and of certain neurons.[11] Circulating IgG antiheart sarcolemma antibody activity has been shown by immunofluorescence[10] and by ELISA techniques.[8,69] Antibodies directed against SRA calcium pump preparations have been measured in sera of animals immunized with *T. cruzi* small membranes[122] and in sera of patients with documented cardiomyopathy associated with *T. cruzi* infection.[69] Finally, adoptive transfer

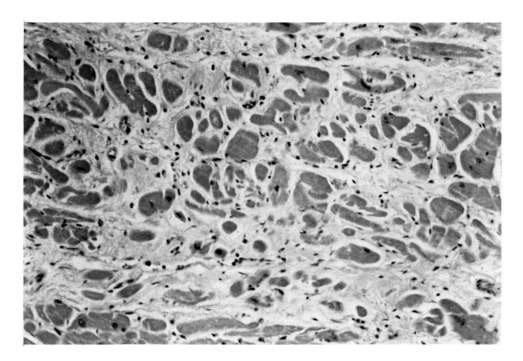

FIGURE 8.   Fibrous replacement of the myocardium and interstitial fibrosis in chronic Chagas' disease. (Hematoxylin and eosin.)

of splenic lymphocytes from *T. cruzi*-infected Balb/c mice resulted in the production of lymphocyte cytotoxicity to monolayers of syngeneic myofibers.[70] In spite of the accumulated evidence from experimental and clinical studies which support the hypothesis that mononuclear cell injury of target cell systems has an immunopathogenic origin, there is no published study to date broaching this question in the field with populations at risk of *T. cruzi* infection.

2. Gross Pathology
a. Cardiomyopathy: Congestive Type

It is estimated that 15 to 20% of individuals without pathophysiologic injury and with positive xenodiagnosis tests of *T. cruzi* parasitemia develop cardiomyopathy usually in the third and fourth decades of life.[1,21] There is no predilection for either sex. The mortality rate once the cardiomyopathy is established approaches 90% within 5 years of its onset.[176] The association of achalasia of the esophagus or colon with *T. cruzi*-induced cardiomyopathy is relatively infrequent (see Section IX.B.2.b below).

The prevalence of *T. cruzi* parasitosis of myocardial cells is low in Chagas' cardiomyopathy. In cases from the northeast of Brazil, Andrade and Andrade[42] found amastigotes in myocardial pseudocysts in 38 out of 126 hearts. A more dramatic finding is the study of Suarez et al.[73] from Venezuela where none of 160 hearts with characteristic *T. cruzi* cardiomyopathy showed intramyocardial cell or intracardiac neuron parasitosis. Koberle and Alcantara[157] showed that only 12 out of 89,722 intracardiac neurons were parasitized and concluded that this is an irregular occurrence. Mott and Hagstrom,[47] in an elegant study, showed that all 12 hearts with *T. cruzi*-associated cardiomyopathy in their study from the northeast of Brazil had mononuclear cell lesions with interrupted and broken axis cylinders and perineuronal inflammation. Of 12 hearts, 10 showed neuronophagia of intracardiac ganglioneurons.[47] In sharp contrast, no such findings are found in Chagas' cardiomyopathy studied in Venezuela[158] and, in a more recent study, 24 of 28 hearts showed only minimal

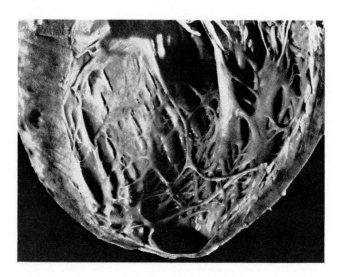

FIGURE 9.   Chagas' cardiomyopathy showing a globular, dilated heart with thinning of the left ventricle without mural thrombosis. (From Suarez, J. A., Puigbo, J. J., Nava Rhode, J. R., Valero, J. A., and Yepez, C. G., *Miocardiopatias*, Acquatella, H. and Pulido, P. A., Eds., Salvat Editores, Barcelona, 1982, 5. With permission.)

mononuclear inflammation of the intracardiac ganglioneurons, but no neuronophagia nor fibrosis or a reduction in the number of neuroganglion cells was seen in any of these hearts.[73] Notwithstanding the studies of Koberle,[41,74] a critical review of the published data obtained from autopsy of humans with long-standing *T. cruzi* infection does not properly support the notion that chagasic cardiomyopathy is significantly associated with replacement fibrosis of the cardiac ganglioneurons or with an important parasitosis of either ganglioneurons or myocardial cells.

b. Apical Lesion

Two types of heart change are seen in Chagas' cardiomyopathy. One type is found in *T. cruzi*-infected patients without cardiomyopathy who come to autopsy after otherwise unexplained sudden-death, usually as a result of medicolegal investigations. These hearts are of normal weight or show a slight increase in weight. The other type of heart change is clearly associated with long-standing and progressive congestive heart failure and shows marked cardiomegaly with dilatation of all chambers. Both types do not show significant coronary artery disease nor remarkable changes of small arteries and arterioles. Importantly, both types show a characteristic apical aneurysm or thinning of the myocardium in a large proportion of cases.[42,73] The prevalence in Venezuela of apical thinning or aneurysms in *T. cruzi*-infected individuals who have no reduction of intracardiac ganglioneurons is reported in 17 out of 118 hearts in the right ventricle (14.4%) and in 108 out of 118 (91.5%) instances and in the left ventricle (Figures 9 to 11). In the northeast of Brazil, Andrade and Andrade[42] reported a lower prevalence of left ventricular apical lesions (32 of 208) and no aneurysms of the apex of the right ventricle have been seen in their autopsy material. Lopes et al.[159] reported from central Brazil that more than half of their cases showed apical aneurysms of the left ventricle.[159] Barring thrombosis, myocardial fiber loss without significant endocardial or epicardial changes is characteristically found in the apical lesions, but this histological change is not limited to the apex of the heart and can simultaneously occur in other focal areas of the left ventricle, particularly in the posterior and lateral walls.[73,146] Both the apical lesions and the thinned-out, segmental lesions of the left ventricle can be detected by M-

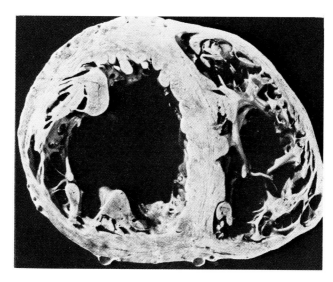

FIGURE 10. Cross-section of a heart from a patient with Chagas' cardiomyopathy showing enlarged chambers, thinning of the lateral wall, and localized endocardial fibrosis. (From Suarez, J. A., Puigbo, J. J., Nava Rhode, J. R., Valero, J. A., and Yepez, C. G., *Miocardiopatias,* Acquatella, H. and Pulido, P. A., Eds., Salvat Editores, Barcelona, 1982, 5. With permission.)

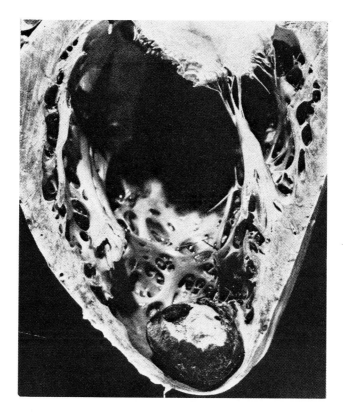

FIGURE 11. Chagas' cardiomyopathy showing characteristic left ventricular apical thinning with mural thrombosis. Normal mitral valve. (From Suarez, J. A., Puigbo, J. J., Nava Rhode, J. R., Valero, J. A., and Yepez, C. G., *Miocardiopatias,* Acquatella, H. and Pulido, P. A., Eds., Salvat Editores, Barcelona, 1982, 5. With permission.)

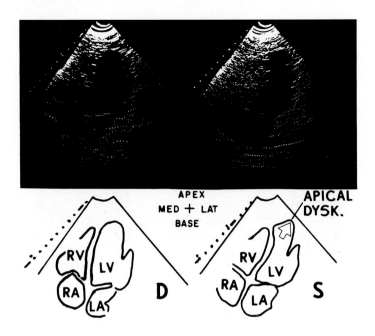

FIGURE 12.   Two-dimensional echocardiograph of a patient with Chagas' disease showing systolic apical dyskinesia (arrow). Electrocardiogram was normal. (D) Diastole, (S) systole, (LA) left auricle, (LV) left ventricle, (RA) right auricle, (RV) right ventricle. (From Acquatella, H., Schiller, N. B., Puigbo, J. J., Giordano, H., Suarez, J. A., Casal, H., Arreaza, N., Valecillos, R., and Hirschhaut, E., *Miocardiopatias*, Acquatella, H. and Pulido, P. A., Eds., Salvat Editores, Barcelona, 1982, 89. With permission.)

mode echocardiography[146] and a proper diagnosis with significant measurements of the ejection fraction can be made clinically[146] (Figure 12). At autopsy, transillumination can accurately delineate areas of significant loss of myocardial cells.

Cardiomyopathy associated with long-standing *T. cruzi* infection is almost impossible to differentiate from findings seen in idiopathic congestive cardiomyopathy.[42,73] Even the apical lesion or aneurysm is not specific for Chagas' heart disease since similar apical lesions are sometimes described associated with tropical idiopathic cardiomyopathy of Africa[42] and not with the congestive idiopathic cardiomyopathy seen in Western Europe and in North America.

The primary lymph nodes accepting the lymphatics that drain the heart show reactive hyperplasia and edema associated to the degree of chronic myocarditis seen histologically with chronic Chagas' heart disease.[42]

c. Achalasia of Esophagus and Colon: Acquired Loss of Parasympathetic Innervation

The prevalence of achalasia of the esophagus and colon associated with long-standing *T. cruzi* infection is low. Chapadeiro et al.[160] and Barbosa et al.[161] found a prevalence of approximately 17% among over 900 *T. cruzi*-infected individuals with cardiomyopathy. Andrade and Andrade[42] reported a prevalence of achalasia of the esophagus and/or colon of 2.6% among 68 autopsied patients with Chagas' heart disease. Macedo[162] has also reported a low incidence of achalasia of the gastrointestinal tract in San Felipe, northeast Brazil, an area endemic for *T. cruzi* infections. No achalasia of the esophagus nor of the colon was seen in 160 cases of Chagas' heart disease who came to autopsy at the Institute of Pathology, Universidad Central de Venezuela.[73] De Rezende[163] reviewed the literature, tabulated the data, and determined that the prevalence of achalasia of the gastrointestinal tract among patients from *T. cruzi* endemic areas of Argentina to be 15 of 426 (3.5%). These prevalences are somewhat lower than the results reported by Koberle[41] who reported that approximately

20% of the cases from central Brazil with Chagas' heart disease showed achalasia of the esophagus and/or colon. The experience in Venezuela, Argentina, and Brazil appears to indicate, therefore, that the principal injury associated with *T. cruzi* infection of long duration is cardiomyopathy. There are only anecdotal reports which document the conversion of achalasia following *T. cruzi* inoculation.[2]

The prevalence of achalasia of the esophagus and colon appears to peak in the second, third, and fourth decades of life and males appear to be at a higher risk of developing the disease.[148] While the esophagus and colon appear to be likely targets of achalasia associated with long-standing *T. cruzi* infection, the stomach, the small intestine, the biliary tree, and even the ureters are sometimes affected.[42,148]

In 1930, Hurst and Rake,[164] who coined the term achalasia, also described the characteristic fibrous replacement of the ganglioneurons of Auerbach's plexus seen in megaesophagus and megacolon. Shortly thereafter, Amorim and Correia Neto[165] in 1932 and Correia Neto and Etzel[166] in 1934 extended their original observations in patients with *T. cruzi* infection. In 1955, Koberle and Nador[167] published their classic measurements showing a generalized reduction of ganglioneurons of Auerbach's plexus of the gastrointestinal tract in *T. cruzi*-infected patients. Achalasia of the esophagus or colon is first associated with a significant hypertrophic thickening of the circular smooth muscle layer accompanied by a similar hypertrophic change in the muscularis mucosa, accompanied by a slight fusiform dilation of the entire esophagus or of a segment of the colon.[42]

Importantly, focal mononuclear cell infiltrates are associated, here and there, with destruction of smooth muscle fibers and, occasionally, involve components of Auerbach's plexus.[42] As the disease progresses, gradual dilatation of the viscus develops resulting in the formation of the "mega" phenomenon (Figure 13). Fibrous replacement of the smooth muscle layer is not as pronounced as that seen in the myocardium in Chagas' heart disease nor as collagenous as seen in the gastrointestinal tract in scleroderma.

C. Complications
1. Anatomic Basis of Sudden Death

In South America, it is not unusual for a patient to die suddenly while hospitalized for other reasons than heart disease, and at autopsy *T. cruzi* amastigotes and diffuse myocarditis are found.[47] The presence of inflammatory cells and/or fibrosis in the heart conduction system in the absence of coronary artery disease has been cited as cause of apparently inexplicable sudden death in *T. cruzi* infection of long duration.[42] Rosenbaum et al.[46] and later Andrade et al.[44] have provided evidence from study of the conduction system of heart from chagasic patients which suggests that the fibers of the conduction system are susceptible to injury in *T. cruzi* infection. In experimentally infected dogs, *T. cruzi* amastigotes were detected in atrioventricular conduction fibers with no particular predilection in distribution.[42] The reason for this targeted injury is not known, but the answer may partly exist on the fetal-like properties of the conduction fibers per se. The fibers differ in their ultrastructural,[168-171] biochemical,[172-174] and immunologic composition[175] from the working myocardium. Andrade et al.[44] have delineated four fundamental lesions of the atrioventricular conduction fibers found in *T. cruzi*-associated cardiomyopathy: (1) complete right bundle branch block and left anterior hemiblock; (2) complete block of left bundle branch; (3) complete right bundle branch block and left posterior hemiblock; and, (4) complete atrioventricular block. The lesions are characterized by fibrous replacement of conduction fibers and vascularization of the tracts with dilatation of the blood vessels. These morphologic changes correlate closely with some of the characteristic arrhythmias and conduction defects observed in patients with *T. cruzi* infection of long duration and may explain the high frequency of sudden death and Chagas' disease.[42]

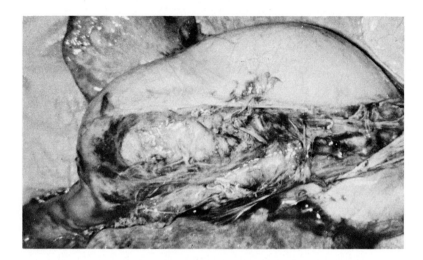

FIGURE 13.   Megaesophagus as a result of achalasia induced by loss of neurons of Auer-bach's plexus. (Surgical field prior to resection; 32-year-old male patient, Hospital Edgard Santos, Salvador, Bahia, Brazil. Patient studied by Dr. Zilton Andrade, Department of Pathology, Universidade Federal da Bahia, Brazil.) (From Santos-Buch, C. A., *Int. Rev. Exp. Pathol.*, 19, 63, 1979. With permission.)

2. Thromboembolic Phenomena and Congestive Heart Failure

Chronic Chagas' cardiomyopathy is very similar to idiopathic cardiomyopathy of nonendemic areas and the prevalence of intracardiac thrombosis and thromboembolic episodes are nearly identical. Andrade and Andrade[42] reported that the mean weight of the heart with Chagas' cardiomyopathy was 506 g (380 to 760 g, n = 208), whereas idiopathic cardiomyopathy was 586 g (380 to 950 g, n = 21) and endomyocardial fibrosis 373 g (200 to 670 g, n = 12). The prevalence of intracardiac thrombosis in chronic Chagas' cardiomyopathy was 76.0% (158/208), idiopathic cardiomyopathy 80.9% (17/21), and endomyocardial fibrosis 58.3% (7/12).

Thromboembolic episodes occur frequently. In the northeast of Brazil nearly three out of four patients with chronic Chagas' cardiomyopathy have emboli to the lungs and kidneys,[42] whereas two out of five patients had thromboembolic episodes principally in the brain and lungs in Venezuela.[73] Andrade and Andrade[42] stress that in their series of cases thromboembolic phenomena occurred in a few patients with chronic Chagas' cardiomyopathy without signs of congestive heart failure and/or significant ventricular tachyarrhythmias. However, congestive heart failure is the most frequent cause of death (97/118, 82%) with an average duration of 13 months. The majority of the remainder of deaths are usually caused by cardiac arrest, probably following significant runs of ventricular tachyarrhythmias, since ventricular premature contractions are frequently associated with chronic Chagas' cardiomyopathy (43 to 60%).[42] Dilatation of the rings of the atrioventricular valves occurs associated with the enlargement of the chambers of the heart. Cardiac insufficiency is a prominent finding (48/118, 41%) which also contributes to intractable heart failure.[42]

3. Dysphagia, Cardiospasm, Obstipation, and Fecal Impaction. Volvulus

Achalasia affecting the esophagus and colon predictably leads to complications related to motility of the bolus of food. Thus, dysphagia, cardiospasm, and esophageal stasis are frequently found associated with megaesophagus, whereas chronic obstipation, formation of "fecalomas", and fecal impaction may present associated with megacolon. Even though parasympathetic denervation of Auerbach's plexus in the gastrointestinal tract is a fundamental lesion seen in some cases of chronic Chagas' disease, no dysfunctions are described of pupillary, laryngeal, or vesical sphincters. Rarely megacolon may produce intestinal obstruction associated with volvulus.

ACKNOWLEDGMENTS

The authors are indebted to Drs. Moyses Sadigursky and Zilton Andrade (Universidade Federal da Bahia, Brazil), Drs. Roberto Arana and Patricio Cossio (Centro de Educacion Medica e Investigaciones Clinicas, Buenos Aires, Argentina), Dr. Rodney Hoff (School of Public Health, Harvard University), Dr. Antonio Teixeira (Universidade de Brasilia, Brazil), Drs. John Ellis, Robert Cody, and Michael Ferenc (The New York Hospital, Cornell University Medical Center), and Dr. Quintus Chess (Memorial-Sloan Kettering Cancer Center) for their direct and indirect contributions to this manuscript. Special thanks are due to Mr. Douglas Weston and Ms. Dorothy Goldman for their invaluable assistance in the preparation of this manuscript. The support of the National Institute of Health, U.S. Public Health Service (Grant #HL-27493) is gratefully acknowledged. We are especially indebted to our students Betsy von Kreuter, Adam Soyer, Jonathan Cohen, and Daniel George, without whose enthusiasm and perseverance little would have been accomplished.

REFERENCES

1. **Laranja, F. S., Diaz, E., Nobrega, G., and Miranda, A.,** Chagas' disease: a clinical, epidemiologic and pathologic study, *Circulation,* 14, 1035, 1956.
2. **Rassi, A., De Rezende, J. M., and Doles, J.,** Caso da doenca de Chagas observada desde periodo inicial da infeccao con aparicimento precoce de megaesofago e megacolo, *Rev. Soc. Bras. Med. Trop.,* 2, 303, 1968.
3. **Prata, A. R.,** Formas clinicas da doenca de Chagas, in *Doenca de Chagas,* Cancado, J. R., Ed., Oficina de Estado de Minais Gerais, Belo Horizonte, Brasil, 1968, 344.
4. **Santos-Buch, C. A.,** American trypanosomiasis, *Int. Rev. Exp. Pathol.,* 19, 63, 1979.
5. **Cossio, P. M., Damilano, G., de la Vega, M. T., Laguens, R. P., Cabeza-Meckert, P., Diez, C., and Arana, R. M.,** *In vitro* interaction between lymphocytes of chagasic individuals and heart tissue, *Medicina (Buenos Aires),* 36, 287, 1976.
6. **Teixeira, A. R. L., Teixeira, G., Macedo, V., and Prata, A.,** *Trypanosoma cruzi*-sensitized T-lymphocyte mediated ^{51}Cr release from human heart cells in Chagas' disease, *Am. J. Trop. Med. Hyg.,* 27, 1097, 1978.
7. **Acosta, A. M., Sadigursky, M., and Santos-Buch, C. A.,** Putative pathogenic cross-reacting striated muscle-*T. cruzi* antigen in chagasic heart disease (abstract), *Fed. Proc., Fed. Am. Soc. Exp.,* 40, 701, 1981.
8. **Cody, R. J., Acosta, A. M., and Santos-Buch, C. A.,** Anti-striated muscle antibodies in idiopathic cardiomyopathy (abstract), *Clin. Res.,* 30, 179A, 1982.
9. **Santos-Buch, C. A.,** American trypanosomiasis: Chagas' disease, in *Immunopathology: 7th Int. Symp.,* Miescher, P. A., Ed., Schwabe, Basel/Stuttgart, 1977, 205.
10. **Sadigursky, M., Acosta, A. M., and Santos-Buch, C. A.,** Muscle sarcoplasmic reticulum antigen shared by a *Trypanosoma cruzi* clone, *Am. J. Trop. Med. Hyg.,* 31, 934, 1982.
11. **Wood, J. N., Hudson, L., Jessell, T. M., and Yamamoto, M.,** A monoclonal antibody defining antigenic determinants on subpopulations of mammalian neurons and *Trypanosoma cruzi* parasites, *Nature (London),* 296, 34, 1982.
12. **Szarfman, A., Terranova, V. P., Rennard, S. I., Foidart, J. M., Fatima-Lima, M., Scheinman, J. I., and Martin, G. R.,** Antibodies to laminin in Chagas' disease, *J. Exp. Med.,* 155, 1161, 1982.
13. **Chess, Q., Acosta, A. M., and Santos-Buch, C. A.,** Reversible acquisition of a host cell surface membrane antigen by *Trypanosoma cruzi, Infect. Immun.,* 40, 299, 1983.
14. Report of a Study Group on Chagas' Disease, Scientific Publ. 195, Pan American Health Organization, Washington, D.C., 1970, 29.

15. **Zeledon, R.,** Epidemiology, modes of transmission and reservoir hosts of Chagas' disease, in *Trypanosomiasis and Leishmaniasis with Special Reference to Chagas' Disease, CIBA Foundation Symp. 20,* Elsevier, Amsterdam, 1974, 51.

16. **Faust, E. C., Beaver, P. C., and Jung, R. C.,** *Animal Agents and Vectors of Human Disease,* 4th ed., Lea & Febiger, Philadelphia, 1975, 54.

17. **Zeledon, R., Solano, G., Zuniga, A., and Swartzwelder, J. C.,** Biology and ethology of *Triatoma dimidiata* (Latreille, 1811). III. Habitat and blood sources, *J. Med. Entomol.,* 10, 363, 1973.

18. **Gomez-Nunez, J. C.,** Resting places, dispersal, and survival of Co$_{60}$-tagged adult *Rhodnius prolixus, J. Med. Entomol.,* 6, 83, 1969.

19. Immunology of Chagas' disease, *Bull. WHO,* 50, 459, 1974.

20. **Wood, S. F. and Wood, F. D.,** Observations on vectors of Chagas' disease in the United States. III. New Mexico, *Am. J. Trop. Med. Hyg.,* 10, 155, 1961.

21. **Maekelt, G. A.,** Seroepidemiology of Chagas' disease, *J. Parasitol.,* 56 (2), 557, 1970.

22. **Barreto, M. P.,** Epidemiologia, in *Trypanosoma Cruzi e Doenca de Chagas,* Brener, Z. and Andrade, Z., Eds., Guanabara Koogan, Rio de Janeiro, 1979, 89.

23. **Burkholder, J. E., Allison, T. C., and Kelly, V. P.,** *Trypanosoma cruzi* (Chagas) (Protozoa: Kinetoplastida) in invertebrate, reservoir and human hosts of the lower Rio Grande valley of Texas, *J. Parasitol.,* 66, 305, 1980.

24. **Walton, B. C., Bauman, P., Diamond, L., and Herman, C.,** The isolation and identification of *Trypanosoma cruzi* from raccoons in Maryland, *Am. J. Trop. Med. Hyg.,* 7, 603, 1958.

25. **Woody, N. C. and Woody, H. B.,** Possible Chagas' disease in United States, *N. Engl. J. Med.,* 290, 749, 1974.

26. **Chagas, C.,** Nova tipanosomiase humana. Estudos sobre a morfologia e o ciclo evolutivo do *Schizotrypanum cruzi;* n. gen., n. sp., ajente etiologico de nova entidade morbida do homen, *Mem. Inst. Oswaldo Cruz,* 1, 159, 1909.

27. **Bittencourt, A. L.,** Congenital Chagas' disease, *Am. J. Dis. Child.,* 130, 97, 1976.

28. **Delgado, M. A. and Santos-Buch, C. A.,** Transplacental transmission and fetal parasitosis of *Trypanosoma cruzi* in outbred white Swiss mice, *Am. J. Trop. Med. Hyg.,* 27, 1108, 1978.

29. **Cerisola, J. A., Rabinovich, A., Alvarez, M., DiCarleto, C. A., and Pruneda, J.,** Enfermedad de Chagas y la transfusion de sangre, *Bol. Of. Sanit. Panam.,* 63, 203, 1972.

30. **Guerra, F.,** American trypanosomiasis. An historical and a human lesson, *J. Trop. Med. Hyg.,* 73, 83, 1970.

31. **Sherlock, I. A.,** Vetores, in *Trypanosoma Cruzi de Doenca de Chagas,* Brener, Z. and Andrade, Z., Eds., Guanabara Koogan, Rio de Janeiro, 1979, chap. 2.

32. **Darwin, C.,** *Natural History and Geology of the Countries Visited During the Voyage of H.M.S. Beagle Round the World,* Appleton, New York, 1882, 330.

33. **Adler, S.,** Darwin's illness, *Nature (London),* 184, 1102, 1959.

34. **Lewinsohn, R.,** Carlos Chagas (1879—1934): the discovery of *Trypanosoma cruzi* and of American trypanosomiasis, *Trans. R. Soc. Trop. Med. Hyg.,* 73, 513, 1979.

35. **Vianna, G.,** Contribucao para o estudo da anatomia patologica da "Molestia de Carlos Chagas", *Mem. Inst. Oswaldo Cruz,* 3, 276, 1911.

36. **Brumpt, A. J. E.,** Le *Trypanosoma cruzi* evolue chez *Conorhinus megistus, Cimex lectularius, Cimex boueti* et *Ornithodorus moubata.* Cycle evolutif de ce parasite., *Bull Soc. Pathol. Exotique,* 5, 360, 1912.

37. **Brumpt, A. J. E.,** Le xenodiagnostic application au diagnostic de quelques infections parasitaires et en particulier a la trypanosomose de Chagas, *Bull. Soc. Pathol. Exotique,* 7, 706, 1912.

38. **Guerreiro, C. and Machado, A.,** Da reaccao de Bordet e Gengou na molestia de Carlos Chagas como elemento diagnostico, *Bras. Med.,* 27, 225, 1913.

39. **Kean, B. H., Mott, K. E., and Russell, A. J.,** *Tropical Medicine and Parasitology,* Vol. 1, Cornell University Press, Ithaca, New York, 1978, 223.

40. **Villela, G.,** A transmissao intrauterine da molestia da Chagas; encefalite congenita pelo *Trypanosoma cruzi* (nota previa), *Folha Med.,* 4, 41, 1923.

41. **Koberle, F.,** Chagas' disease and Chagas' syndromes: the pathology of American trypanosomiasis, *Adv. Parasitol.,* 6, 63, 1968.

42. **Andrade, Z. A. and Andrade, S. G.,** Patolojia, in *Trypanosoma cruzi e Donenca de Chagas,* Brener, Z. and Andrade, Z. A., Eds., Guanabara Koogan, Rio de Janeiro, 1979, chap. 6.

43. **Andrade, Z. A.,** Lesao apical do coracao na miocardite cronica chagasica, *Hospital (Rio de Janeiro),* 50, 803, 1956.

44. **Andrade, Z. A., Andrade, S. G., Oliveira, G. B., and Alonso, D. R.,** Histopathology of the conducting tissue of the heart in Chagas' myocarditis, *Am. Heart J.,* 93, 316, 1978.

45. **Andrade, Z. A. and Andrade, S. G.,** Estudo immunocitoquimico da doenca de Chagas experimental, *Rev. Inst. Med. Trop. Sao Paulo,* 11, 44, 1969.

46. **Rosenbaum, M. B. and Alvarez, A. J.,** The electrocardiogram in chronic chagasic myocarditis, *Am. Heart J.,* 50, 492, 1955.
47. **Mott, K. E. and Hagstrom, J. W. C.,** The pathologic lesions of the cardiac autonomic nervous system in chronic Chagas' myocarditis, *Circulation,* 31, 273, 1965.
48. **Cossio, P. M., Laguens, R. P., Diez, C., Szarfman, A., Segal, A., and Arana, R. M.,** Chagasic cardiopathy: antibodies reacting with the plasma membrane of striated muscle and endothelial cells, *Circulation,* 50, 1252, 1974.
49. **Cossio, P. M., Laguens, R. P., Kreutzer, E., Diez, C., Segal, A., and Arana, R. M.,** Chagasic cardiopathy: immunopathologic and morphologic studies in myocardial biopsies, *Am. J. Pathol.,* 86, 533, 1977.
50. **Khoury, E. L., Diez, C., Cossio, P. M., and Arana, R. M.,** Heterophil nature of EVI antibody in *Trypanosoma cruzi* infection, *Clin. Immunol. Immunopathol.,* 27, 283, 1983.
51. **Santos-Buch, C. A. and Teixeira, A. R. L.,** Immunology of experimental Chagas' disease. III. Rejection of allogeneic heart cells in vitro, *J. Exp. Med.,* 140, 38, 1974.
52. **Budzko, D. B., Pizzimenti, M. C., and Kierszenbaum, F.,** Effects of complement depletion in experimental Chagas' disease: immune lysis of virulent forms of *Trypanosoma cruzi, Infect. Immun.,* 11, 86, 1975.
53. **Rimoldi, M. T., Cardoni, R. L., Olabuenaga, S. E., and de Bracco, M. M.,** *Trypanosoma cruzi:* sequence of phagocytosis and cytotoxicity by human polymorphonuclear leukocytes, *Immunology,* 42, 521, 1981.
54. **Okabe, K., Kipnis, T. L., Calich, V. L. G., and Dias da Silva, W.,** Cell-mediated cytoxicity to *Trypanosoma cruzi.* I. Antibody-dependent cell mediated cytotoxicity to trypomastigote bloodstream forms, *Clin. Immunol. Immunopathol.,* 16, 344, 1980.
55. **Hoff, R.,** Killing *in vitro* of *Trypanosoma cruzi* by macrophages from mice immunized with *Trypanosoma cruzi* or BCG and absence of cross-immunity on challenge *in vivo, J. Exp. Med.,* 142, 299, 1975.
56. **Trischmann, T. M., Tanowitz, H., Wittner, M., and Bloom, B.,** *Trypanosoma cruzi:* role of the immune response in the natural resistance of inbred strains of mice, *Exp. Parasitol.,* 45, 160, 1978.
57. **Trischmann, T. M. and Bloom, B. R.,** Genetics of murine resistance to *Trypanosoma cruzi, Infect. Immun.,* 35, 546, 1982.
58. **Ribeiro dos Santos, R. and Hudson, L.,** *Trypanosoma cruzi:* binding of parasite antigens to mammalian cell membranes, *Parasite Immunol.,* 2, 1, 1980.
59. **Ribeiro dos Santos, R. and Hudson, L.,** *Trypanosoma cruzi:* immunological consequences of parasite modification of host cells, *Clin. Exp. Immunol.,* 40, 36, 1980.
60. **Ribeiro dos Santos, R. and Hudson, L.,** Denervation and the immune response in mice infected with *Trypanosoma cruzi, Clin. Exp. Immunol.,* 44, 349, 1981.
61. **Santos-Buch, C. A.,** Autoimmunity and Chagas' disease: demonstration of a common immunogen of heart and *Trypanosoma cruzi,* in *The Menarini Series on Immunopathology, Vol. I: Proc. 1st Symp. on Organ Specific Autoimmunity,* Miescher, P. A., Ed., Schwabe, Basel/Stuttgart, 1978, 101.
62. **Cerisola, J. A., Rohwedder, R., Segura, E. L., del Prado, C. E., Alvarez, M., and Wynne de Martini, J.,** *Xenodiagnostico: Normalizacion — Utilidad,* Ministerio de Bienestar Social, Buenos Aires, Argentina, 1974.
63. **Andrade, Z. A. and Ramalho, L. M. P.,** Miocardite chagasica. Estudo morfologico de 38 casos comprovados pelo encontro de parasitos nas seccoe histologicas, *Gaz. Med. Bahia.,* 66, 55, 1966.
64. **Mott, K. E., Lehman, J. S., Hoff, R., Morrow, R. H., Muniz, T., Sherlock, I., Draper, C. C., Pugliese, C., and Guimaraes, A. C.,** The epidemiology and household distributions of seroreactivity to *Trypanosoma cruzi* in a rural community in northeast Brazil, *Am. J. Trop. Med. Hyg.,* 25, 552, 1976.
65. **Teixeira, A. R. L., Teixeira, G., Macedo, V., and Prata, A.,** Acquired cell-mediated immunodepression in acute Chagas' disease, *J. Clin. Invest.,* 62, 1132, 1978.
66. **Cerisola, J. A., Alvarez, A., Lugones, H., and Rebolsan, J. B.,** Evolucion serologica de pacientes con enfermedad de Chagas aguda tratados con Bayer 2502, *Bol. Chil. Parasitol.,* 24, 54, 1969.
67. **Marsden, P. D.,** personal communication, 1983.
68. **Andrade, Z. and Andrade, S.,** American trypanosomiasis, in *Pathology of Protozoan and Helminthic Disease,* Marcial-Rojas, R. A., Ed., Williams & Wilkins, Baltimore, 1971, 69.
69. **Acosta, A. M., Sadigursky, M., Cody, R. J., Sadigursky, C., Brodsky, C. I., and Santos-Buch, C. A.,** Anti-striated muscle membrane calcium pump antibody activity in cardiomyopathies, submitted.
70. **Acosta, A. M. and Santos-Buch, C. A.,** Autoimmune anti-heart lymphocyte cytotoxicity produced by adoptive transfer of *Trypanosoma cruzi* sensitized lymphocytes, submitted.
71. **Acosta, A. M. and Santos-Buch, C. A.,** Induction of experimental autoimmune myocarditis in Balb/c mice, submitted.
72. **Allison, A. C.,** The pathogenesis of autoimmune disease, in *The Menarini Series on Immunopathology. Vol. 1. Proc. 1st Symp. on Organ Specific Autoimmunity,* Miescher, P. A., Ed., Schwabe, Stuttgart/Basel, 1978, 283.

73. **Suarez, J. A., Puigbo, J. J., Nava Rhode, J. R., Valero, J. A., and Yepez, C. G.,** Pathologic study of 210 cases of cardiomyopathies in Venezuela, in *Miocardiopatias,* Acquatella, H. and Pulido, P. A., Eds., Salvat Editores, Barcelona, 1982, 5.
74. **Koberle, F.,** Pathogenesis of Chagas' disease, in *Trypanosomiasis and Leishmaniasis with Special Reference to Chagas Disease. CIBA Foundation Symp. 20,* Elsevier, Amsterdam, 1974, 137.
75. **Guevara, J. F., Blandon, R., Johnson, C. M., Sousa, O., and Leandro, I.,** Aspectos clinicos anatomo-pathologicos y terapeuticos de la enfermedad de Chagas en Panama, *Arq. Bras. Cardiol.,* 30 (Suppl. 2), 140, 1979.
76. **Koberle, F.,** Uber das neurotoxin des *Trypanosoma cruzi, Z. Allg. Pathol. Pathol. Anat.,* 95, 408, 1956.
77. **Oliveira, J. S. M.,** Cardiopatia chagasica experimental, *Rev. Goianna Med.,* 15, 77, 1969.
78. **Seneca, H. and Peer, P. M.,** Immunobiological properties of chagastoxin (lipopolysaccharide), *Trans. R. Soc. Trop. Med. Hyg.,* 60, 610, 1966.
79. **Eichbaum, F. W.,** Pesquisas sobre a presenca de substancias toxicas em culturas do *Trypanosoma cruzi, An. Cong. Internal. Sobre Doenca Chagas,* 2, 479, 1961.
80. **Musacchio, J. and Meyer, H.,** Acao do *Schizotrypanum cruzi* degenerado ou em suspensao de trypano-somos mortos sobre celulas nervosas em cultura de tecido de embriao de galinhas, *An. Cong. Internal. Doenca Chagas,* 3, 1065, 1962.
81. *Physicians' Desk Reference,* 37th ed., Medical Economics, Oradell, 1983, 709.
82. **Lucchesi, B. R.,** Inotropic agents and drugs used to support the failing heart, in *Cardiovascular Pharmacology,* Antonaccio, M., Ed., Raven Press, New York, 1977, 337.
83. **Gould, S. E. and Ioannides, G.,** Ischemic heart disease, in *Pathology of the Heart and Blood Vessels,* Gould, S. E., Ed., Charles C Thomas, Springfield, Ill., 1968, 601.
84. **Campbell, W. G., Jr. and Santos-Buch, C. A.,** Widely distributed necrotizing arteritis induced in rabbits by experimental renal alterations. II. Relationship of the arterial lesions to perirenal inflammation, *Am. J. Pathol.,* 35, 769, 1959.
85. **Dammin, G. J., Goldman, M. L., Schroeder, H. A., and Pace, M. G.,** Arterial hypertension in dogs. II. The effects of neurogenic hypertension with a study of periodic renal biopsies over a seven year period, *Lab. Invest.,* 5, 72, 1956.
86. **Weiner, N.,** Atropine, scopolamine and related anti-muscarinic drugs, in *The Pharmacological Basis of Therapeutics,* Gilman, A. G., Goodman, L. S., and Gilman, A., Eds., Macmillan, New York, 1980, 120.
87. **Margarino-Torres, C.,** Patogenia de la miocarditis cronica en la enfermedad de Chagas, *Soc. Argen. Patol. Reg. Norte Quinta Reun.,* 2, 902, 1930.
88. **Chagas, C.,** Estado actual da trypanosomiase Americana, *Rev. Biol. Hyg. Sao Paulo,* 5, 58, 1934.
89. **Tejada-Valenzuela, C. and Castro, F.,** Miocarditis cronica en Guatemala, *Rev. Col. Med. Guatemala,* 9, 124, 1958.
90. **Jaffe, R., Jaffe, W. G., and Kozma, C.,** Experimentelle herzeranderungen durch organ-spezifische auto antikorper, *Frankfurt Z. Pathol.,* 70, 235, 1959.
91. **Kozma, C. and Drayer, B.,** Estudios immunopathologicos en diversas cardiopatias, *Gaz. Med. Caracas,* 70, 251, 1961.
92. **Cossio, P. M., Diez, C., Szarfman, A., Kreutzer, E., Candiolo, B., and Arana, R. M.,** Chagasic cardiopathy. Demonstration of a serum gamma globulin factor which reacts with endocardium and vascular structures, *Circulation,* 49, 13, 1974.
93. **Szarfman, A., Cossio, P. M., Diez, C., Arana, R. M., and Sadun, E.,** Antibodies against endocardium, vascular structures, and interstitium of striated muscle that cross-react with *Trypanosoma cruzi* and *T. rhodesiense, J. Parasitol.,* 60, 1024, 1974.
94. **Szarfman, A., Khoury, E. L., Cossio, P. M., Arana, R. M., and Kagen, I. G.,** Investigation of the EVI antibody in parasitic diseases other than American trypanosomiasis. An anti-skeletal muscle antibody in leischmaniasis, *Am. J. Trop. Med. Hyg.,* 24, 19, 1975.
95. **Szarfman, A., Cossio, P. M., Arana, R. M., Urman, J., Kreutzer, E., Laguens, R. P., Segal, A., and Coarasa, L.,** Immunologic and immunopathologic studies in congenital Chagas' disease, *Clin. Immunol. Immunopathol.,* 4, 489, 1975.
96. **Laguens, R. P., Cossio, P. M., Diez, C., Segal, A., Vasquez, C., Kreutzer, E., Khoury, E., and Arana, R. M.,** Immunopathologic and morphologic studies of skeletal muscle in Chagas' disease, *Am. J. Pathol.,* 80, 153, 1975.
97. **Trezza, E., Tucci, P. J. F., Buffollo, E., and Montenegro, M. R.,** Anticorpos antimiocardio na doenca de Chagas cronica. Correlacao entre a serologia e a electrocardiografia, *Arq. Bras. Cardiol.,* 28, 327, 1975.
98. **Hubsch, R. M., Sulzer, A. J., and Kagan, I. G.,** Evaluation of an autoimmune type antibody in the sera of patients with Chagas' disease, *J. Parasitol.,* 62, 523, 1976.
99. **Szarfman, A., Cossio, P. M., Schmunis, G. A., and Arana, R. M.,** The EVI antibody in acute Chagas' disease, *J. Parasitol.,* 63, 149, 1977.

100. **Szarfman, A., Laranja, F. S., Souza, W., Quintao, L. G., Gerecht, D., and Schmunis, G. A.,** Tissue reacting antibodies in a rhesus monkey with long-term *Trypanosoma cruzi* infection, *Am. J. Trop. Med. Hyg.,* 27, 832, 1978.

101. **Schmunis, G. A., Cossio, P. M., Szarfman, A., Coarasa, L., and Arana, R. M.,** Tissue reacting antibodies (EVI antibodies) in nitrofurtimox treated patients with Chagas' disease, *J. Infect. Dis.,* 138, 401, 1978.

102. **Khoury, E. L., Cossio, P. M., Szarfman, A., Marcos, J. C., Garcia Morteo, O., and Arana, R. M.,** Immunofluorescent vascular pattern due to EVI antibody of Chagas' disease. Its diagnostic value, *Am. J. Clin. Pathol.,* 69, 62, 1978.

103. **Lenzi, H. L., Lenzi, J. G., and Andrade, Z. A.,** Experimental production of EVI antibodies, *Am. J. Trop. Med. Hyg.,* 31, 48, 1982.

104. **Nicholson, R. L., Dawkins, R. L., McDonald, B. L., and Wetherall, J. D.,** A classification of anti-heart antibodies: differentiation between heart-specific and heterophil antibodies, *Clin. Immunol. Immunopathol.,* 7, 349, 1977.

105. **Cabral, H. R. A., de Paolasso, E. W., and Iniguez-Montenegro, C.,** Valoracion clinica de reaccion de Rose-Ragan en la enfermedad de Chagas aguda, *Prensa Med. Argent.,* 54, 1713, 1967.

106. **Szarfman, A., Cossio, P. M., Laguens, R. P., Segal, A., de la Vega, M. T., Arana, R. M., and Schmunis, G. A.,** Immunologic studies of Rockland mice infected with *Trypanosoma cruzi.* Development of anti-nuclear antibodies, *Biomedicine,* 22, 489, 1975.

107. **Khoury, E. L., Ritacco, V., Cossio, P. M., Laguens, R. P., Szarfman, A., Diez, C., and Arana, R. M.,** Circulating antibodies to peripheral nerve in American trypanosomiasis (Chagas' disease), *Clin. Exp. Immunol.,* 36, 8, 1979.

108. **Khoury, E. L. and Fields, K. L.,** Chagas' disease and autoimmunity, *Lancet,* 1088, 1980.

109. **Cabral, H. R. A., Segura-Seco, E., and de Paolosso, E. R. W.,** Enfermedad de Chagas aguda y autoimmunidad, *Rev. Fac. Clen. Med. (Cordoba),* 25, 419, 1967.

110. **Santos-Buch, C. A. and Teixeira, A. R. L.,** The immunology of experimental Chagas' disease. IV. Production of lesions in rabbits similar to those of chronic Chagas' disease in man, *Am. J. Pathol.,* 80, 163, 1974.

111. **Acosta, A. M. and Santos-Buch, C. A.,** Autoimmune myocarditis produced by *Trypanosoma cruzi,* submitted.

112. **Boyum, O.,** Separation of leukocytes from blood and bone marrow, *Scand. J. Clin. Lab. Invest.,* 21 (Suppl. 97), 1, 1968.

113. **Shah, S. A. and Dickson, J. A.,** Lymphocyte separation from blood, *Nature (London),* 249, 168, 1974.

114. **Bollon, A. P., Nath, K., and Shay, J. W.,** Establishment of contracting heart muscle cell cultures, *Tiss. Cult. Assoc. Man.,* 3, 637, 1977.

115. **Gardner, I., Bowern, N. A., and Blanden, R. V.,** Cell mediated cytotoxicity against ectromelia virus-infected target cells. I. Specificity and kinetics, *Eur. J. Immunol.,* 4, 63, 1974.

116. **Doherty, P. C., Zinkernagel, R. M., and Ramshaw, I. A.,** Specificity and development of cytotoxic thymus-derived lymphocytes in lymphocytic choriomeningitis, *J. Immunol.,* 112, 1548, 1974.

117. **Shearer, G. M., Rehn, T. G., and Schmitt-Verhulst, A. M.,** Role of murine major histocompatibility complex in the specificity of *in vitro* T-cell-mediated lympholysis against chemically-modified autologous lymphocytes, *Transplant. Rev.,* 29, 222, 1976.

118. **Naor, D.,** Unresponsiveness to modified self antigens — a censorship mechanism controlling autoimmunity?, *Immunol. Rev.,* 50, 187, 1980.

119. **Battisto, J. R., Butler, L. D., and Wong, H.,** Use of hapten-altered self moieties to probe the cell-mediated lympholytic response and immunotolerance interface, *Immunol. Rev.,* 50, 47, 1980.

120. **Marshall-Clarke, S. and Playfair, J. H. L.,** B cells: subpopulations, tolerance, autoimmunity, and infection, *Immunol. Rev.,* 43, 110, 1979.

121. **Santos-Buch, C. A. and Acosta, A. M.,** Immunology of chagasic heart disease, in *Clinical Immunology of the Heart,* Zabriskie, J. B., Engle, M. A., and Villareal, H., Jr., Eds., John Wiley & Sons, New York, 1981, 143.

122. **Acosta, A. M., Sadigursky, M., and Santos-Buch, C. A.,** Anti-striated muscle antibody activity produced by *Trypanosoma cruzi, Proc. Soc. Exp. Biol. Med.,* 172, 364, 1983.

123. **Martonosi, A.,** The regulation of sarcoplasmic Ca^{2+} concentration in cardiac muscle, in *Current Topics in Membranes and Transport,* Brauner, F. and Kleinzeller, A., Eds., Academic Press, New York, 1972, 126.

124. **Caroni, P. and Carafoli, E.,** An ATP-dependent Ca^{2+} pumping system in dog heart sarcolemma, *Nature (London),* 283, 765, 1980.

125. **Pessoa, S. B. and Cardosa, F. A.,** Nota sobre a immunidade cruzada na leishmaniase tegumentar e na molestia de Chagas, *Hospital,* 21, 187, 1942.

126. **Howard, J. E. and Rubio, M.,** Enfermedad de Chagas congenita. I. Estudio clinico y epidemiologico de 30 casos, *Bol. Chil. Parasitol.,* 23, 107, 1968.

127. **Bittencourt, A. L., Sadigursky, M., and Barbosa, H. S.,** Doenca de Chagas congenita: estudo de 29 casos, *Rev. Inst. Med. Trop. Sao Paulo,* 17, 146, 1975.

128. **Saleme, A., Yanicelli, G. L., and Ingo, L. A.,** Enfermedad de Chagas-Mazza congenita en Tucuman, *Arch. Argent. Pediatr.,* 69, 162, 1971.

129. **Bittencourt, A. L.,** The congenital transmission of Chagas disease as a cause of abortion, *Gaz. Med. Bahia,* 69, 118, 1969.

130. **Bittencourt, A. L. and Barbosa, H. A.,** Incidencia da transmissao congenita da doenca de Chagas em abortos, *Rev. Inst. Med. Trop. Sao Paulo,* 14, 131, 1972.

131. **Rassi, A., Borges, C., and Koberle, F.,** Sobre a transmissao congenita da doenca de Chagas, *Rev. Goiana Med.,* 4, 319, 1958.

132. **Andrade, S., Bittencourt, A. L., and Figueira, R. M.,** Estudo experimental de amostras de *Trypanosoma cruzi* isoladas de gestantes chagasicas, *Rev. Patol. Trop.,* 2, 301, 1973.

133. **Brito, T. and Vasconcelos, E.,** Necrotizing arteritis in megaesophagus: histopathology of ninety-one biopsies taken from the cardia, *Rev. Inst. Med. Trop. San Paulo,* 1, 195, 1959.

134. **Okumura, M., Brito, T., and Silva, L. H. R.,** The pathology of experimental Chagas' disease in mice. I. Digestive tract changes with reference to necrotizing arthritis, *Rev. Inst. Med. Trop. San Paulo,* 2, 17, 1960.

135. **Decourt, L. V., Sosa, E. A., and Pileggi, F.,** Estudos electrofisiologicos cardiacos na forma indeterminada da doenca de Chagas, *Arq. Bras. Cadiol.,* 36, 227, 1981.

136. **Friedmann, A. A., Armelin, E., Garcez Leme, L. E., Faintuch, J. J., Gansul, R. C., Diament, J., and De Serro Azul, L. G.,** Desempenho ventricular na doenca de Chagas. Relacoes ecocardiograficas na miocardiopatia com disturbio dromotropo e na fase pre-clinica, *Arq. Bras. Cardiol.,* 36, 23, 1981.

137. **Mady, C., Pereira Barretto, A. C., Stolf, N., Lopes, E. A., Dauar, D., Wajngarten, M., Martinelli Filho, M., Macruz, R., and Pileggi, F.,** Biopsia endomiocardica na forma indeterminada da doenca de Chagas, *Arq. Bras. Cardiol.,* 36, 387, 1981.

138. **Carrasco, H. A., Palacios, E., Scorza, C., Rangel, A., Inglesis, G., Sanoja, C. L., Molina, C., and Fuenmajor, A.,** La biopsia miocardica en la enfermedad de Chagas (experiencia clinica in 56 pacientes), in *Miocadiopatias,* Acquatella, H. and Pulido, P. A., Eds., Salvat Editores, Barcelona, 1982, 19.

139. **Valecillos, R.,** Aspecto radiologico de la miocardiopatia cronica chagasica, in *Miocardiopatias,* Acquatella, H. and Pulido, P. A., Eds., Salvat Editores, Barcelona, 1982, 53.

140. **Chagas, C. and Villelal, E.,** Cardiac form of American trypanosomiasis, *Mem. Inst. Oswaldo Cruz,* 14, 3, 1922.

141. **Porto, C. C.,** O electrocardiograma no pronostico e evalucao de doenca de Chagas, *Arq. Bras. Cardiol.,* 17, 313, 1964.

142. **Rosenbaum, M. B.,** Chagasic myocardiopathy, *Prog. Cardiovasc. Dis.,* 7, 199, 1964.

143. **Hirschhaut, E., Aparicio, J. M., Acquatella, H., Arreaza, N., Puigbo, J. J., Combellas, I., Giordano, M., and Mendoza, I.,** Prueba de esfuerzo en el diagnostico de la miocardiopatia chagasica cronica, in *Miocardiopatias,* Acquatella, H. and Pulido, P. A., Eds., Salvat Editores, Barcelona, 1982, 61.

144. **de Hernandez, M. I. R.,** Contribucion de la electrocardiografia dinamica en el estudio dela miocardiopatia chagasica cronica, in *Miocardiopatias,* Acquatella, H. and Pulido, P. A., Eds., Salvat Editores, Barcelona, 1982, 71.

145. **Mendoza, I., Moleiro, F., Casal, H., Puigbo, J. J., Acquatella, H., Combellas, I., Giordano, H., Hirschhaut, E., and Pifano, F.,** Correlacion entre el electro y vectorcardiograma y las anormalidades contractiles en la miocarditis cronica chagasica, in *Miocardiopatias,* Acquatella, H. and Pulido, P. A., Eds., Salvat Editores, Barcelona, 1982, 57.

146. **Acquatella, H., Schiller, N. B., Puigbo, J. J., and Giordano, H., Suarez, J. A., Casal, H., Arreaza, N., Valecillos, R., and Hirschhaut, E.,** Estudio ecocardiografico en la enfermedad de Chagas: miocardiopatia cronica con lesiones segmentarias, in *Miocardiopatias,* Acquatella, H. and Pulido, P. A., Eds., Salvat Editores, Barcelona, 1982, 89.

147. **Arreaza, N., Puigbo, J. J., Acquatella, H., Casal, H., Giordano, H., Valecillos, R., Hirschhaut, E., and Combellas, I.,** La ventriculografia radionuclear en la miocardiopatia cronica chagasica, in *Miocardiopatias,* Acquatella, H. and Pulido, P. A., Eds., Salvat Editores, Barcelona, 1982, 107.

148. **de Rezende, J. M.,** Formas digestivas de enfermedad de Chagas, in *Primer Congreso Argentino de Parasitologia: Simp. Int. de Enfermedad de Chagas, Buenos Aires, Dieciembre 1982,* Soc. Arg. Parasitol., Buenos Aires, 1972, 232.

149. **Raia, A. and Campos, O. M.,** Megacolon: contribucao ao estudo de sua patogenia e tratemento, *Rev. Med. Cir. Sao Paulo,* 15, 391, 1955.

150. **Koberle, F.,** Zur frage der entstehung sog. "Idiopathischer Dilatationem" muskular der hohlorgan, *Virchows Arch.,* 329, 337, 1956.

151. **Raizman, R. E.,** Chagasic megaesophagus: similarity to achalasia by manometrics, radiography, and response to pneumatic dilatation, *Am. J. Dig. Dis.,* 20, 882, 1975.

152. **Taliaferro, W. H. and Pizzi, T.,** Connective tissue reactions in normal and immunized mice to a reticulotropic strain of *Trypanosoma cruzi, J. Infect. Dis.,* 96, 199, 1955.

153. **Andrade, S. G. and Andrade, Z. A.,** Estudo histopatologico comparativo das lesoes produzidas por duas cepas de *Trypanosoma cruzi, Hospital,* 70, 101, 1966.

154. **Andrade, S. G., Carvalho, M. L., and Figueira, R. M.,** Caracterizacao morfobiologica e histopatologica de diferentes cepas do *Trypanosoma cruzi, Gaz. Med. Bahia,* 70, 32, 1970.

155. **Amaral, C. F. S., Tafuri, W. L., and Brener, Z.,** Frequencia do parasitismo encefalico em camundongos experimentalmente inoculados com diferentes cepas do *Trypanosoma cruzi, Rev. Soc. Bras. Med. Trop.,* 9, 243, 1975.

156. **Dvorak, J. A.,** New *in vitro* approach to quantitation of *Trypanosoma cruzi* — vertebrate cell interactions, in *New Approaches in American Trypanosomiasis Research: Proc. Int. Symp.,* Pan American Health Organization, Washington, D.C., 1976, 109.

157. **Koberle, F. and Alcantara, F. G.,** Mechanismo da destruicao neuronal do sistema nervoso periferico na molestia de Chagas, *Hospital,* 57, 1057, 1960.

158. **Mijares, M. S.,** Contribucion al estudio de la patologia de la miocarditis cronica chagasica en Venezuela. Revision de 130 autopsias, *Arch. Hosp. Vargas,* 7, 117, 1965.

159. **Lopes, E. R., Chapadeiro, E., Almeida, H. O., and Abraao, D.,** Peso do coracao e tipo de morte no chagasico cronico, *Rev. Inst. Med. Trop. Sao Paulo,* 12, 293, 1970.

160. **Chapadeiro, E., Lopes, E. R., Mesquita, P. M., and Pereira, F. E. L.,** Incidencia de "megas" associados a cardiopatia chagasica, *Rev. Inst. Med. Trop. Sao Paulo,* 6, 287, 1964.

161. **Barbosa, A. J. A., Pitella, J. E. H., and Tafuri, W. L.,** Incidencia de cardiopatia chagasica em 15,000 necropsias consecutivas e sua associacao com os "megas", *Rev. Soc. Bras. Med. Trop.,* 4, 219, 1970.

162. **Macedo, V. O.,** Influencia da exposicao a reinfeccao na evolucao da doenca de Chagas, Tese. Rio de Janeiro, 1973.

163. **De Rezende, J. M.,** Clinica: manifestacoes digestivas, in *Trypanosoma Cruzi de Doenca de Chagas,* Brener, Z. and Andrade, Z. A., Eds., Guanabara Koogan, Rio de Janeiro, 1979, chap. 9.

164. **Hurst, A. F. and Rake, G. W.,** Achalasia of the cardia (so-called cardiospasm), *Q. J. Med.,* 23, 491, 1930.

165. **Amorim, M. and Correia Neto, A.,** Histopatologia e patogene do megaesofago e megarreto, *An. Fac. Med. Univ. Sao Paulo,* 8, 101, 1932.

166. **Correia Neto, A. and Etzel, E.,** Le mega-oesophage et le megacolon devant la theorie de l'achalasie. Etude clinique et anatomopatologique, *Rev. Sud. Am. Med. Chir.,* 7, 395, 1934.

167. **Koberle, F. and Nador, E.,** Etiologia e patogenia do megaesofago no Brasil, *Rev. Paul. Med.,* 47, 643, 1955.

168. **Bojsen-Moller, F. and Tranum-Jensen, J.,** Rabbit heart nodal tissue, sinuatrial ring bundle and atrioventricular connections identified as a neuromuscular system, *J. Anat.,* 112, 367, 1972.

169. **James, T. N. and Spence, C. A.,** Ultrastructure of the human atrioventricular node, *Circulation,* 37, 1049, 1968.

170. **Kawamura, K. and James, T. N.,** Comparative ultrastructure of cellular junctions in working myocardium and the conduction system under normal and pathological conditions, *J. Mol. Cell. Cardiol.,* 3, 31, 1971.

171. **Legato, M. J.,** Ultrastructure of the atrial, ventricular and Purkinje cell, with special reference to the genesis of arrhythmias, *Circulation,* 47, 1035, 1956.

172. **Helander, E.,** Studies on the chemical components of the conducting system of the heart. II. The water soluble protein, *Cardiologia,* 47, 146, 1965.

173. **Helander, E.,** Studies on the chemical components of the conducting system of the heart. III. The contracting protein, *Cardiologia,* 49, 359, 1966.

174. **Helander, E.,** Studies on the chemical components of the conducting system of the heart. IV. Contractility of the atrioventricular conducting system, *Cardiologia,* 49, 362, 1966.

175. **Szabo, S., Lapohos, E., Lukacs, E., Kapusi, A., and Reichel, C.,** Immunological properties of the heart conducting system, *Z. Immunitartsfursch.,* 130, 252, 1966.

176. **Diez, C.,** personal communication.

Chapter 9

IMMUNOLOGY OF CHAGAS' DISEASE*

Rodney Hoff and Markley H. Boyer

TABLE OF CONTENTS

*   Supported by Charles A. King Trust, Boston and U.S. Public Health Service Grants AI 16305, AI 16479, and
    AI 18680.

I. INTRODUCTION

In the preceding chapter, Santos-Buch et al.[1] reviewed the clinical, pathologic, and epidemiologic features of Chagas' disease. In this chapter, we review recent developments in the immunology of *Trypanosoma cruzi* and Chagas' disease. Immunity influences many aspects of human Chagas' disease. Most individuals are able to suppress or control the acute infection with *T. cruzi* and, once recovered, do not experience relapse of the acute disease. However, despite the lack of symptoms and the appearance of humoral and cellular reactivity to parasite antigens, the infection persists at chronic low levels, probably for life. Months to years after the acute phase, some infected individuals develop a chronic progressive disease of the heart and alimentary tract that appears to be the result of an immunopathologic process.

Recent immunologic research on Chagas' disease has focused on: (1) identifying the *host immune* mechanisms responsible for resistance to the parasite, (2) delineating the parasite antigens which are targets for immune destruction and are capable of eliciting protective immune responses, (3) determining the mechanisms whereby *T. cruzi* evades host immunity, and (4) characterizing the immune mechanisms and the parasite antigens involved in the pathogenesis of the chronic disease. The ultimate objectives of these separate, but related, goals have been to develop safe immunoprophylactic measures to prevent the infection and perhaps to modify the progression of the chronic disease. The immunology of *T. cruzi* infection and Chagas' disease has also been reviewed recently by Brener,[2] Scott and Snary,[3] Kuhn,[4] Miles,[5] and Santos-Buch.[6]

A. Life Cycle of *T. cruzi* and Immunologic Features of Human Infection and Disease

The immunology of *T. cruzi* is complicated by the multiple developmental stages of the parasite found in both mammalian and insect hosts.[2] The three basic morphologic forms or stages of the parasite — the trypomastigote, amastigote, and epimastigote — have distinct physiologic and antigenic features. Initially, humans and reservoir hosts are exposed to the infective metacyclic trypomastigotes transmitted with the feces of the triatomine vector. Entering through the bite wound or mucosal tissues, the metacyclic trypomastigotes quickly penetrate cells and transform into nonflagellate amastigotes which multiply by binary fission in the host cell cytoplasm. When a host cell is about to burst, the amastigotes transform into nondividing, flagellated trypomastigotes. Released into intracellular spaces and into the blood, the trypomastigotes infect other cells or are taken up by the insect vector when it feeds. In the insect's midgut, trypomastigotes transform into epimastigotes which multiply by binary fission. After several days, some epimastigotes escape the midgut and enter the bug's hindgut where they complete transformation to infective metacyclic trypomastigotes which pass out with the feces.

In humans, primary infection with *T. cruzi* is usually mild or inapparent. Only a small proportion of infected individuals develop an acute illness prompting them to seek medical attention. The common acute symptoms include a persistent fever lasting several weeks, malaise, generalized lymphadenopathy, and hepatosplenomegaly. In some cases there are signs at the portal of entry of the parasite, on which an indurated erythematous area of the skin (chagoma) or bipalpebral edema (Romana's sign) develops.[1] During the acute stage, trypomastigotes are present in microscopically detectable numbers in the peripheral blood, and amastigotes are found in muscle cells, macrophages, and connective tissue cells. Specific immune responses are indicated by the intense infiltration of infected tissues with lymphocytes and macrophages, the appearance of IgM and IgG antibodies to *T. cruzi*, and by in vitro lymphocyte reactivity and delayed skin hypersensitivity to *T. cruzi* antigens. About 10% of acute cases, primarily infants, develop meningoencephalitis and/or acute myocarditis with congestive failure which are usually fatal. However, in the majority of patients, the acute disease resolves without treatment.[1,7-11]

The acute phase is followed by a chronic asymptomatic or indeterminate phase that continues for years. Parasites can be detected in the blood and in the tissues, but at extremely low numbers that usually require culture or xenodiagnosis for detection.[12] The chronic infection is usually diagnosed by detection of specific IgG antibodies using a variety of serologic tests.[2,3,12] Months to years after the primary infection, approximately 20 to 40% of infected individuals develop a progressive chronic disease affecting primarily the heart and the gastrointestinal tract.[1,13] The pathogenesis of the chronic disease has not been fully resolved, but the extent of the chronic inflammatory lesions and fibrosis, which is out of proportion to the few organisms persisting in the blood and tissues, has prompted speculation that immune mechanisms are responsible.[1,14] Whatever the underlying pathologic mechanism, there is a perplexing regional difference in the target organs affected by Chagas' disease. In Venezuela, the cardiac form predominates, and megaesophagus and megacolon are extremely rare. In Chile, the cardiac disease is less common and mega-disease, particularly megacolon, is seen more frequently. In northeast Brazil, both cardiac and gastrointestinal disease occur although the cardiac form predominates. The variable clinical expression of Chagas' disease is believed to be related to inherent differences in the pathogenicity of *T. cruzi* strains circulating in the endemic countries.[5]

B. Heterogeneity of *T. cruzi* and Animal Models of Acute and Chronic Chagas' Disease

T. cruzi isolated from different patients, and even clones of a parasite stock, often display marked heterogeneity in virulence, histotropism, morphology, antigenic make-up, isoenzymes, kinetoplast DNA, growth rates in liquid culture and tissue culture, temperature-dependent regulation of growth, and in morphogenesis and infectivity for vectors.[2,5,15-17] This inherent heterogeneity complicates definition of animal models and makes it difficult to evaluate experimental findings when different parasite strains are used. Therefore, for immunologic studies, it is best to use cloned stocks of *T. cruzi* with defined biologic characteristics.

Because of convenience and the availability of a wide variety of genetically defined strains, the mouse has become the standard model for immunologic study of Chagas' disease. Like humans, mice develop immunity to *T. cruzi* during the primary infection. This is reflected by (1) recovery from the acute disease, (2) resistance of recovered mice to an otherwise lethal challenge infection, and (3) immune reactivity to *T. cruzi* as indicated by the production of specific antibodies and specifically sensitized lymphocytes. The effect of experimental manipulations on host immunity is usually monitored by changes in the level of parasitemia and tissue parasitism and by changes in the timed mortality rate. As with humans, mice do not develop a sterile immunity to *T. cruzi*. During the chronic phase, the organisms can usually be recovered from the blood by culture or by xenodiagnosis, and with thorough searching, intracellular parasites can be found in organ tissues. Therefore, the presence of viable organisms and the effect of premunition on immunity needs to be considered in experimental manipulation. The age and sex of mice also affect their innate resistance to *T. cruzi;* young mice have higher parasitemia and mortality than adult mice, and males are more susceptible than females.[2-6]

In the mouse, the histotropism of the infecting strain of *T. cruzi* has an important influence on the outcome of infections. In general, strains have a preference for either muscle cells (musculotropic) or macrophages of the spleen, liver, bone marrow, and central nervous system (macrophagotropic or reticulotropic).[2] Both histotropic types are able to parasitize muscle cells, although the former type does so to a much greater degree. Macrophagotropic strains usually produce a fulminant acute disease with peaks of parasitemia and mortality occurring during the first 14 days of infection; a more chronic course lasting 20 to 40 days is characteristic for musculotropic strains. Macrophagotropism appears to be related to a property of the parasite's membrane that prevents or facilitates uptake by macrophages. In vitro, uptake by macrophages of bloodstream trypomastigotes of the macrophagotropic Y strain is at least 40 times greater than with the musculotropic CL strain. In vivo, CL strain trypomastigotes injected intravenously keep circulating for many hours without penetrating host cells, in contrast to Y strain trypomastigotes which are very quickly removed from the circulation by macrophages.[18]

II. IMMUNOLOGY OF HOST RESISTANCE

A. Role of T Cells and B Cells in Immunity

The mouse model has been used extensively to study the relative importance of humoral and cell-mediated immunity in resistance to acute *T. cruzi* infection. The dependence of immunity on B cells and antibody is demonstrated by the ability to passively transfer resistance to recipients with serum from chronically infected donors.[19-22] Further evidence for humoral factors in immunity to *T. cruzi* is the increased susceptibility in mice genetically selected to give low antibody responses[23] and in rats made B cell deficient by treatment with anti-μ serum.[24] The protective antibodies that passively transfer resistance in mice have been identified by Takehara et al.[25] to be IgG_{2a} and IgG_{2b} immunoglobulins. McHardy[22] has shown that the antibodies protect against challenge with either bloodstream or insect-derived trypomastigotes.

The involvement of T cells in immunity to *T. cruzi* is indicated by the increased susceptibility of nude mice and mice made deficient in T cells,[26-30] and by adoptive transfer of resistance to recipients with inoculations of immune thymocytes and spleen cells.[20,29-32] These experiments, however, fail to delineate the relative importance of T cells as helper cells in the production of protective antibodies[31] and as effector cells in cell-mediated immunity. Scott[20] and Trischmann and Bloom[32] have found that immune spleen cell preparations depleted of T cells retain the ability to passively protect mice against challenge infection, while B cell-depleted preparations lose this activity. This suggests that T cells function primarily as helper cells for B cell responses, and that lymphokines and cytotoxic T lymphocytes are not essential for immunity to challenge infection. On the other hand, Burgess and Hanson[33] have found that prior depletion of T cells from immune spleen cell preparations reduces the passive protection conferred, and that adoptive transfers of purified immune T cells fully protect irradiated recipients. With these divergent results, further studies are needed to clarify the specific roles of T cells in immunity to acute *T. cruzi* infection.

B. Genetics of Host Resistance in the Mouse

Susceptibility to acute infection varies dramatically among different inbred strains of mice. The spectrum ranges from highly resistant C57BL/10 and DBA/1 to highly sensitive C3H/He, DBA/2, and strain A mice.[30] Experiments with congenic mice and with F_1 hybrids of resistant and sensitive parents indicate that resistance is primarily controlled by genes outside the H-2 major histocompatibility complex.[29,30] How genetic factors affect resistance (or susceptibility) is not understood. It is known that during *T. cruzi* infection, susceptible mouse strains have lower antibody responses to TNP and sheep red blood cells and produce less macrophage-activating factors and lymphotoxin than resistant strains.[34-37] Wrightsman et al.[29] note that multiple genes may be involved as the level of parasitemia and mortality appears to be controlled separately, the gene controlling for low parasitemia response being dominant and the gene-promoting survival of B10 strain mice being partially influenced by H-2^s-linked genes.

Strains of mice which spontaneously develop autoimmune disease have been found to be highly susceptible to *T. cruzi* infection.[38,39] In congenic BXSB and MRL/1pr strains, susceptibility appears to be linked to the single gene-controlling autoimmunity. Transfer of the *1pr* (lymphoproliferative) gene to mice with C3H, C57, and AKR backgrounds has been shown to greatly enhance susceptibility to infection. In BXSB mice, replacement of the YSB chromosome with a YBL/6 chromosome from a resistant C57BL/6 strain renders the hybrid BXSB mice resistant to infection. The immunologic mechanisms, whereby these genes influence either autoimmunity or susceptibility to *T. cruzi*, have not been resolved.

C. Immune Effector Mechanisms in Chagas' Disease

In the mammalian host the parasite life cycle can be interrupted by (1) preventing establishment of intracellular infection by metacyclic trypomastigotes, (2) preventing cell-to-cell spread of the infection by neutralization or destruction of circulating trypomastigotes, and (3) destruction of host cells containing the obligate intracellular amastigotes. Because extracellular trypomastigotes are more easily studied in vitro, much is known about the immune mechanisms affecting this stage. In vitro, trypomastigotes are destroyed or neutralized through the action of antibody and complement, antibody-dependent cell-mediated cytotoxicity, macrophages, natural killer cells, and lymphotoxin. Destruction of amastigotes, which gain a measure of protection from their intracellular habitat, probably requires prior destruction of the infected host cell.

1. Complement-Mediated Destruction of Trypomastigotes

In the mouse, the presence of antibodies to *T. cruzi* that are capable of mediating complement lysis of trypomastigotes in vitro is associated with protective immunity.[21,40] These lytic antibodies, which coat the circulating parasites, appear during the acute phase and persist throughout the chronic infection. Their maintenance requires active infection; the antibodies are lost when the infection is drug cured, and it has not proved possible to induce lytic antibodies by immunization with killed or fractionated organisms.[40] The dependence of immunity on complement is indicated by the increased susceptibility of mice that have been treated with cobra venom factor to deplete complement,[42] however, not all complement components may be required; Krettli[43] found no difference in the level of parasitemia in normal and C5-deficient mice.

Although initiated by antibody, in vitro lysis of trypomastigotes by human complement is achieved primarily through activation of the alternative pathway as indicated by the complete dependence of the reaction on the presence of factor B and properdin.[41,44] However, some components of the classical pathway may contribute, as the degree of lysis with C2-deficient serum or with chelation of Ca^{2+} is less. Given the predominance of alternative pathway activation in antibody-dependent lysis of trypomastigotes, the role antibody plays in initiation of complement activation is not understood. Kipnis et al.[45] have speculated that antibodies somehow modify the trypomastigote membrane components that protect it from activating the alternative pathway. These components are apparently absent from epimastigotes, which activate the alternative complement sequence in absence of antibody.

Krettli et al.[44] have shown that the musculotropic CL strain of *T. cruzi* is relatively resistant to complement lysis mediated by antibodies present during the acute phase of infection. Although antibody binds to their surface, CL strain trypomastigotes appear to be able to escape lysis either by shedding the antibodies or by producing "fabulation" enzymes that cleave the Fc portion of surface-bound antibodies.[46] The antibodies minus the Fc fragment would be incapable of activating complement, and their presence would block further binding of lytic antibodies.

2. Cell-Mediated Cytotoxicity to Trypomastigotes

In vitro, bloodstream trypomastigotes can be lysed independently of complement by contact with eosinophils, neutrophils, and lymphoid cells and by exposure to lymphotoxin. With eosinophils and neutrophils, the cytotoxicity to trypomastigotes is dependent on the presence of specific antibodies (ADCC) as immune serum is required and the lysis can be inhibited by protein A and aggregated IgG.[47,49] How ADCC causes destruction of trypomastigote targets has not been resolved, but ultrastructural studies with epimastigote targets suggest that the sequence of damage consists first of specific attachment to the granulocyte, followed by phagocytosis, and later release of parasite debris into the extracellular medium;[50] active oxygen reduction products and myeloperoxidase are apparently involved in the intracellular destruction.[51] Kierszenbaum et al.[52] have shown that purified basic protein from granules of human eosinophils is cytotoxic to trypomastigotes in vitro, and Nogueira et al.[53] have shown that a peroxidase purified from granules of horse eosinophils is capable of sensitizing trypomastigotes for killing by normal mouse macrophages. Interestingly, the CL strain of *T. cruzi*, which is resistant to antibody-dependent lysis by complement, is sensitive to ADCC; however, for reasons not understood, ADCC with immune spleen cells is blocked when target trypomastigotes are coated with antibody.[47]

Mouse lymphoid cells with the characteristic phenotype of NK cells (NK 1.2) have been shown to kill trypomastigotes in vitro independently of antibody.[54] During *T. cruzi* infection, NK cell numbers increase coincidently with serum levels of interferon, a lymphokine known to stimulate these cells.[55-57] The increased NK cell activity that results from treating mice with interferon or interferon-inducer drugs such as Tilerone® or poly(I.C) has been correlated with enhanced resistance to acute *T. cruzi* infection.[54,57] Since interferon itself has no direct effect on trypomastigotes or their ability to infect cells,[58] the in vivo resistance has been attributed to either increased NK cell activity or macrophage activation.[54,57] Further evidence for involvement of NK cells in immunity is suggested by the increased susceptibility of the beige mutant of C57 mice which are deficient in NK cell activity.[54,57] Krassner et al.[37] have recently described a lymphotoxin that may be important in enhancing survival in acute infection with *T. cruzi*; in vitro, the lymphotoxin neutralizes the ability of trypomastigotes to infect host cells.

3. Uptake and Killing of Trypomastigotes by Macrophages

Macrophages are host cells for *T. cruzi* during the early acute phase of infection, but as immunity develops histologic studies indicate that they no longer support growth of the parasite.[59] Experimentally it has been shown that mice selectively depleted of macrophages by silica treatment are highly susceptible to *T. cruzi*,[60] while treatment with *Corynebacterium parvum* to stimulate macrophages is protective.[61] During primary *T. cruzi* infection in the mouse, macrophages become activated and are able to kill trypomastigotes in vitro, whereas macrophages from normal mice support infection and intracellular growth of the parasite.[62-64] Enhanced parasiticidal activity to *T. cruzi* in vitro is also present in macrophages from BCG-infected mice indicating that this mechanism is nonspecific.[62,65] Macrophage activation is achieved through lymphokines produced by specifically sensitized lymphocytes; mouse spleen cells or human peripheral lymphocytes sensitized by *T. cruzi* infection, by BCG infection, or by streptococcal infection produce lymphokines in vitro when stimulated with the homologous antigen.[66-68] Nathan et al.[69] have shown that the increased parasiticidal capacity of activated macrophages is related to their increased generation of superoxide radicals, while in normal macrophages, trypomastigotes survive by escaping from the hostile environment of the phagocytic vacuoles.[64,70,71]

Specific antibodies have been shown to enhance the uptake of *T. cruzi* by macrophages, but they are not essential, as blockage of macrophage Fc and C3b receptors does not impair phagocytosis. Opsonization with antibody per se does not affect the growth of *T. cruzi* in normal or unstimulated macrophages; however, by enhancing uptake, antibodies amplify the capacity of activated macrophages to kill the parasite.[18,72] Specific antibody may be particularly important in overcoming an antiphagocytic substance present on the surface of bloodstream trypomastigotes.[73]

In addition to its effector function, macrophages are probably essential for processing antigen and for cooperation with lymphocytes. During *T. cruzi* infection, there is a dramatic increase in the proportion of Ia antigen-bearing macrophages present in the peritoneal cavity of mice and in vitro stimulation with lymphokines from infected mice has been shown to increase the expression and synthesis of Ia antigens on macrophages.[74] Since Ia-positive macrophages also regulate T cell function, their increased number during primary infection may strongly influence the mode of immune responses to the parasite.

4. Cell-Mediated Destruction of Intracellular Amastigotes

During its intracellular phase, *T. cruzi* is believed to be inaccessible to the effector mechanisms that kill extracellular trypomastigotes. Analogous to viral immunity, elimination of intracellular amastigotes, particularly those in nonphagocytic cells, requires prior destruction of the parasitized cell;[75] then exposed to the extracellular environment, amastogotes are probably vulnerable to the same effector mechanisms that kill trypomastigotes. In order to be susceptible to immune destruction, the infected host cell surface membranes must either express appropriate parasite antigens, or be altered in such a way so as to appear as nonself. Thus far, attempts to identify *T. cruzi* antigens on the surface of infected cells in tissue culture by means of anti-*T. cruzi* antiserum have been unsuccessful.[76,77] Interestingly, in the course of these experiments it was found that parasite antigens liberated during host cell rupture adhere to the surface of adjacent normal cells. In vitro, these antigen-coated host cells are susceptible to lysis by sensitized lymphocytes and by immune serum and complement, indicating that these mechanisms may be involved in pathogenesis.[77]

Although antisera does not detect parasite-elaborated antigens on host cells, in vitro studies by Kuhn and Murane[78] suggest that cytotoxic lymphocytes are able to specifically recognize and destroy syngeneic infected cells. There is, however, considerable controversy about the selectivity of the cytotoxic lymphocytes. Experiments by Santos-Buch and Teixeira[79] and Teixeira et al.[80] indicate that sensitized lymphocytes from infected rabbits and humans seem to indiscriminately kill either normal or *T. cruzi*-infected allogeneic heart cells, but not allogeneic kidney cells, indicating a degree of organ specificity. If cell-mediated cytotoxicity to *T. cruzi* is highly destructive to target tissues, as the Santos-Buch and Teixeira[79] experiments suggest, it would be to the host's advantage to suppress this immunologic response. There is some evidence that delayed-type sensitivity to *T. cruzi* antigens and heart antigens is, indeed, suppressed during the chronic phase of infection in man and experimental animals.[81,82] The nature of the antigens that are recognized on host cells by cytotoxic T cells and the restriction of recognition by antigens of the major histocompatibility complex have not been determined.

III. ANTIGENS OF *T. CRUZI*

Incorporated into a variety of serologic assays, *T. cruzi* antigens have been the basis for specific immunodiagnosis of the human infection (reviewed by Scott and Snary[3] and Miles[5]). In addition to specific antibodies, the infection can also be diagnosed by detecting circulating parasite antigens with specific antisera,[83-86] or through the use of species-specific monoclonal antibodies to the parasite.[87] The immunologic and pathologic implications of circulating antigens have yet to be considered, however, their presence may provide the means for monitoring the level of infection and evaluating chemotherapy. Recently, attention has also been focused on identification of the parasite antigens that are recognized by the host's parasiticidal mechanisms and that are capable of evoking protective immunity. The major surface antigen of bloodstream trypomastigotes recognized by immune serum is a 90-kilodalton (kd) glycoprotein.[73,88] This glycoprotein, which is also present on amastigotes and epimastigotes, is sensitive to trypsin and binds to *Len culinaris* lectin. Because trypsinization facilitates the uptake of trypomastigotes by macrophages, Nogueira et al. have speculated that the 90-kd glycoprotein is responsible for the parasite's ability to resist phagocytosis by macrophages.[73] Mice immunized with the 90-kd glycoprotein and saponin adjuvant are partially protected against challenge infection,[89] although they fail to develop the lytic antibodies associated with acquired immunity.[40] Preliminary evidence indicates that the *T. cruzi* neuraminidase described by Pereira[90] is identical to the 90-kd glycoprotein.

The major surface antigen of metacyclic trypomastigotes appears to be a 72-kd glycoprotein.[40,91] This antigen is also present on epimastigotes, but is absent from bloodstream trypomastigotes and intracellular amastigotes. A monoclonal antibody to the 72-kd antigen (WIC 29.26) has been prepared;[92] immunization with the purified glycoprotein protects mice against challenge with metacyclic trypomastigotes, but not against challenge with bloodstream trypomastigotes.[93] Interestingly, the WIC 29.26 monoclonal antibody inhibits transformation of epimastigotes to metacyclic trypomastigotes in subcutaneously implanted Millipore® chambers in mice, indicating that the 72-kd glycoprotein may be involved in morphogenesis of the parasite in the insect vector.[94] The structure of the 72-kd glycoprotein is somewhat unusual in that it is comprised of more than 50% carbohydrate.[92]

A variety of *T. cruzi* antigens have been extracted or fractionated from epimastigotes and some have been shown to protect mice against challenge infection;[86,95-99] however, these antigens have not been well characterized and their relationships to the 90 and 72-kd glycoproteins have not been established. The development of monoclonal antibodies to additional surface antigens of *T. cruzi* should facilitate further antigenic analysis of the parasite.[87,89,100-102]

IV. EVASION OF IMMUNE DESTRUCTION

The fact that low levels of parasites persist in both the blood and tissues during the chronic phase suggests that *T. cruzi* possesses multiple means to evade acquired immune responses of the host. *T. cruzi* apparently lacks the unique ability of African trypanosomes which evade host immunity by continually varying their surface antigens.[103] Trypomastigotes of *T. cruzi* are probably able to evade antibody-dependent mechanisms either by quickly capping and sloughing antigen-antibody complexes[104,105] or by producing fabulation enzymes that cleave the Fc portion of surface-bound antibodies.[46] In the latter case, the antibodies minus the Fc fragment would be incapable of mediating complement lysis, opsonization, and ADCC, and their presence would block further attachment of functionally intact antibodies. Because infected cells fail to express parasite antigens that can be recognized by immune mechanisms,[76,77] amastigotes are probably protected during the intracellular replication cycle. The duration of this protection would be extended indefinitely if the amastigotes stopped multiplying and became latent before destroying host cells; however, the existence of such latent forms during chronic infection, although postulated, has yet to be demonstrated.[106] Survival of intracellular amastigotes may also be enhanced by specific suppression of cell-mediated responses that are cytotoxic for parasitized cells.[81]

Evasion of immune destruction may be aided by the ability of *T. cruzi* infection to disrupt immunologic function. In the mouse, acute *T. cruzi* infection is accompanied by marked suppression of T and B cell responses to unrelated antigens and mitogens,[107-112] by polyclonal B cell activation,[113] and by the inability to produce and respond to interleukin 2.[114] However, the relative susceptibility of various strains of inbred mice to acute *T. cruzi* infection does not appear to be related to the degree of immunosuppression,[112,115] and, with recovery from the acute phase, mice regain normal immunologic function.[116] Thus, the extent to which generalized immunosuppression contributes to maintenance of chronic infection remains to be established.

V. IMMUNOPATHOLOGY

The chronic inflammatory lesions of chronic Chagas' disease, which appear out of proportion to simple mechanical disruption of host cells, are currently believed to have an immunopathologic basis.[1] A major difficulty in delineating the causal mechanisms has been the lack of a suitable experimental animal model of the chronic disease. Immune destruction of host tissues in chronic Chagas' disease are postulated to result either from hypersensitivity reactions to the parasite or from induction of autoimmunity. Because delayed-type hypersensitivity reactions are common features of chronic intracellular infections with viruses, bacteria, and protozoa,[117] it has been postulated that neighboring uninfected cells (innocent bystanders) may be destroyed in the attempt to eliminate the intracellular infection. In the case of *T. cruzi*, in vitro studies suggest that the destructive process may be aided by the ability of parasite antigens to adhere to normal tissue cells;[76,77] as a consequence, these cells may be destroyed by the host's antiparasitic immune responses. Therefore, it may be the host's advantage to suppress cell-mediated cytotoxicity which produces excessive tissue damage.[81] If this hypothesis is correct, the development of severe disease in a proportion of individuals after a long latent period could result from a gradual loss of specific suppression (changes related to age, nutritional status, incidental disease, etc.) permitting an increased level of cell-mediated immunity.[81]

The fact that chronically infected individuals develop cell-mediated and antibody reactivity to heart and skeletal muscles, blood vessels and peripheral nerves has led to speculation that tissue damage is caused by autoimmunity induced by *T. cruzi* antigens which cross-react with host antigens.[1,2,6] Putative cross-reactive antigens include an ATPase of sarcoplasmic reticulum,[118] laminin,[119] and a variety of proteins from heart and neuronal cells identified by the monoclonal antibody CE5.[120] The in vivo experiments of Laguens et al.,[121] showing that chronic heart lesions can be induced in recipient mice by adoptive transfer of sensitized spleen cells from chronically infected animals, lend additional support to an autoimmune pathogenesis. However, recent attempts to prove an association between clinical heart disease and humoral and cellular autoreactivity to heart tissue in humans infected with *T. cruzi* have not been successful.[122,123]

VI. PROSPECTS FOR VACCINATION

Even though *T. cruzi* seemingly evades host immune responses, several factors favor the eventual development of an effective immunization for human Chagas' disease:

1. Infection of mice with avirulent strains of *T. cruzi* or inoculation of radiation- or drug-attenuated organisms results in significant protection (but not sterile immunity) to otherwise lethal challenge[124-126] and reduces the pathologic manifestation of chronic disease.[127] Vaccines consisting of parasite extracts or purified components are also protective but usually require the use of adjuvants.[89,93,128]
2. There is no evidence that *T. cruzi* is capable of antigenic variation comparable to that descibed in African trypanosomiasis.[103]
3. There appears to be cross-immunity between *T. cruzi* strains of wide geographical origin and between strains obtained from humans and animals.[129]

There are, however, several important problems to overcome in developing a safe and effective vaccine for human Chagas' disease.[130] First, the vaccine must either block primary infection with metacyclic trypomastigotes or prevent the establishment of the chronic infection, something that naturally acquired immunity fails to do. To date, experimental vaccines in animals have failed to induce a sterile immunity to challenge with either bloodstream trypomastigotes or metacyclic trypomastigotes. With partial protection, the exposed host may avoid the acute phase of the disease but remains at risk to the chronic Chagas' disease. Second, there is the danger that the vaccine itself could stimulate autoimmunity if it contained cross-reacting antigens to heart or other host tissues. These problems, potential or otherwise, may limit the options for vaccination. Conceptually, it seems logical to concentrate on directing the immune attack on the more vulnerable stages of the parasite. As mentioned previously, the intracellular multiplicative phase of *T. cruzi* in nonphagocytic cells is probably least susceptible to immune attack, while extracellular trypomastigotes are, theoretically at least, more vulnerable. Destruction of the invading metacyclic forms would totally protect the host, while destruction of bloodstream forms would prevent cell-to-cell spread and eventually halt the progression of the infection.

REFERENCES

1. **Santos-Buch, C. A. and Acosta, A. M.,** Pathology of Chagas' disease, in *Immunology and Pathogenesis of Trypanosomiasis,* Tizard, I., Ed., CRC Press, Boca Raton, Fla., 1985.
2. **Brener, Z.,** Immunity to *Trypanosoma cruzi, Adv. Parasitol.,* 18, 247, 1980.
3. **Scott, M. T. and Snary, D.,** American trypanosomiasis (Chagas' disease), in *Immunology of Parasitic Infections,* 2nd ed., Cohen, S. and Warren, K. S., Eds., Blackwell Scientific, Edinburgh, 1982, chap. 11.
4. **Kuhn, R. E.,** Immunology of *Trypanosoma cruzi* infection, in *Advances in Parasitic Disease,* Vol. 1, Mansfield, J., Ed., Marcel Dekker, New York, 1981, chap. 3.
5. **Miles, M. A.,** Transmission cycles and the heterogeneity of *Trypanosoma cruzi,* in *Biology of the Kinetoplastida,* Vol. 2, Lumsten, W. H. R. and Evans, D., Eds., Academic Press, New York, 1979, chap. 2.
6. **Santos-Buch, C. A.,** American trypanosomiasis: Chagas' disease, *Int. Rev. Exp. Pathol.,* 19, 63, 1979.
7. **Rassi, A.,** Clinica: fase aguda, in *Trypanosoma cruzi e Doenca de Chagas',* Brener, Z. and Andrade, Z., Eds., Guanabara Koogan, Rio de Janeiro, 1979, chap. 7.
8. **Schmunis, G. A., Szarfman, A., Coarasa, L., and Vainstok, C.,** Immunoglobulin concentration in treated human acute Chagas' disease, *Am. J. Trop. Med. Hyg.,* 27, 473, 1978.
9. **Teixeira, A. R. L., Roters, F. A., and Mott, K. E.,** Acute Chagas' disease, *Gaz. Med. Bahia,* 70, 176, 1970.
10. **Teixeira, A. R. L., Teixeira, G., Macedo, V., and Prata, A.,** Acquired cell-mediated immunodepression in acute Chagas' disease, *J. Clin. Invest.,* 62, 1132, 1978.
11. **Hoff, R., Teixeira, R. S., Carvalho, J. S., and Mott, K. E.,** *Trypanosoma cruzi* in the cerebrospinal fluid during acute Chagas' disease, *N. Engl. J. Med.,* 298, 604, 1978.
12. **Hoff, R., Mott, K. E., Franca Silva, J., Menezes, V., Hoff, J. N., Barrett, T. V., and Sherlock, I.,** Prevalence of parasitemia and seroreactivity to *Trypanosoma cruzi* in a rural population of northeast Brazil, *Am. J. Trop. Med. Hyg.,* 28, 461, 1979.
13. **Maguire, J. H., Mott, K. E., Lehman, J. S., Hoff, R., Muniz, T. M., Guimaraes, A. C., Sherlock, I., and Morrow, R. H.,** Relationship of electrocardiographic abnormalities and seropositivity to *Trypanosoma cruzi* within a rural community in northeast Brazil, *Am. Heart J.,* 105, 287, 1983.
14. **Andrade, Z. A.,** Chagas' disease (American trypanosomiasis), in *Pathology of Protozoal and Helminthic Diseases,* Marcial Rojas, R. A., Ed., Williams & Wilkins, Baltimore, 1971, chap. 2.
15. **Engel, J. C., Dvorak, J. A., Segura, E. L., and Crane, M. St.,** *Trypanosoma cruzi:* biological characterization of 19 clones derived from two chronic chagasic patients. I. Growth kinetics in liquid medium, *J. Protozool.,* 29, 555, 1982.
16. **Postan, M., Dvorak, J. A., and McDaniel, J. P.,** Studies of *Trypanosoma cruzi* clones in inbred mice. I. A comparison of the course of infection of C3H/HEN⁻ mice with two clones isolated from a common source, *Am. J. Trop. Med. Hyg.,* 32, 497, 1983.
17. **Brener, Z.,** Biology of *Trypanosoma cruzi, Annu. Rev. Microbiol.,* 27, 347, 1973.
18. **Alcantara, A. and Brener, Z.,** *Trypanosoma cruzi:* role of macrophage membrane components in the phagocytosis of bloodstream forms, *Exp. Parasitol.,* 50, 1, 1980.
19. **Kierszenbaum, F.,** Protection of congenitally athymic mice against *Trypanosoma cruzi* infection by passive antibody transfer, *J. Parasitol.,* 66, 673, 1980.

20. **Scott, M. T.,** The nature of immunity against *Trypanosoma cruzi* in mice recovered from acute infection, *Parasite Immunol.,* 3, 209, 1981.
21. **Krettli, A. U. and Brener, Z.,** Protective effect of specific antibodies in *Trypanosoma cruzi* infections, *J. Immunol.,* 116, 755, 1976.
22. **McHardy, N.,** Passive protection of mice against infection with *Trypanosoma cruzi* with plasma: the use of blood- and vector bug-derived trypomastigote challenge, *Parasitology,* 80, 471, 1980.
23. **Kierzenbaum, F. and Howard, J. G.,** Mechanisms of resistance against experimental *Trypanosoma cruzi* infections: the importance of antibodies and antibody-forming capacity in the Biozzi high and low responder mice, *J. Immunol.,* 116, 1208, 1976.
24. **Rodriguez, A., Santoro, F., Afchain, D., Bazin, H., and Capron, A.,** *Trypanosoma cruzi* infection in B-cell-deficient rats, *Infect. Immun.,* 31, 524, 1981.
25. **Takehara, H. A., Perini, A., DaSilva, M. H., and Mota, I.,** *Trypanosoma cruzi:* role of different antibody classes in protection against infection in the mouse, *Exp. Parasitol.,* 52, 137, 1981.
26. **Kierszenbaum, F. and Pienkowski, M. M.,** Thymus-dependent control of host defense mechanisms against *Trypanosoma cruzi* infection, *Infect. Immun.,* 24, 117, 1979.
27. **Schmunis, G. A., Gonzalez Capa, S. M., Traversa, O. C., and Janovsky, J. F.,** The effect of immuno-depression due to neonatal thymectomy on infections with *Trypanosoma cruzi* in mice, *Trans. R. Soc. Trop. Med. Hyg.,* 65, 89, 1971.
28. **Roberson, E. L., Hanson, W. L., and Chapman, W. L., Jr.,** *Trypanosoma cruzi:* effects of anti-thymocyte serum in mice and neonatal thymectomy in rats, *Exp. Parasitol.,* 34, 168, 1973.
29. **Wrightsman, R., Krassner, S., and Watson, T.,** Genetic control of responses to *Trypanosoma cruzi* in mice: multiple genes influencing parasitemia and survival, *Infect. Immun.,* 36, 637, 1982.
30. **Trischmann, T. M., Tanowitz, H., Wittner, M., and Bloom, B.,** *Trypanosoma cruzi:* role of the immune response in the natural resistance of inbred strains of mice, *Exp. Parasitol.,* 45, 160, 1978.
31. **Burgess, D. E., Kuhn, R. E., and Carlson, K. S.,** Induction of parasite-specific helper T lymphocyte during *Trypanosoma cruzi* infections in mice, *J. Immunol.,* 127, 2092, 1981.
32. **Trischmann, T. M. and Bloom, B. R.,** *Trypanosoma cruzi:* ability of T-cell-enriched and -depleted lymphocyte populations to passively protect mice, *Exp. Parasitol.,* 49, 225, 1980.
33. **Burgess, D. E. and Hanson, W. L.,** *Trypanosoma cruzi:* the T-cell dependence of the primary immune response and the effects of depletion of T cell and Ig-bearing cells on immunological memory, *Cell. Immunol.,* 52, 176, 1980.
34. **Cunningham, D. S., Kuhn, R. E., Tarleton, R. L., and Dunn, R. S.,** *Trypanosoma cruzi:* effect on B-cell-responsive and responding clones, *Exp. Parasitol.,* 51, 257, 1981.
35. **Tanowitz, H. B., Minato, N., Lalonde, R., and Wittner, M.,** *Trypanosoma cruzi:* correlation of resistance and susceptibility in infected inbred mice with the *in vivo* primary antibody response to sheep red blood cells, *Exp. Parasitol.,* 52, 233, 1981.
36. **Nogueira, N., Ellis, J., Chaplan, S., and Cohn, Z.,** *Trypanosoma cruzi: in vivo* and *in vitro* correlation between T-cell activation and susceptibility in inbred strains of mice, *Exp. Parasitol.,* 51, 325, 1981.
37. **Krassner, S. M., Granger, B., Morrow, C., and Granger, G.,** *In vitro* release of lymphotoxin by spleen cells from C3H/HEJ and C57BL/6 mice infected with *Trypanosoma cruzi, Am. J. Trop. Med. Hyg.,* 31, 1080, 1982.
38. **Boyer, M. H., Hoff, R., Kipnis, T. L., Murphy, E. D., and Roths, J. B.,** *Trypanosoma cruzi:* susceptibility in mice carrying mutant gene 1pr (lymphoproliferation), *Parasite Immunol.,* 5, 135, 1983.
39. **Boyer, M. H., Holburt, E., and Hoff, R.,** Susceptibility to *T. cruzi* infection in three murine strains with autoimmune syndromes, presented at 31st Annual Meeting American Society of Tropical Medicine and Hygiene, Cleveland, Ohio, November 7 to 11, 1982.
40. **Krettli, A. U. and Brener, Z.,** Resistance against *Trypanosoma cruzi* associated to anti-living trypomas-tigote antibodies, *J. Immunol.,* 128, 2009, 1982.
41. **Krettli, A. and Nussenzweig, R. S.,** Presence of Immunoglobulins on the Surface of Circulating Try-pomastigotes of *T. cruzi* Resulting in Activation of the Alternative Pathway of Complement and Lysis, PAHO Sci. Publ. No. 347, Pan American Health Organization, Washington, D.C., 1977, 71.
42. **Budzko, D. B., Pizzimenti, M. C., and Kierszenbaum, F.,** Effects of complement depletion in exper-imental Chagas' disease: immune lysis of virulent blood forms of *Trypanosoma cruzi, Infect. Immun.,* 11, 86, 1975.
43. **Krettli, A. U.,** Efeito de Anticorpos e do Complemento Sobre Triopmastigotas Sanguineas de Camundongos Infectados com *Trypanosoma cruzi,* thesis, Universidade Federal de Minas Gerais, Brasil, 1978, 71.
44. **Krettli, A. U., Weisz-Carrington, P., and Nussenzweig, R. S.,** Membrane-bound antibodies to blood-stream *Trypanosoma cruzi* in mice: strain differences in susceptibility to complement-mediated lysis, *Clin. Exp. Immunol.,* 37, 416, 1979.
45. **Kipnis, T. L., David, J. R., Alper, C. A., Sher, A., and Dias da Silva, W.,** Enzymatic treatment transforms trypomastigotes of *Trypanosoma cruzi* into activators of alternative complement pathway and potentiates their uptake by macrophages, *Proc. Natl. Acad. Sci. U.S.A.,* 78, 602, 1981.

46. **Krettli, A. U. and Eisen, H.,** Escape mechanisms of *Trypanosoma cruzi* from the host immune system, in Seminaire INSERM: Relations Hote-Parasite dans les Affections Parasitaire Naturelles et Experimentales, Seillac, France, July 1980.

47. **Okabe, K., Kipnis, T. L., Calich, V. L. G., and Dias da Silva, W.,** Cell-mediated cytotoxicity to *Trypanosoma cruzi*. I. Antibody-dependent cell-mediated cytotoxicity to trypomastigote bloodstream forms, *Clin. Immunol. Immunopathol.,* 16, 344, 1980.

48. **Kierzenbaum, F. and Hayes, M. M.,** Mechanisms of resistance against experimental *Trypanosoma cruzi* infection, *Immunology,* 40, 61, 1980.

49. **Kipnis, T. L., James, S. L., Sher, A., and David, J. R.,** Cell-mediated cytotoxicity to *Trypanosoma cruzi*: II. Antibody-dependent killing of bloodstream forms by mouse eosinophils and neutrophils, *Am. J. Trop. Med. Hyg.,* 30, 47, 1981.

50. **Rimoldi, M. T., Cardoni, R. L., Olabuenaga, S. E., and DeBracco, M. M.,** *Trypanosoma cruzi*: sequence of phagocytosis and cytotoxicity by human polymorphonuclear leucocytes, *Immunology,* 42, 521, 1981.

51. **Cardoni, R. L., Docampo, R., and Casellas, A. M.,** Metabolic requirements for the damage of *Trypanosoma cruzi* epimastigotes by human polymorphonuclear leukocytes, *J. Parasitol.,* 68, 547, 1982.

52. **Kierszenbaum, F., Ackerman, S. J., and Gleich, G.,** Destruction of bloodstream forms of *Trypanosoma cruzi* by eosinophil granule major basic protein, *Am. J. Trop. Med. Hyg.,* 30, 775, 1981.

53. **Nogueira, N. M., Klebanoff, S. J., and Cohn, Z. A.,** *T. cruzi*: sensitization to macrophage killing by eosinophil peroxidase, *J. Immunol.,* 128, 1705, 1982.

54. **Hatcher, F. M. and Kuhn, R. E.,** Destruction of *Trypanosoma cruzi* by natural killer cells, *Science,* 218, 295, 1982.

55. **Sonnenfeld, G. and Kierszenbaum, F.,** Increased serum levels of interferon-like activity during the acute period of experimental infection with different strains of *Trypanosoma cruzi, Am. J. Trop. Med. Hyg.,* 30, 1189, 1981.

56. **Hatcher, F. M., Kuhn, R. E., Cerrone, M. C., and Burton, R. C.,** Increased natural killer cell activity in experimental American trypanosomiasis, *J. Immunol.,* 127, 1126, 1981.

57. **James, S. L., Kipnis, T. L., Sher, A., and Hoff, R.,** Enhanced resistance to acute infection with *Trypanosoma cruzi* in mice treated with an interferon inducer, *Infect. Immun.,* 35, 588, 1982.

58. **Kierszenbaum, F. and Sonnenfeld, G.,** Characterization of the antiviral activity produced during *Trypanosoma cruzi* infection and protective effects of exogenous interferon against experimental Chagas' disease, *J. Parasitol.,* 68, 194, 1982.

59. **Taliaferro, W. H. and Pizzi, T.,** Connective tissue reactions in normal and immunized mice to a reticulotropic strain of *Trypanosoma cruzi, J. Infect. Dis.,* 96, 199, 1955.

60. **Kierszenbaum, F., Knecht, E., Budzko, D. B., and Pizzimenti, M. C.,** Phagocytosis: a defense mechanism against infection with *Trypanosoma cruzi, J. Immunol.,* 112, 1839, 1974.

61. **Brener, Z. and Cardoso, J. E.,** Nonspecific resistance against *Trypanosoma cruzi* enhanced by *Cornyebacterium parvum, J. Parasitol.,* 62, 645, 1976.

62. **Hoff, R.,** Killing *in vitro* of *Trypanosoma cruzi* by macrophages from mice immunized with *T. cruzi* or BCG, and absence of cross-immunity on challenge *in vivo, J. Exp. Med.,* 142, 299, 1975.

63. **Nogueira, N., Gorden, S., and Cohn, Z.,** *Trypanosoma cruzi*: modification of macrophage function during infection, *J. Exp. Med.,* 146, 157, 1977.

64. **Kress, Y., Bloom, B. R., Wittner, M., Rowen, A., and Tanowitz, H.,** Resistance of *Trypanosoma cruzi* to killing by macrophages, *Nature (London),* 257, 394, 1975.

65. **Kress, Y., Tanowitz, H., Bloom, B., and Wittner, M.,** *Trypanosoma cruzi*: infection of normal and activated mouse microphages, *Exp. Parasitol.,* 41, 66, 1977.

66. **Nogueira, N. and Cohn, Z.,** *Trypanosoma cruzi*: *in vitro* induction of macrophage microbicidal activity, *J. Exp. Med.,* 148, 288, 1978.

67. **Williams, D. M. and Remington, J. S.,** Effect of human monocytes and macrophages on *Trypanosoma cruzi, J. Immunol.,* 19, 1977.

68. **Nogueira, N., Chaplan, S., Reesink, M., Tydings, J., and Cohn, Z. A.,** *Trypanosoma cruzi*: induction of microbicidal activity in human mononuclear phagocytes, *J. Immunol.,* 128, 2142, 1982.

69. **Nathan, C., Nogueira, N., Juangbhanich, C., Ellis, J., and Cohn, Z.,** Activation of macrophages *in vivo* and *in vitro*: correlation between hydrogen peroxide release and killing of *Trypanosoma cruzi, J. Exp. Med.,* 149, 1056, 1979.

70. **Nogueira, N. and Cohn, Z.,** *Trypanosoma cruzi*: mechanism of entry and intracellular fate in mammalian cells, *J. Exp. Med.,* 143, 1402, 1976.

71. **Milder, R. and Kloetzel, J.,** The development of *Trypanosoma cruzi* in macrophages *in vitro*. Interaction with lysosomes and host cell fate, *Parasitology,* 80, 139, 1980.

72. **Alcantara, A. and Brener, Z.,** The *in vitro* interaction of *Trypanosoma cruzi* bloodstream forms and mouse peritoneal macrophages, *Acta Trop.,* 35, 209, 1978.

73. **Nogueira, N., Chaplan, S., Tydings, J. D., Unkeless, J., and Cohn, Z.,** *Trypanosoma cruzi:* surface antigens of blood and culture forms, *J. Exp. Med.,* 153, 629, 1981.

74. **Behbehani, K., Pan, S., and Unanue, E. R.,** Marked increase in Ia-bearing macrophages during *Trypanosoma cruzi* infection, *Clin. Immunol. Immunopathol.,* 19, 190, 1981.

75. **Zinkernagel, R. M. and Doherty, P. C.,** MHC restricted cytotoxic T cells: studies on the biologic role of polymorphic major transplantation antigens determining T-cell restriction-specificity function and responsiveness, *Adv. Immunol.,* 27, 61, 1979.

76. **Abrahamsohn, I. A. and Kloetzel, J.,** Presence of *Trypanosoma cruzi* antigen on the surface of both infected and uninfected cells in tissue culture, *Parasitology,* 80, 147, 1980.

77. **Ribeiro dos Santos, R. and Hudson, L.,** *Trypanosoma cruzi:* binding of parasite antigens to mammalian cell membranes, *Parasite Immunol.,* 2, 1, 1980.

78. **Kuhn, R. E. and Murane, J. E.,** *Trypanosoma cruzi:* immune destruction of parasitized mouse fibroblasts *in vitro, Exp. Parasitol.,* 41, 66, 1977.

79. **Santos-Buch, C. A. and Teixeira, A. R. L.,** The immunology of experimental Chagas' disease. III. Rejection of allogeneic heart cells *in vitro, J. Exp. Med.,* 140, 38, 1974.

80. **Teixeira, A. R. L., Teixeira, G., Macedo, U., and Prata, A.,** *Trypanosoma cruzi*-sensitized T-lymphocyte-mediated ^{51}Cr release from human heart cells in Chagas' disease, *Am. J. Trop. Med. Hyg.,* 27, 1097, 1978.

81. **Scott, M. T.,** Delayed hypersensitivity to *Trypanosoma cruzi* in mice: specific suppressor cells in chronic infection, *Immunology,* 44, 409, 1981.

82. **Todd, C. W., Todd, N. R., and Guimaraes, A. C.,** Do lymphocytes from chagasic patients respond to heart antigens?, *Infect. Immun.,* 40, 832, 1983.

83. **Araujo, F. G.,** Detection of circulating antigens of *Trypanosoma cruzi* by enzyme immunoassay, *Ann. Trop. Med. Parasitol.,* 76, 25, 1982.

84. **Araujo, F. G., Chiari, E., and Dias, J. C. P.,** Demonstration of *Trypanosoma cruzi* antigen in serum from patients with Chagas' disease, *Lancet,* 2, 246, 1981.

85. **Bongertz, V., Hungerer, K. D., and Galvao-Castro, B.,** *Trypanosoma cruzi:* circulating antigens, *Mem. Inst. Oswaldo Cruz,* 76, 71, 1981.

86. **Gottlieb, M.,** A carbohydrate-containing antigen from *Trypanosoma cruzi* and its detection in the circulation of infected mice, *J. Immunol.,* 119, 465, 1977.

87. **Araujo, F. G., Sharma, S. D., Tsai, V., Cox, P., and Remington, J. S.,** Monoclonal antibodies to stages of *Trypanosoma cruzi:* characterization and use for antigen detection, *Infect. Immun.,* 37, 344, 1982.

88. **Snary, D. and Hudson, L.,** *Trypanosoma cruzi* cell surface proteins: identification of one major glycoprotein, *FEBS Lett.,* 100, 166, 1979.

89. **Scott, M. T. and Snary, D.,** Protective immunization of mice using cell surface glycoprotein from *Trypanosoma cruzi, Nature (London),* 282, 73, 1979.

90. **Pereira, M. E. A.,** A developmentally regulated neuraminidase activity in *Trypanosoma cruzi, Science,* 219, 1444, 1983.

91. **Nogueira, N., Unkeless, J., and Cohn, Z.,** Specific glycoprotein antigens on the surface of insect and mammalian stages of *Trypanosoma cruzi, Proc. Natl. Acad. Sci. U.S.A.,* 79, 1259, 1982.

92. **Snary, D., Ferguson, M. A. J., Scott, M., and Allen, A. K.,** Cell surface antigens of *Trypanosoma cruzi:* use of monoclonal antibodies to identify and isolate an epimastigote-specific glycoprotein, *Mol. Biochem. Parasitol.,* 3, 343, 1981.

93. **Snary, D.,** Cell surface glycoproteins of *Trypanosoma cruzi:* protective immunity in mice and antibody levels in human chagasic sera, *Trans. R. Soc. Trop. Med. Hyg.,* 77, 126, 1983.

94. **Sher, A. and Snary, D.,** Specific inhibition of the morphogenesis of *Trypanosoma cruzi* by a monoclonal antibody, *Nature (London),* 300, 639, 1982.

95. **Lederkremer, R. M., Tanaka, C. T., Alves, J. M., and Colli, W.,** Lipeptidophosphoglycan from *Trypanosoma cruzi, Eur. J. Biochem.,* 74, 263, 1977.

96. **Piras, M. M., Osorio de Rodriguez, O., and Piras, R.,** *Trypanosoma cruzi:* antigenic composition of axonemes and flagellar membranes of epimastigotes cultured *in vitro, Exp. Parasitol.,* 51, 59, 1981.

97. **Pereira, N. M., Timm, S. L., daCosta, S. C. G., Rebello, M. A., and deSouza, W.,** *Trypanosoma cruzi:* isolation and characterization of membrane and flagellar fractions, *Exp. Parasitol.,* 46, 225, 1978.

98. **Fruit, J., Afchain, D., Petitprez, A., and Capron, A.,** *Trypanosoma cruzi:* location of a specific antigen on the surface of bloodstream trypomastigotes and culture epimastigote forms, *Exp. Parasitol.,* 45, 183, 1978.

99. **Gonzalez-Cappa, S. M., Bronzina, A., Katzin, A. M., Golfera, H., DeMartini, G. W., and Segura, E. L.,** Antigens of subcellular fractions of *Trypanosoma cruzi.* II. Humoral immune response and histopathology of immunized mice, *J. Protozool.,* 27, 467, 1980.

100. **Alves, M. J. M., Aikawa, M., and Nussenzweig, R. S.,** Monoclonal antibodies to *Trypanosoma cruzi* inhibit motility and nucleic acid synthesis of culture forms, *Infect. Immun.,* 39, 377, 1983.

101. **Anthony, R. L., Cody, J. S., and Constantine, N. T.,** Antigenic differentiation of *Trypanosoma cruzi* and *Trypanosoma rangeli* by means of monoclonal-hybridoma antibodies, *Am. J. Trop. Med. Hyg.,* 30, 1192, 1981.

102. **Miles, M. A.,** The epidemiology of South American trypanosomiasis — biochemical and immunological approaches and their relevance to control, *Trans. R. Soc. Trop. Med. Hyg.,* 77, 5, 1983.

103. **Snary, D.,** *Trypanosoma cruzi:* antigenic invariance of the cell surface glycoprotein, *Exp. Parasitol.,* 49, 68, 1980.

104. **Schmunis, G. A., Szarfman, A., Langerbach, T., and deSouza, W.,** Induction of capping in blood stage trypomastigotes of *Trypanosoma cruzi* by human anti-*T. cruzi* antibodies, *Infect. Immun.,* 20, 567, 1978.

105. **Kloetzel, J. and Deane, M. P.,** Presence of immunoglobulins on the surface of bloodstream *Trypanosoma cruzi* capping during differentiation in culture, *Rev. Inst. Med. Trop. S. Paulo,* 19, 397, 1977.

106. **Chagas, C.,** The discovery of *Trypanosoma cruzi* and of American trypanosomiasis, *Mem. Inst. Oswaldo Cruz,* 15, 1, 1922.

107. **Clinton, B. A., Ortiz-Ortiz, L., Garcia, W., Martine, T., and Capin, R.,** *Trypanosoma cruzi:* early immune responses in infected mice, *Exp. Parasitol.,* 37, 417, 1975.

108. **Cunningham, D. S. and Kuhn, R. E.,** *Trypanosoma cruzi*-induced suppression of the primary immune response in murine cell cultures to T-cell-dependent and independent antigens, *J. Parasitol.,* 66, 16, 1980.

109. **Ramos, C., Lamoyi, E., Feoli, M., Rodriguez, M., Perez, M., and Ortiz-Ortiz, L.,** *Trypanosoma cruzi:* immunosuppressed response to different antigens in the infected mouse, *Exp. Parasitol.,* 45, 190, 1980.

110. **Kierszenbaum, F.,** On evasion of *Trypanosoma cruzi* from the host immune response. Lymphoproliferative responses to trypanosomal antigens during acute and chronic experimental Chagas' disease, *Immunology,* 44, 641, 1981.

111. **Kierszenbaum, F.,** Immunologic deficiency during experimental Chagas' disease (*Trypanosoma cruzi* infection): role of adherent, nonspecific esterase positive splenic cells, *J. Immunol.,* 129, 1295, 1982.

112. **Cunningham, D. S., Kuhn, R. E., and Rowland, E. C.,** Suppression of humoral responses during *Trypanosoma cruzi* infections in mice, *Infect. Immun.,* 22, 155, 1978.

113. **Ortiz-Ortiz, L., Parks, D. E., Rodriguez, M., and Weigle, W. O.,** Polyclonal B lymphocyte activation during *Trypanosoma cruzi* infection, *J. Immunol.,* 124, 121, 1980.

114. **Harel-Bellan, A., Joskowicz, M., Fradelizi, D., and Eisen, H.,** Modification of T-cell proliferation and interleukin 2 production in mice infected with *Trypanosoma cruzi, Proc. Natl. Acad. Sci. U.S.A.,* 80, 3466, 1983.

115. **Corsini, A. C., Oliveira, O. L. P., and Costa, M. G.,** Unimpaired delayed type hypersensitivity reactions in mice infected with *Trypanosoma cruzi* strain Y, *Z. Parasitenkd.,* 61, 179, 1980.

116. **Hayes, M. M. and Kierszenbaum, F.,** Experimental Chagas' disease: kinetics of lymphocyte responses and immunological control of the transition from acute to chronic *Trypanosoma cruzi* infection, *Infect. Immun.,* 31, 1117, 1981.

117. **Warren, K. S.,** Mechanisms of immunopathology in parasitic infections, in *Immunology of Parasitic Infections,* 2nd ed., Cohen, S. and Warren, K. S., Eds., Blackwell Scientific, Oxford, 1982, chap. 5.

118. **Sadigursky, M., Acosta, A. M., and Santos-Buch, C. A.,** Muscle sarcoplasmic reticulum antigen shared by a *Trypanosoma cruzi* clone, *Am. J. Trop. Med. Hyg.,* 31, 934, 1982.

119. **Szarfman, A., Terranova, V. P., Rennard, S. L., Foidart, J. M., Lima, M. F., Scheinman, J. I., and Martin, G. R.,** Antibodies to laminin in Chagas' disease, *J. Exp. Med.,* 155, 1161, 1982.

120. **Wood, J. N., Hudson, L., Jessell, T. M., and Yamamoto, M.,** A monoclonal antibody defining antigenic determinants on subpopulations of mammalian neurons and *Trypanosoma cruzi* parasites, *Nature (London),* 296, 34, 1982.

121. **Laguens, R. P., Meckhert, P. C., Chambo, G., and Gelpi, R. J.,** Chronic Chagas' disease in the mouse. II. Transfers of the heart disease by means of immunocompetent cells, *Medicina (Buenos Aires),* 41, 40, 1981.

122. **Szarfman, A., Luggetti, A., Rassi, A., Rezende, M., and Schmunis, G. A.,** Tissue reacting immunoglobulins in patients with different clinical forms of Chagas' disease, *Am. J. Trop. Med. Hyg.,* 30, 43, 1981.

123. **Mosca, W. and Plaja, J.,** Delayed hypersensitivity to heart antigens in Chagas' disease as measured by *in vitro* lymphocyte stimulation, *J. Clin. Microbiol.,* 14, 1, 1981.

124. **Hanson, W. L., Chapman, W. L., and Waits, V. B.,** Immunization of mice with irradiated *Trypanosoma cruzi* grown in cell culture: relation of numbers of parasites, immunizating injections, and route of immunization to resistance, *Int. J. Parasitol.,* 6, 341, 1981.

125. **Hungerer, K. D., Enders, B., and Zwister, O.,** On the immunology of infection with *T. cruzi.* II. The preparation of an apathogenic living vaccine, *Behring Inst. Mitteil.,* 60, 84, 1976.

126. **Kierszenbaum, F. and Budzko, D. B.,** Immunization against experimental Chagas' disease by using culture forms of *Trypanosoma cruzi* killed with a solution of sodium perchlorite, *Infect. Immun.,* 12, 461, 1975.

127. **Basombrio, M. A. and Besuchio, S.,** *Trypanosoma cruzi* culture used as vaccine to prevent chronic Chagas' disease in mice, *Infect Immun.,* 36, 351, 1982.

128. **Neal, R. A. and Johnson, P.,** Immunization against *Trypanosoma cruzi* using killed antigens with saponin as adjuvant, *Acta Trop.,* 34, 87, 1977.

129. **McHardy, N. and Elphick, J. P.,** Immunization of mice against infection with *Trypanosoma cruzi:* cross-immunization between five strains of the parasite using freeze thawed vaccine containing epimastigotes of up to five strains, *Int. J. Parasitol.,* 8, 25, 1978.

130. **Brener, Z. and Camargo, E. P.,** Perspectives of vaccination in Chagas' disease, in Working Group on: Perspectives of Immunization in parasitic diseases, *Pontif. Acad. Sci. Scripta Varia,* 47, 145, 1982.

Chapter 10

IMMUNOLOGY OF NONPATHOGENIC TRYPANOSOMES OF RODENTS

Pierre Viens

TABLE OF CONTENTS

I. INTRODUCTION

In the case of trypanosomiasis, relatively little human or veterinary field data are available to support our present immunological vision of host-parasite relationships which, as a result, is based mainly on experimental in vivo or in vitro phenomena. Animal models themselves are sometimes questioned as to their relevance, but can be considered, so to speak, as a better-than-nothing affair, a "zoo-like representation of the bush."

In the past, insufficient attention has been paid to the natural host-parasite relationships in readily available, well-studied laboratory rodents (namely, mice). Such studies, on natural models, may be regarded as highly valid tests of some of the sophisticated concepts of modern trypanosome immunology.[1] Of course, neither *Trypanosoma lewisi* of the rat nor *T. musculi* of the mouse shall ever have any human or veterinary (economical) importance.* The biological uniqueness of these rodent trypanosomes lies in the fact that they constitute rare examples of naturally occurring laboratory models. In these diseases long-established host-parasite relationships have led to a state of low pathogenicity, complex biological and immunological equilibria, and strict host restriction.[3-7] A better understanding of the methods of adaptation of both host and parasite might clarify some of the reasons for the failures of host defenses in infections due to salivarian and other stercorarian pathogenic trypanosomes.

Immunoparasitologists studying *T. lewisi* and *T. musculi* have now reached a point where the assumption that both parasites behave similarly in their respective hosts is questioned. From the pioneer work of Laveran and Mesnil[8] through the extensive studies of Taliaferro and collaborators (comprehensively reviewed by D'Alesandro in 1970[9]) and that of Targett and Viens,[10] *T. lewisi* has monopolized the stage to the point of being considered representative of the group. Most other rodent trypanosomes of the *Herpetosoma* subgenus have not been studied in sufficient detail for useful consideration here. Perhaps this is due to the high degree of host specificity of these parasites which, on one hand, demonstrates their adaptativeness, but, on the other, complicates laboratory studies.

Recent reviews on the general biological aspects of rodent trypanosomes[3-7] provide a useful source of complementary relevant information.

II. COURSE OF INFECTION, BASIC IMMUNE REACTIONS OF THE RODENT HOST, AND GENERAL INFORMATION

A. Course of Infection and Basic Immune Reactions

T. lewisi and *T. musculi* are, under natural conditions, transmitted by fleas.[4,6,7] Understandably, it has been more convenient in the laboratory to use syringe-passaged blood parasites rather than metacyclic forms harvested from the flea vectors, but we do not know

* On the world-wide importance of trypanosomiasis, see Ormerod.[2]

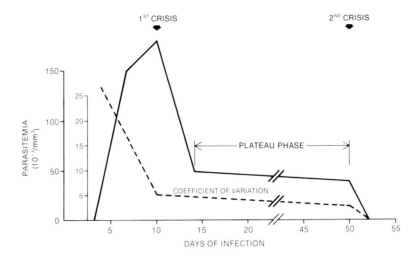

FIGURE 1. *T. lewisi* infection in the rat (schematic). (———): Parasitemia; (----): coefficient of variation.

whether and to what extent such a biological shortcut artificially alters the infectious process. Although patterns of parasitemia appear generally similar in both *T. lewisi* and *T. musculi* infections, recent reports suggest that even minor variations might reflect differences in basic host-parasite relationships and should, therefore, not be overlooked.

1. T. lewisi

Intraperitoneal or intravenous injection of *T. lewisi* blood forms into a rat is followed by a prepatent period after which parasitemia increases rapidly, up to about the tenth day, when it is abruptly checked (Figure 1). This event was named the "first crisis".[11] The number of dividing and newly formed parasites may be assessed using the coefficient of variation (C.V.). This is considered a more accurate measure of reproductive activity than merely estimating the number of parasites in division.[9] The C.V. is high in the early stage of the infection, but it falls rapidly at the time of the first crisis. The decline in the number of these dividing forms has been attributed to the antibody "ablastin" (discussed below) whereas the first crisis itself is mediated by a (first) trypanocidal antibody specific for the young and dividing forms.[11] Parasitemia then reaches a plateau phase of variable duration and consists solely of adult trypomastigotes. The infection is terminated progressively, or more suddenly, after a variable period of time due to the activities of a ("second" or "late") trypanocidal antibody affecting adult trypanosomes. This has been designated as the "second crisis".[9] Other, namely, cellular, immune mechanisms may also be involved in the second crisis[9] and, for that matter, at the time of the first crisis, also.[12] The state of immunity that follows is absolute, specific, and probably lifelong.[13] Dividing parasites have been observed in the kidney capillaries during the early course of infection, but not after the first crisis.[14] Trypanosomes were not found in the peritoneal cavity.[15]

Experimental manipulation of the rat immune system has generated varied and sometimes conflicting results.[9] Some of them shall be summarized briefly, for little new information has accumulated since 1970. Early findings that splenectomy and blockade of the reticuloendothelial system interfered with ablastin or trypanocidal responses[16] were probably the results of concomitant *Bartonella* infections.[9] Sublethal (300 to 500 rad) irradiation increased the parasitemia through impairment of trypanocidal antibody synthesis but ablastin synthesis was not altered. This led D'Alesandro to conclude that the rat had no natural resistance to the proliferation of *T. lewisi*.[9] I would tend to be not so definitive since irradiation causes complex and still undefined lesions not necessarily related to resistance.

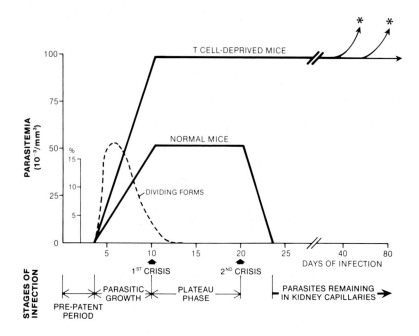

FIGURE 2.   *T. musculi* infection in normal or T cell-deprived mice (schematic). Parasitemia in normal and T cell-deprived (——) mice are illustrated, together with the percentage of dividing forms (----) in normal mice. (*): Death of one infected mouse.

Hanson and Chapman[17] reported that neonatal thymectomy did not influence the course of *T. lewisi* infection. On the other hand, fulminating infections were reported in rats treated with antithymocyte serum which interfered with ablastin production.[18,19] Early and difficult to explain findings of Marmoston-Gottesman[20] were attributed to the persistence of T cells in adult, thymectomized, but not irradiated animals.[9] Due to inherent practical difficulties linked to selective T cell deprivation of the adult rat, little has been published on thymus dependency of *T. lewisi* infection. This lack of information is unfortunate since T cell deprivation constitutes an exquisitely sensitive and useful tool to dissect the host immune response.

Cortisone treatment has received more attention, but dosage and treatment schedules have been the source of conflicting results.[9,21] Cortisone increased the severity of *T. lewisi* infection[22-25] but authors disagree as to whether this was due to inhibition of ablastin[24] or trypanocidal antibodies.[24,25] Established immunity resisted cortisone treatment.[9,25,26] Cyclophosphamide inhibited specific IgG synthesis and increased the severity of the infection (see below).[27,28]

2. T. musculi

The time course of *T. musculi* infection in CBA mice, as well as in various inbred strains of mice,[29,30] is illustrated schematically in Figure 2. As was described with *T. lewisi*, initial stages consist of a prepatent period followed by a rapidly increasing parasitemia in which parasites are seen to divide in the blood. Parasite reproductive forms are maximal around day 7 of infection, but decrease rapidly to disappear completely from the peripheral blood at the time (day 10) when parasite numbers plateau. This has been termed the "first crisis" by analogy with *T. lewisi* infection; but the great difference must be emphasized in the pattern of onset of the plateau phase between the two parasites (Figures 1 and 2) and a proposal will be made later in this review that this apparently minor difference may, in fact, signify basic differences in the mechanisms used by the host to control the initial parasitemia.

The plateau phase, relatively stable and consisting solely of trypomastigotes, terminated abruptly within 24 to 48 hr around the 20th day after inoculation.[31] The resulting immunity is absolute, specific, and probably life-long,[32] yet permits a most unusual feature: the persistence of infective (to naive host) dividing and adult forms of the parasite in the *vasa recta* of the kidney.[33] This constitutes a fundamental difference from the pathogenesis of *T. lewisi* in the rat, and its biological implications will be discussed below. Dividing trypanosomes are found in great numbers in the peritoneal cavity of infected mice throughout the course of parasitemia, even after such dividing forms have disappeared from the peripheral blood at the time of the first crisis.[34] This, again, differs strikingly from the situation in *T. lewisi*-infected rats.[15,35]

By analogy with the concept of *T. lewisi* infection in the rat and based on experimental data published in 1936 by Taliaferro,[36] it was suggested that the control of *T. musculi* infection was also mediated by ablastin and the first and second trypanocidal antibody complex.[9] The author feels however, that the pattern of parasitemia described in *T. musculi* by Taliaferro[36] barely justifies this conclusion, particularly at the time of the first crisis when ablastin and the early trypanocidal antibody were postulated to be acting synergically. Earlier studies[10,32,37] partially supported this assumption, but recent evidence[38,39] has tended to revive the longstanding controversy over ablastin, at least as it relates to *T. musculi* in the mouse. This matter will be discussed in greater detail in the following section.

Adult mice were T cell deprived by thymectomy, followed by 850 rad irradiation and reconstituted with syngeneic bone marrow cells.[40] In these T cell-deprived hosts, the initial control of infection was still effective (Figure 2). The resulting plateau phase extended for up to 200 days. After some 40 or more days of infection, it flared up abruptly in some mice causing rapid death in association with parasitemias exceeding 1×10^{-9} organisms per milliliter.[40] Among thousands of mice that have been thus T cell deprived and infected in our laboratory in the past decade, not a single animal recovered from *T. musculi* infection, although the level of parasitemia was maintained at a very low level in some of them. This thymus dependency of *T. musculi* was maintained in genetically resistant or sensitive strains of mice[30] (see following sections). When T cell-deprived mice received thymus grafts during the plateau phase of infection (day 14), a marked reconstitution of immune competence (associated with great individual variation) was observed after 60 to 200 days.[41] This specific immune reconstitution, generated by the newly implanted thymus in a state of very heavy antigenic load (parasitemias averaging 1×10^8 organisms per milliliter), was rather unexpected. Experiments involving neonatally athymic (nude) mice along with thymus-grafted reconstituted controls[42] confirmed the important role of this organ in recovery from *T. musculi* infection.[10,31,40,43]

B. Somatic and Exo-Antigens

Somatic and exo-antigens of both *T. lewisi*[44] and *T. musculi*[45] have been demonstrated in the plasma of immunosuppressed hosts. During *T. musculi* infection, antibodies directed against these antigens may be detected up to 341 days after infection and the persistence of this humoral response is linked to the presence of parasites in the kidneys.[33,45] An exo-antigen can be defined as any trypanosome-derived molecule released into the plasma of the infected host, that can induce a specific immune reaction (humoral or cellular) against the parasite shedding those molecules. The subject of exo-antigens has been previously reviewed,[9,10] particularly for *T. lewisi*. D'Alesandro[46] was unable to demonstrate any relationship between the presence of exo-antigens, ablastin, and(or) the trypanocidal antibodies. It has to be remembered that the presence of exo-antigens may be derived from several different sources, for example: (1) normal parasite metabolites, (2) accidentally or purposely released surface coat components, or (3) liberation of normal or modified somatic components following parasite death. It is obvious that these exo-antigens may modulate, in some ways, the host immune reactions to the living parasite itself. But until more precise knowledge is available on the biochemical nature of these substances and their relation to the physiology of the parasite, particularly their attachment as part of the parasite outer coat, the author feels that hypotheses and speculations should be kept to a minimum in order not to add undue confusion to the literature.

C. In Vitro Cultivation

In the past decade, reports of successful in vitro cultivation of the blood forms of both *T. lewisi* and *T. musculi* hold promise of opening up new methods for the investigation of immune mechanism involved in the control of infection with these parasites (reviewed by Molyneux[7]). D'Alesandro,[47] in 1962, described a medium which successfully supported *T. lewisi* blood form growth and division long enough to serve as an in vitro assay for ablastin.[47-51] D'Alesandro's medium has also been adapted[39,52,53] for in vitro assay of ablastin during *T. musculi* infection. Long-term maintenance of *T. lewisi* blood forms has been achieved in rat kidney[54] and other mammalian tissue cultures.[55] *T. musculi* has been successfully maintained for many weeks in the trypomastigote infective form in a medium containing rat or mouse peritoneal cells[56] or spleen cells,[57,58] however, immune spleen cells inhibited this growth.[58] The requirements for cell-containing media in order to achieve long-term cultivation have prompted Albright and Albright[59] to attempt to identify the factor(s) responsible for parasite survival. They observed that cell-free medium had to be conditioned with rodent macrophages or cell extract in order to support growth of *T. musculi*.

Providing that constant attention is paid to ensure that these cultured forms, even if resembling trypomastigotes, are, in fact, structurally similar to the blood form parasites, these in vitro systems should prove useful in future research. At this time, however, this cannot be assured since the surface coat antigens of the various trypanosome populations of *T. lewisi* or *T. musculi* are still ill-defined. Another approach that should prove rewarding is the use of metacyclic forms of the parasites to induce infection.[7]

D. Ultrastructural Studies and Antigenic Variation
1. T. lewisi

Ultramicroscopic analysis of both *T. lewisi*[60] and *T. musculi*[61,62] has revealed typical trypanosome structures (for review, see Molyneux[7]). Since, however, the parasites meet the host's milieu at and through their surface membranes, a better definition of these is essential for a complete understanding of immune interactions. In a series of reports, Dwyer[63-65] described the major polysaccharide components of the surface membrane of *T. lewisi*. Avidly bound host serum proteins consisting of albumin, α_2-macroglobulins, and IgG formed 5% of the total surface coat. Accumulation of antigen-specific host IgG was shown by fluorescein-conjugated antirat immunoglobulin.[66,67] This accumulation did not occur in immunosuppressed rats; and it was suggested that these IgGs were, in fact, ablastin.[67]

Binding of ferritin-conjugated antirat IgG demonstrated a high concentration of antigens in the desmosomal region and the flagellar pocket of the parasite,[68] suggesting mobility of surface antigens in live trypanosomes. Capping of *T. lewisi* surface antigens has been achieved after incubation of the parasite with a rabbit antirat whole immunoglobulin preparation at 37°C but not at 0°C;[69] such capping could also be observed at 0°C if purified antirat IgG was used instead. It has to be remembered that ablastin of the rat is an IgG (see below). Unlike that of *T. brucei*,[70-72] the surface coat of *T. lewisi* is loose and diffuse,[66] and immunologically triggered stripping of surface antigens should not occur in vivo since an additional ligand is needed. This also implies that rational analysis of *T. lewisi* and *T. musculi* surface antigens in vivo will require the use of highly specific (monoclonal?) labeled antibodies* in order to avoid the need for a conjugated extra ligand which might induce capping.

---

* For a recent review of the use and pitfalls of monoclonal antibodies in parasitic research, see Cross.[73]

These results clearly establish that, while interacting in ways now generally accepted for many mammalian or parasitic cells[74] including *T. brucei*,[75] the interactions between *T. lewisi* surface coat components and host antibodies are fundamentally different from those described for the African trypanosomes. The possibility of antigenic variation occurring at the surface membrane of rodent trypanosomes, therefore, has to be considered in a different way. The analysis of the pellicular membrane revealed a network of subpellicular microtubules attached to the membrane, and the recent availability of these trypanosome membrane preparations in a reasonably purified state should facilitate a rapid development of knowledge in this field.[76]

2. T. musculi

The cell surface of *T. musculi* also consists of membrane-bound carbohydrates or polysaccharides.[77,78] Nonspecific IgG is adsorbed onto *T. musculi* surfaces as a result of their negative charge, and this seems to be different from the specific (ablastin) related mechanism described for *T. lewisi*.[67] The binding of plasma proteins to the parasite surface interfered with ^{51}Cr-binding.[79] It is not yet possible to demonstrate progressive build-up of either specific IgM, IgG_1, or IgG_2 on the surface of *T. musculi* during the course of infection,[15] contrary to what has been reported with *T. lewisi*.[80]

E. Pathology

Rodent trypanosomes are notoriously nonpathogenic. Nevertheless, important histological modifications of the immuno-committed organs or tissues such as the spleen, thymus, and blood cells have been described as well as changes in the liver and the kidney[81-83] (review[7]).

1. Anemia, Thrombocytopenia, and Splenomegaly

These are characteristic features of both *T. lewisi*[83] and *T. musculi*[15,82] infections, all occurring at peak parasitemia. Cox,[84] in a review, suggested that anemia, splenomegaly, glomerulonephritis, and a thrombocytopenic syndrome, associated with hemoprotozoan infections such as trypanosomiasis, were due to immunoconglutininins raised through immune-complex stimulation. He hypothesized that these nonspecific immunoconglutinins would enhance both erythrocyte and trypanosome elimination by splenic phagocytes, while immune complexes would bind to the glomerular membrane of the kidney. His hypothesis has been reinforced by the observation that administration of *Corynebacterium parvum* to infected rodents enhances the hemoprotozoan infection.[84]

2. Glomerulonephritis

Glomerulonephritis has been described in both *T. lewisi*[83-85] and *T. musculi*[7,15] infections and was thought[84] to result from the deposition of autoantibodies:[83] or antigen-antibody complexes on basal membranes of glomerular capillaries. Molyneux[7] infected mice with metacyclic forms of cultured *T. musculi* and observed cellular infiltrates in the glomeruli, later evolving into glomerulonephritis. However, he observed relevantly that unless mice are infected with pure, cultured metacyclic forms of the parasites, the similarity of the observed lesions to those produced by viral infection should ensure only a tentative interpretation of such results, since viral particles can easily be transferred by blood-passaged parasites.[7]

3. Hematopoietic Organs (Spleen and Thymus)

Splenomegaly is a recognized feature of both *T. lewisi*[50,83,86] and *T. musculi*[82,87] infections (reviewed[7,9,10]). In *T. lewisi*-infected rat spleens, reticular cells proliferate early and are soon surrounded by lymphocytes and plasmacytes.[86] This is followed by a rapid expansion in the size of lymphoid follicles which return to a normal size after recovery from the infection.[50,83]

The *T. musculi*-infected mouse spleen shows a similar lymphoreticular hyperplasia with IgG-producing cells proliferating in the center of T cell-dependent areas.[82,88] Hirokawa et al.[82] noted a temporary thymic involution during *T. musculi* infection.

4. Liver

Simaren[89] and Lee and Barnabas[90] studied the ultrastructural changes in *T. lewisi*-infected rat liver, and this was reviewed by Molyneux.[7] Although *T. musculi*-infected mouse liver was enlarged, light microscopy revealed no obvious histological changes.[82]

III. HUMORAL FACTORS OF IMMUNITY

A. Ablastin and the Early Trypanocidal Antibody
1. T. lewisi

Since Taliaferro[91] in 1924 described this "reaction product" (which he later named ablastin[11]) whose properties were to inhibit selectively *T. lewisi* reproduction without affecting it in other ways, there has been a continuous controversy[92,93] about this most unusual antibody (reviewed[9,10]). Indeed, early results suggested that ablastin could not be adsorbed by antigen and showed little affinity for its theoretical antigenic determinant.[9] Alternative mechanisms to the ablastin theory have been proposed from time to time[12,94] but have not found significant experimental support.

Taliaferro's original description of ablastin[11] drew a distinction between ablastin and the first (early) trypanocidal antibody response. He suggested that a joint effect of both antibodies would be necessary to cause the first crisis. Briefly, ablastin would be synthetized in response to the presence of young and dividing forms of *T. lewisi*, thus resulting in a cessation of the parasite replication. The organisms would then be eliminated by the trypanocidal activity of the first antibody.[9] In his studies, however, the in vivo measurements were performed in such a way that an objective interpretation of experimental results was difficult.

Subsequently, D'Alesandro's[96] studies strongly strengthened the presumptive existence of both ablastin and trypanocidal antibodies. In 1959, an immunochemical analysis of these humoral factors revealed that both ablastin and the first trypanocidal antibody were, in fact, IgG molecules, while the late (second) trypanocidal antibody was an IgM. However, it was not until 1962 that, following the availability of a specific in vitro assay, a clear distinction could be established between ablastin and the early (first) trypanocidal antibody.[9,47,97] This same in vitro assay was later used in the demonstration that active incorporation of H^3-thymidine by *T. lewisi* could be inhibited by treatment with a specific antiserum.[49]

Since then, further characterizations of both ablastin[98,99] and its related ablastinogen were reported. Ouabain, which inhibits ATPase, Na^+, and K^+ membrane transport[100] and ^{14}C incorporation into thymidine, thus mimics the effect of ablastin;[101] and this suggested to Patton[102] that ablastinogen could be part of the transport mechanisms located in the membrane of the trypanosome.[103] Interestingly enough, such a hypothesis had been postulated previously by Chandler[92] in 1958.

Plasma from hydrocortisone-treated *T. lewisi*-infected rats has been used to immunize normal rats which respond by ablastin synthesis.[103] Unfortunately, specific adsorption of this plasma was not carried out and the earlier reservations concerning both the nature and relevance of exo-antigens must be emphasized in the interpretation of such results. The nature of ablastinogen still remains largely speculative, and while dividing and nondividing parasites display different biochemical processes,[104] this has not yet been used experimentally for improving its characterization.

Discussions on the nonadsorbability and low affinity of ablastin for its putative antigen has always tended to provoke some concern among immunologists. It was recently observed, however, that IgG molecules (as detected by fluorescein-labeled [FAT] antirat IgG) do accumulate on the surface of *T. lewisi* during the course of infection in normal, but not in immunosuppressed, animals.[80] The presence of these surface immunoglobulins, apparently nonopsonic and unable to fix complement, has been used to explain the persistence of *T. lewisi* in the blood stream of infected rats.[105]

In addition, ablastin activity can be adsorbed by trypanosomes from immunosuppressed rats more effectively than by trypanosomes from normal rats.[80] These results could not be repeated by Drew and Jenkin[178] who further questioned the existence of ablastin because they were unable to induce its production by immunization with fractions from *T. lewisi*, or to remove it when 90% of serum immunoglobulins had been eliminated. These arguments appear to me to be invalid: immunization in this way is clearly not the best way of presenting "ablastinogen" to the immune system, and it is conceivable that ablastic activity can reside in the residual 10% immunoglobulin.

It might be of interest here to stress that this accumulation of specific immunoglobulin on the parasite's surface has not been reported either after electron microscopic examination[67] or treatment of *T. musculi* with fluorescein-tagged antibodies.[15]

Chandler[92] believed that ablastin alone was responsible for the neutralization of the enzymatic apparatus necessary to active parasitic replication. Ormerod[93] criticized the duality of this ablastin-first trypanocidal antibody concept and he, therefore, proposed that dividing and adult trypanosomes were different, this based on the presence of "cytoplasma granules" (which still remain to be defined). He suggested that when the number of dividing parasites increase, a first trypanocidal antibody destroyed them without the need for ablastin until a second set of trypanocidal antibodies cleared the blood of adult trypomastigotes. The plateau phase would, thus, be due to an automatic killing of newly formed parasites fed into the bloodstream through kidney capillaries. Unfortunately, in the case of *T. lewisi* infection of the rat, parasites were neither found in kidneys after the first crisis[9,14] nor in the peritoneal cavity throughout the infection,[35] and Ormerod's hypothesis could not be experimentally verified for *T. lewisi* infection. Ormerod was, nevertheless, probably correct as far as *T. musculi* infection of the mouse is concerned as will be seen later.

At the present time a dual ablastin-trypanocidal antibody interaction during the first crisis responsible for the initial control of *T. lewisi* infection of the rat seems to be fairly well accepted by a majority of investigators.[106] Alternative or complementary mechanisms have been proposed,[94] especially involving cellular immune interactions,[12] and these are worth further investigation.[10] For example, when *T. lewisi*-infected rat spleen cells were cultured in vitro, Greenblatt and Tyroler[107] noticed ablastic activity associated with clusters of cells surrounding activated macrophages to which young trypanosomes were observed to adhere.

2. T. musculi

In 1938, Taliaferro repeated the protocols that had led to the definition of ablastin and the early trypanocidal antibody in *T. lewisi*, and concluded that a similar set of events explained the initial control of *T. musculi* infection of the mouse.[36] Although the abrupt crisis in *T. lewisi* parasitemia was best explained by the joint action of ablastin and a trypanocidal antibody, the ill-defined, bell-shape curve of parasitemia in the reported *T. musculi* infection[36] made the evidence rather slim (author's opinion). The conclusions that *T. musculi* followed a pattern of host-parasite relationship similar to that of *T. lewisi* were, nevertheless, accepted.[9] Recent data, however, suggest that the ablastin concept is not necessary to explain the initial control of *T. musculi* parasitemia.[38,39]

Early reports from this laboratory have demonstrated that T cell-deprived mice could control the initial *T. musculi* parasitemia[31,40] as efficiently as either newborns,[108] antithymocyte serum,[40] or cyclophosphamide-treated[88] mice. Total body irradiation (350 rad or more) was the only treatment that prevented this initial phase of control.[40] Antibody class analysis coupled to passive serum transfer experiments led to the proposal that ablastin in the mouse was a thymus-dependent IgG_1, while the early trypanocidal antibody response was due to a thymus-independent IgM.[32] This differed significantly from the *T. lewisi* model, where both ablastin and the early trypanocidal antibody were shown to belong to the IgG class.[97] Results from in vitro experiments using a modified cell-free d'Alesandro's medium failed to demonstrate any significant ablastic activity of mouse serum sampled at various intervals, both during infection and after recovery.[39] However, Dusanic[52] observed that if a culture medium containing 20% antiserum was used in a similar in vitro assay, only 30 to 50% of the parasites consisted of dividing forms as compared to 50 to 95% in control groups. This, the author feels, was not proof of biologically significant ablastic activity when it is compared to the complete inhibition of *T. lewisi* replication observed under similar conditions.[39,47] Brooks and Reed[109] repeated D'Alesandro and Clarkson's experiments on *T. lewisi* infection of the rat,[80] and claimed that they could selectively absorb ablastin from mouse serum with *T. musculi* populations rich in dividing forms. However, reexamination of their experimental data suggests that the absolute number of dividing forms in the experimental group was comparable to the number observed in the control group. The activities of a trypanocidal antibody, rather than ablastin alone, would have fitted their experimental results equally well.[38]

It is possible that the ablastic phenomenon in vivo is mediated through complex humoral-cellular interactions as suggested by Greenblatt[12] and others?[110] This hypothesis could explain the little, if any, effect of so-called ablastic mouse sera in in vitro cell-free assays.[39] It would also explain why *T. musculi* reproduces very actively throughout the course of infection in the peritoneal cavity[34] where cell populations are different from those of the circulating blood compartment; and, also, the persistence of parasitic divisions in the *vasa recta* of the kidney despite the presence of antibodies.[33] To investigate this, we injected large amounts of dividing parasites, harvested from the peritoneal cavity, intravenously into mice already infected for various periods of time. In mice infected for 10 days or longer, including T cell-deprived mice (where the initial control of infection had been achieved), the injected dividing parasites were cleared within minutes. The elimination of dividing forms was detectable in 5-day-infected mice and became progressively more efficient until day 10 of infection.[38] This was clearly a trypanocidal effect but it should be remembered that it is not operative in the peritoneal cavity until the last day of infection[34] nor does it act in the *vasa recta* of the kidney.[33] It is attractive to think of it in terms of a complex set of interactions rather than a merely humoral phenomenon. Our hypothesis, therefore, is that the humoral component of the initial control is due to a trypanocidal IgM molecule[32] (almost or completely absent from the peritoneal cavity). This would explain, in part, the very active trypanoblastic activity taking place in this site. I shall comment later on the second (late) trypanocidal effect of *T. musculi*, which is now thought to be mediated by high-affinity IgG. The recent report by Brooks et al.[111] of the IgM-IgG shift of the humoral response to *T. musculi* in infected normal or nude mice corroborates this hypothesis.

B. Late (Second) Trypanocidal Antibody

In *T. lewisi* infection, it was proposed that this second antibody was an IgM.[9,99,112] Interestingly, lactating rats produce a protective anti-*T. lewisi* rheumatoid-like factor (IgM), which stimulates the IgG-mediated ablastic response.[113] Such a nonspecific IgM molecule is, however, different from the late trypanocidal IgM antibody.

In contrast to *T. lewisi*, Viens et al.[32] suggested some years ago that IgG antibodies were the cause of the late trypanocidal effect against *T. musculi*. Pouliot used cyclophosphamide as a means of differentiation between T and B cell populations involved in the final control of *T. musculi* infection and his findings strengthened this view.[88]

C. Complement
1. T. lewisi

Complement activation by the classical pathway usually results in trypanolysis. There are circumstances where this does not occur such as, for example, with *T. brucei* where the density of surface antigens constitute a protective barrier[71] or when *T. cruzi* can cleave the antibodies bound at their surface into Fab fragments ("fabulation"),[1,114] thus, preventing complement fixation to Fc receptors.[115] The late trypanocidal antibody (IgM) causes agglutination of *T. lewisi*[9,99,112] and activates the complement cascade.[116] Nielsen et al.[117-120] showed that a heat-stable, glycolipid extract of *T. lewisi* could also activate complement. This was suggested as another route by which the parasite could escape lytic destruction[120] or to increase the rat's susceptibility to heterologous infections.[121]

2. T. musculi

Agglutination has not been reported to occur with *T. musculi*.[10,32] This is an unusual finding in any known trypanosome infection. Deficiency in C5 such as occurs in B10.D2/oSn mice does not influence the course of *T. musculi* infection.[122,123] Complement-mediated lysis was not considered as a mechanism of major importance in *T. musculi* elimination by Jarvinen and Dalmasso[123,124] who believed that genetic factors (see below) are more important than complement in controlling *T. musculi* parasitemia. However, treatment of C3H mice with cobra venom factor to eliminate C3, when parasites were in the adult stage, resulted in prolonged *T. musculi* infections which were attributed to impairment of phagocytosis.[123] We recently obtained evidence that lysis of *T. musculi* parasite at the end of the infection period required fresh, complement-containing plasma.[125] The emerging picture is, thus, far from being clear.

D. Other Humoral Factors

Serum transfer experiments have provided strong evidence that immunity to *T. lewisi*[97] and *T. musculi*,[37,40] for both its ablastic and/or trypanocidal aspects, was at least, in part, humoral. As presented before, reasonable characterization of the immunoglobulins involved has been achieved for *T. lewisi*,[42,97] whereas their nature remains largely speculative in the case of *T. musculi*.

The most puzzling aspect of the problem lies in the initial control of *T. musculi* parasitemia: although not influenced by most immunosuppressive treatments, it is, nevertheless, transferred by serum.[37,40] Serum factors other than immunoglobulins, such as hormones and acute phase proteins,[126] could possibly be implicated. We have shown recently the emergence of MW 27,200 and MW 52,800 proteins in the serum of mice from the tenth day of infection with *T. musculi*.[179] This suggests a direction for future research.

IV. THYMUS DEPENDENCY AND SOME CELLULAR FACTORS OF IMMUNITY

A. *T. lewisi*

The previous sections clearly showed that the rat immune reponse to *T. lewisi* is essentially antibody mediated (see D'Alesandro[9]). The thymus dependency concept in *T. lewisi* infections is obscured by discordant results ranging from the ineffectiveness of neonatal thymectomy[17] to the fulminating parasitemias that occur in ATS-treated rats.[18,19] With the exception of Greenblatt et al.[12,86] and Ferrante et al.[50] who suggested that the spleen (and its resident macrophages) could provide an architectural network favorable to ablastic activity, most published literature on the cellular response to *T. lewisi* has dealt with macrophage phagocytosis[51,127] and the proliferation of phagocytic cells.[8,50,128] Peritoneal macrophages activated by either carrageenan[129] or lysozyme[130] act to reduce *T. lewisi* parasitemia. Normal spleen cell transfers did not modify the course of infection, nor did immune cells injected at day 7 of infection.[131] Spleen cells from infected rats were not able to mount a secondary response to SRBC and this inhibition was attributed to the presence of exo-antigens.[132] In contrast to the frequently reported phenomenon of immunosuppression described with *T.*

musculi,[57,87,133-136] which is reviewed below, *T. lewisi* extracts failed to show any inhibitory activity on the mouse immune response.[134]

B. *T. musculi*

Due to the recent availability of a great variety of well-characterized mouse strains, much insight has been gained in the past decade on the role of cellular immunity in the course of *T. musculi* infection. Originally, our knowledge of the role of cell-mediated immunity came from studies on the thymus dependency of the infection through the experimental use of T cell-deprived mice.[31,137]

1. Role of T, B, and Other Cells

The initial control over the parasitemia appears to be resistant to all immunosuppressive measures with the exception of irradiation.[31,32,40,41,88] As previously stated, recent data suggest that ablastin is of little significance in *T. musculi* infections,[38] rather it seems that trypanocidal activity controls the parasitemic growth. The mechanisms involved are not purely humoral, as suggested by incomplete destruction of parasites in in vitro (cell-free) assays[39] as compared to their extremely rapid elimination when dividing parasites were injected in vivo.[38] Pouliot et al.[138] stressed that T cells may affect very early events in the infectious process. Experimental transfer of T- (treated or not with anti-θ serum) and B-enriched spleen cell populations, derived from normal or immune mice, into T cell-deprived infected hosts led to the conclusions that the primary effector mechanism of the immune response was not directed by a T cell (θ^+). Instead, the thymus could, early in the infection, promote B cell maturation in the bone marrow which eventually leads to active trypanocidal antibody synthesis. Similar conclusions were reached around the same time by other investigators studying host resistance to murine malaria caused by *Plasmodium yoeli* infection.[139] However, direct evidence is still lacking concerning a cellular involvement in the early trypanocidal phenomenon against *T. musculi.*

As shown previously, the late elimination of *T. musculi* from the blood (Figure 2) is clearly a thymus-dependent event.[40,137] Both splenic B and T cell populations[87,88] as well as IgG-secreting cells of the T-dependent zones of the spleen[82] markedly increase in number during this phase of *T. musculi* infection. The conclusion that elimination of *T. musculi* from the blood was antibody-mediated was reinforced when cyclophosphamide was administered to mice at various times before and during *T. musculi* infection.[88] When given prior to infection, the initial parasitemia was more severe and IgG production was delayed. If the drug was given at day 7 when parasitemia was increasing rapidly, the number of parasites was considerably higher than in control animals and immunoglobulin production; especially IgG_1 was delayed. When treatment was given at day 18 when parasite elimination had already started, this elimination was blocked, thus, coinciding with a considerable reduction in both IgG_1 and IgG_2 antibody titers along with an almost complete destruction of lymphoid cell lines.

Macrophages become activated during the course of *T. musculi* infection; their number, size, protein content, and release of peroxides are all augmented.[140] In vitro phagocytosis of *T. musculi* was also enhanced when antiserum was incorporated into culture medium.[53] Although these results support the antibody-mediated nature of *T. musculi* elimination (apparently linked to complement lysis),[125] it must be pointed out that antiserum transferred to infected mice during the plateau phase does not influence the course of parasitemia.[32] In contrast, the transfer of nonadherent immune spleen cells has been reported to accelerate recovery from *T. musculi,*[137,141] but attempts to correlate this possible involvement of in vivo cell-mediated immunity with in vitro studies have been unsuccessful.[142]

C. Platelets

Recently, observations on wet blood smears of mice about to recover from *T. musculi* infections have attracted our attention because of some unusual cellular interactions. Blood platelets were seen to be adhering to these compromised trypanosomes. It is not clear whether this was purely a peripheral phenomenon due to the known attraction of platelets to antibody-complement complexes or whether it suggested a more active role for platelets in parasite elimination.[125] It is interesting to note that platelets are absent from both the peritoneal cavity and the *vasa recta* of the kidney,[143] locations where *T. musculi* can easily survive. In addition, this platelet-adherence phenomenon was not observed until the very end of the infection. As early as 1917, Rieckenberg[144] described a specific platelet-adherence test used for the diagnosis of *T. brucei* infection. It is hoped that a renewed interest will develop in the role of platelets and other cell populations such as granulocytes in resistance to these agents.[145,180]

V. MITOGENICITY AND IMMUNOSUPPRESSION

At the peak of infection with *T. musculi*, the mouse immune response to SRBC[57,87,135,136,146] and other T-dependent antigens[87,133] is depressed. This has been attributed to a negative interference of the parasite on B cell function[133-135] rather than to the induction of typical suppressor cells.[133] Natural killer (NK) cell activity was enhanced early during *T. musculi* infection and then declined to subnormal levels for more than 3 weeks.[181] Paradoxically, it was also observed that the background level of anti-SRBC antibodies is raised during the course of infection,[146] and that an antigenic extract of *T. musculi* was mitogenic for B cells, in vitro. A similar set of observations has been reported for *T. brucei*.[147,148] The precise biological significance of both polyclonal activation and immunosuppression still remains to be established.[146] *T. brucei* infection has been frequently reported to cause immunosuppression[148-153] and it may protect rabbits from allergic neutritis.[154] Malaria infection was shown, on the other hand, to interfere with the immune-mediated protective effect of vaccination.[155]

Although the concept of parasitic modulation of host responses, through immunosuppression, is academically attractive, one should again be very careful in generalizing from such epiphenomena. Most experimental evidence for this has arisen from in vitro manipulations of explanted cell populations and inherent variations, as a result of those manipulations or to the in vitro approach, by itself, should always be kept in mind. The biological significance of parasite-induced depression or activation of the immune system should be reinforced in future by placing more emphasis on in vivo experimental approaches. The analysis of cellular components in this should also call attention to neglected cell populations such as platelets, granulocytes, and macrophages. The great heterogeneity of these populations may further complicate the matter. As with lymphocytes, there is no such thing as "the macrophage", but there rather are macrophages of various origins, functions, and stages of maturation, and all are present at the same time. This exercise, although tedious, should provide a better understanding of the dynamic aspects of the immune response, since we will have to correlate our findings with the naturally occurring host-parasite equilibrium. In addition, we must remember that little progress will be achieved in analyzing immunosuppression until parasite antigens are isolated,[1] purified, and their mode of action on the immune system better characterized.

VI. NATURAL RESISTANCE TO INFECTION

A. Genetic Resistance

Genetic approaches to the study of host defense mechanisms against parasitic infections have gained considerable attention over the past decade, and this subject has recently been extensively reviewed by Wakelin[156] and Bradley.[157] It is important here to define the term "genetic" or "natural" resistance as determined by the expression of several polymorphic loci clearly different from the "acquired" or "immune" resistance related to the expression of Ir genes, which also show polymorphism.[156] Resistance to *T. congolense*[158] and *T. rhodesiense*[159] infection is, in the mouse, controlled by genes clearly different from the H-2 complex. At the present time, no complete study has yet been published on the possible implication of genetic factors in the resistance of rats to *T. lewisi* infection; however, it has been known for some time that the course of parasitemia varies considerably in different inbred strains of rats.

The course of *T. musculi* infection in various inbred strains of mice has been investigated. Both Albright and Albright[29] as well as Magluilo et al.[30] observed, generally, that A/He, C3H, and CBA behaved as susceptible strains whereas C57Bl/6, DEA/2, and BALB/c behaved as resistant strains. This was not linked to the expression of a particular H-2 haplotype.

The phenotypic expression of the genetic differences (between resistant and susceptible hosts) was reflected only by the intensity of the plateau phase of parasitemia and was linked neither to differences in the pattern[29,30] nor to the duration of the infection.[30] Albright and Albright correlated the in vivo susceptibility of the C3H strain, as opposed to the resistant B6, with the ability of C3H cells to support greater replication of *T. musculi* in vitro.[29] Irradiation was observed to increase the severity of *T. musculi* infection in C3H mice to a greater extent than in B6 mice. The authors concluded that genetic resistance was not mediated by macrophages.[29] Magluilo et al.[30] showed that genetically determined resistance to infection was not expressed by T cells. Although the genetic study of resistance is still relatively recent, further research using genetic tools should prove useful in our better understanding of host resistance to these infections.

B. Role of Pregnancy and Lactation
1. T. lewisi
Shaw[161] demonstrated that *T. lewisi* parasitemia in pregnant rats was significantly increased when the pregnant animals were infected at midterm in their pregnancy and could lead to maternal deaths. The viability of the litter varied ranging from fetal resorption to normal delivery according to the time of infection. Apart from this study, the impact of pregnancy on the course of *T. lewisi* seems to have generated little interest. This is surprising since pregnancy is perhaps the most natural and drastic physiological change encountered in all animal species, including rodents, during their lifetime. This lack of attention is even more disappointing in view of the dramatic perturbations in the host-parasite relationship brought about by pregnancy in *T. musculi* infection of the mouse. Recently, Mellow and Clarkson[160] demonstrated that lactation per se could effectively protect both the mother and baby rats from *T. lewisi* infection, and they have identified a rheumatoid factor-like IgM as a possible mediator of this.[113]

2. T. musculi
Krampitz has described previously the effect of pregnancy on *T. musculi* infection in mice,[162-164] and this subject has also been reviewed elsewhere.[21] If infected between day 4 and 14 (of a 20- to 21-day pregnancy period), the parasitemia of these pregnant mice increased tenfold when compared to parasitemia of control nonpregnant groups. This increase in the severity of infection was explained by an uncontrolled proliferation of the trypanosomes in the placenta.[21,164] Krampitz,[21] in order to explain this proliferation, put forward several hypotheses varying from the presence of a "pro-blastin" favoring parasite multiplication to the action of hormonal or strictly local placental factors. We believe that such a major disturbance in the host's ability to control parasite replication might have an important biological significance, especially since it has also been reported to occur in wild mice[21] and is, therefore, not an artifact resulting from the inbreeding process.

Once a mouse has recovered from a *T. musculi* infection, its immunity cannot be abrogated by T cell deprivation, ATS, cyclophosphamide treatment, or by irradiation.[10,32] How, therefore, can *T. musculi* be efficiently transmitted under natural conditions since the parasite is available to the flea vector for only a very limited period of time? We have observed that the forms sequestered in the kidney, which had been proposed as a means of transmission, could not produce infection in naive mice when fed orally.[165] Moreover, colostrum from immune mothers conferred transient but total protection to the offspring.[108]

Recently, we performed a series of experiments in which a group of female mice, which had recovered from *T. muscli* infection, were impregnated and the presence of trypanosomes in their peripheral blood was monitored.[166] (It should be remembered that normally, a total and absolute immunity develops in mice that have recovered from such an infection.[31,32]) At about day 14 of pregnancy, *T. musculi* parasites were observed in the peripheral blood in four out of five pregnant mice. These results confirm that pregnancy of previously infected hosts favors the release into the bloodstream of parasites, which are normally strictly sequestered in the kidney. These findings are in agreement with Krampitz's suggestion that "the reproduction or persistence of hemoflagellates in the host body's (silent corners) present fascinating problems in trypanosome research."[21] Of course, the mechanisms involved in this form of sequestration are not yet understood, but they are of great biological and ecological significance in both the comprehension of parasite transmission and the establishment and maintenance of lifelong immunity to reinfection.

C. Intercurrent Infections

The widespread use of laboratory animals in experimental research has conditioned many investigators to consider a rather restrictive monoinfectious image of the host-parasite relationship as being representative of the natural situation. This probably results from a lack of confrontation or knowledge of the realities of the field environment. The "clean" experimental approach has the obvious advantage of simplifying the interpretation of results, however, it fails to represent adequately the complexity of the interactions between host and parasite that actually define the biological parameters of an infection. Scientists too often mistake their animal room for the ultimate in relevancy. Multiple infections, as they occur in nature, cause immunological and physiological interactions that will inevitably modify the rules of the host-parasite battle. Conceptually, the effect of these modifications, which may be anxiogenic to the aim-oriented investigator, cannot be discarded in a rational experimental approach (even if they often are), and much research would gain in credibility if these challenges were accepted at the start.

What is known about the effect of intercurrent pathogens on the establishment, evolution, and recovery from *T. lewisi* and *T. musculi* infections? D'Alesandro[9] reviewed the subject of *T. lewisi* and *T. musculi* infections in combination with *Bartonella*, *T. brucei*, *B. berghei*, helminth, and *Spirillum minus* infections. Concomitant infection could result in either increased, unchanged, or even lowered trypanosome virulence. Infection with *T. spiralis* decreased the severity of *T. lewisi* infection of the rat.[167] *T. lewisi* infected rats are more susceptible to *Salmonella typhimurium* and this has been explained on the basis of complement depletion by the trypanosome.[121] (See also Chapter 7.) It has been also reported[168,169] that *T. musculi* parasitemia could be enhanced by a simultaneous *P. yoeli* infection. In a broad sense, the research in the field of multiple infection is still largely descriptive and is, therefore, associated with an unlimited freedom to formulate hypothetical mechanisms. Nevertheless, we are confronted here with in vivo situations that may occur in the field. Even if their inherent complexity sometimes leads to puzzling experimental results, they may, perhaps, illuminate the answers to some long-questioned biological phenomena. They should be regarded as a challenge for the adventurous investigator.

D. Environmental Factors

It is very unlikely that natural trypanosomes of rodents are not influenced through modifications of host response, by the severe environmental changes characteristic of field conditions. Attempts to reproduce experimentally the effect of some of these environmental factors have been reported in the literature. The effect of aging is variable, but usually young animals are more susceptible to *T. lewisi* and *T. musculi* than are older animals,[9] although Albright and Albright[170] recently reported significantly increased parasitemias in infected aged mice.

Hypoxia, simulating the effect of altitude, enhanced *T. lewisi* growth.[171] Starvation[172] and fighting[173] increased *T. musculi* parasitemia, while modifications in room temperature produced various effects: cold increased virulence especially if associated with starvation,[172] whereas warmth interfered with parasite growth.[174] Additional information on this subject is available in Molyneux's[7] and Mansfield's[5] reviews. Again, these experiments are still very descriptive and little explanatory information is available.

E. Passive Immunization

Little work has been done since d'Alesandro[9] reviewed the subject in 1970. Using bacterial adjuvants, Tizard and Ringleberg[175] demonstrated that bacterial endotoxin reduced *T. lewisi* parasitemia, while *B. pertussis* vaccination enhanced it. Ablastin could not be demonstrated after immunization of rats with *T. lewisi* products in various adjuvants.[178] BCG treatment had little effect on *T. musculi* infections in various susceptible or resistant inbred strains of mice.[176]

VII. CONCLUSION

This review is aimed at underlining the infection patterns of *T. lewisi* in the rat and *T. musculi* in the mouse and at drawing a clearer distinction between two apparently similar host-parasite relationships.

The author predicts that since *T. musculi* differs from the so-called rodent group representative *T. lewisi*, if other natural hosts for other representative rodent trypanosomes can be bred and used in the laboratory, many new and fascinating discoveries are to be expected. In this regard, he disagrees with D'Alesandro's[9] statement: "Although interesting differences in life histories occur, these are but variations on a basic theme. Therefore, it will probably be found that the considerable information on a few species is generally applicable to the whole group." It is also clear that if natural flea transmission becomes practically feasible under controlled and standardized laboratory conditions, or if more attention is paid to infections induced by metacyclic forms of the parasites, the resulting research might become more relevant.

Nevertheless, some words of caution are still felt necessary: (1) because a cultivated parasite "looks like" a trypomastigote, it is not necessarily one. Two similar makes of cars are not identical because both are painted the same color. When more becomes known about surface antigens of various trypanosome strains or populations, a better and more precise interpretation of the behavior of in vitro-grown parasites will be possible; (2) blood parasites of natural hosts are subjected, in vivo, to a tremendously complicated array of influences which are different from the well-known artificially selected immune reactions. In vitro immune assays for rodent trypanosomes call for the same caution as any other in vitro assay, but in view of the recent availability of those long-awaited tools, the author felt that a "reminder of relevancy" would be useful; (3) natural rodent host-parasite interrelations raise a basic question which is seldom, if at all, mentioned when discussing in vivo experimentally obtained results: to what extent is the inbred mouse, raised in a clean, hygienic animal room, truly representative of *Mus musculus*?; (4) no overemphasis can be placed on the necessity to study the widest possible range of naturally occurring host-parasite relationships using the most sophisticated tools of modern immunology. The author believes that from these types of studies it will be possible, at least partly, to uncover some of mother nature's keys to equilibrium vs. nonequilibrium in the host-microbe interactions. Some of the mechanisms involved, especially those which result from long evolutionary processes, may lead to a greater comprehension of the real, relatively "young" problems that are encountered either in human diseases or in parasitic diseases of domestic animals. Nonpathogenic trypanosomes have developed methods of evading the host immune response. What is known on this subject in other pathogenic trypanosome species[177] is already sufficiently fascinating to stimulate similar research within the rodent trypanosomes.

ACKNOWLEDGMENTS

The author's contribution to the study of *T. musculi* has been supported by the Medical Research Council of Canada and has been carried out in active collaboration with a team of young and enthusiastic investigators whose names can be retrieved from the list of references. Mrs. Andree L'Ecuyer deciphered my tortuous handwriting and I am grateful to her devotion and patience.

REFERENCES

1. **Mitchell, G. F.,** Effector mechanism of host-protective immunity to parasites and evasion by parasites, in *Parasites: Their World and Ours,* Mettrick, D. F. and Desser, S. S., Eds., Elsevier, Amsterdam, 1982, 24.
2. **Ormerod, W. E.,** Human and animal trypanosomiases as world public health problems, *Pharmacol. Ther.,* 6, 1, 1979.
3. **Hoare, C. A.,** Evolutionary trends in mammalian trypanosomes, *Adv. Parasitol.,* 5, 47, 1967.
4. **Hoare, C. A.,** *The Trypanosomes of Mammals. A Zoological Monograph,* Blackwell Scientific, Oxford, 1972.
5. **Mansfield, J. M.,** Nonpathogenic trypanosomes of mammals, in *Parasitic Protozoa,* Kreier, J. P., Ed., Academic Press, New York, 1977, 297.
6. **Molyneux, D. H.,** Development patterns in trypanosomes of the subgenus *Herpetosoma, Ann. Soc. Belge Med. Trop.,* 229, 1970.
7. **Molyneux, D. H.,** Biology of trypanosomes of the subgenus *Herpetosoma,* in *Biology of the Kinetoplastidae,* Lumsden, W. H. R. and Evans, D. A., Eds., Academic Press, New York, 1976, 285.
8. **Laveran, A. and Mesnil, F.,** Recherches morphologiques et expérimentales sur le trypanosome des rats (*Trypanosoma lewisi,* Kent), *Ann. Inst. Pasteur (Paris),* 673, 1901.
9. **D'Alesandro, P. A.,** Non-pathogenic trypanosomes of rodents, in *Immunity to Parasitic Animals,* Vol. 2, Jackson, E. J., Herman, R., and Singer, I., Eds., Appleton-Century-Crofts, New York, 1970, 691.
10. **Targett, G. A. T. and Viens, P.,** Immunity to *Trypanosoma (herpetosoma)* infections in rodents, in *Biology of the Kinetoplastidae,* Vol. 2, Lumsden, W. R. R. and Evans, D. A., Eds., Academic Press, London, 1977, 461.
11. **Taliaferro, W. H.,** Trypanocidal and reproduction inhibition antibodies to *Trypanosoma lewisi* in rats and rabbits, *Am. J. Hyg.,* 16, 32, 1932.
12. **Greenblatt, C. L.,** Nutritional and immunological factors in the control of infections with *Trypanosoma lewisi, Exp. Parasitol.,* 38, 342, 1975.
13. **Lee, C. M. and Lincicome, D. R.,** *Trypanosoma lewisi:* duration of the immune state in the rats, *Z. Parasitenkd.,* 38, 344, 1972.
14. **Wilson, V. C. L. C., Viens, P., Targett, G. A. T., and Edwards, C. I.,** Comparative studies on the persistence of *Trypanosoma (herpetosoma) musculi* and *Trypanosoma (herpetosoma) lewisi* in immune hosts, *Trans. R. Soc. Trop. Med. Hyg.,* 67, 271, 1973.
15. **Viens, P.,** unpublished data, 1982.

16. **Taliaferro, W. H.,** The effect of splenectomy and blockade on the passive transfer of antibodies against *Trypanosoma lewisi, J. Infect. Dis.,* 62, 98, 1938.

17. **Hanson, W. L. and Chapman, W. L., Jr.,** Comparison of the effects of neonatal thymectomy on *Plasmodium berghei, Trypanosoma lewisi* and *Trypanosoma cruzi* infection in the albino rat, *Z. Parasitenkd.,* 44, 227, 1974.

18. **Spira, D. T. and Greenblatt, C. L.,** The effect of antithymocyte serum on *Trypanosoma lewisi* infections, *J. Protozool.,* 17 (Suppl.), 29, 1970.

19. **Tawil, A. and Dusanic, D. G.,** The effects of antilymphocytic serum (ALS) on *Trypanosoma lewisi* infections, *J. Protozool.,* 18, 445, 1971.

20. **Marmoston-Gottesman, J., Perla, D., and Vorzimer, J.,** Immunological studies in relation to the suprarenal gland. VI. *Trypanosoma lewisi* infection in supra renalectomized adult albino rats, *J. Exp. Med.,* 52, 587, 1930.

21. **Krampitz, H. E.,** Ablastin: antigen tolerance and lack of ablastin control of *Trypanosoma musculi* during host's pregnancy, *Exp. Parasitol.,* 38, 317, 1975.

22. **Bawden, M. P. and Stauber, L. A.,** *Trypanosoma lewisi:* characteristics of an antigen which induces ablastic antibody, *Exp. Parasitol.,* 36, 397, 1974.

23. **Clark, D. T. and Patton, C. L.,** *Trypanosoma lewisi* infections in normal rats and rats treated with dexamethasone, *J. Parasitol.,* 51, 27, 1965.

24. **Patton, C. L. and Clark, D. T.,** *Trypanosoma lewisi* infections in normal rats and in rats treated with dexamethasone, *J. Protozool.,* 15, 31, 1968.

25. **Herbert, I. V. and Becker, E. R.,** Effect of cortisone and X-irradiation on the course of *Trypanosoma lewisi* infection in the rat, *J. Parasitol.,* 47, 304, 1961.

26. **Sherman, I. W. and Ruble, J. A.,** Virulent *Trypanosoma lewisi* infections in cortisone treated rats, *J. Parasitol.,* 53, 258, 1967.

27. **El-On, J. and Greenblatt, C. L.,** Cyclophosphamide suppression of antibody synthesis and enhancement of *Trypanosoma lewisi* infections in rats, *J. Protozool.,* 18 (Suppl.), 36, 1971.

28. **El-On, J. and Greenblatt, C. L.,** The effects of the immunosuppressive agent cyclophosphamide on IgG levels and parasite number of experimental trypanosomiasis, *Isr. J. Med. Sci.,* 7, 1294, 1971b.

29. **Albright, J. W. and Albright, J. F.,** Differences in resistance to *Trypanosoma musculi* infection among strains of inbred mice, *Infect. Immun.,* 33, 364, 1981.

30. **Magluilo, P., Viens, P., and Forget, A.,** Immunosuppression during *Trypanosoma musculi* infection in inbred strains of mice, *J. Clin. Lab. Immunol.,* 10, 151, 1983.

31. **Viens, P. and Targett, G. A. T.,** *Trypanosoma musculi* infection in intact and thymectomized CBA mice, *Trans. R. Soc. Trop. Med. Hyg.,* 65, 424, 1971.

32. **Viens, P., Targett, G. A. T., and Lumsden, W. H. R.,** The immunological response of CBA mice to *Trypanosoma musculi:* mechanisms of protective immunity, *Int. J. Parasitol.,* 5, 235, 1975.

33. **Viens, P., Targett, G. A. T., Wilson, V. C. L., and Edwards, C. I.,** The persistence of *Trypanosoma (herpetosoma) musculi* in the kidneys of immune CBA mice, *Trans. R. Soc. Trop. Med. Hyg.,* 66, 669, 1972.

34. **Lajeunesse, M. C., Richards, R., Viens, P., and Targett, G. A. T.,** Persistence of dividing forms of *Trypanosoma musculi* in the peritoneal cavity of infected CBA mice, *IRCS Med. Sci.,* 3, 244, 1975.

35. **Bourbonniere, L.,** personal communication, 1982.

36. **Taliaferro, W. H.,** Ablastic and trypanocidal antibodies against *Trypanosoma duttoni, J. Immunol.,* 35, 303, 1938.

37. **Targett, G. A. T. and Viens, P.,** Ablastin: control of *Trypanosoma musculi* infections in mice, *Exp. Parasitol.,* 38, 309, 1975.

38. **Desbiens, C. and Viens, P.,** *Trypanosoma musculi* in CBA mice: trypanocidal mechanism eliminating dividing forms, *Parasitology,* 83, 109, 1981.

39. **Trudel, L., Desbiens, C., Viens, P., and Targett, G. A. T.,** Ablastin and the control of *Trypanosoma musculi* in mice, *Parasite Immunol.,* 4, 149, 1982.

40. **Viens, P., Targett, G. A. T., Leuchars, E., and Davies, A. J. S.,** The immunological response of CBA mice to *Trypanosoma musculi.* I. Initial control of the infection and the effect of T cell deprivation, *Clin. Exp. Immunol.,* 16, 279, 1974.

41. **Targett, G. A. T., Leuchars, E., Davies, A. J. S., and Viens, P.,** Thymus graft reconstitution of T cell-deprived mice infected with *Trypanosoma musculi, Parasite Immunol.,* 3, 353, 1981.

42. **Brooks, B. O. and Reed, N.,** Thymus dependency of *Trypanosoma musculi* elimination from mice, *J. Reticuloendothel. Soc.,* 22, 605, 1977.

43. **Rank, R. G., Robert, D. W., and Weidanz, W. P.,** Chronic infection with *Trypanosoma musculi* in congenitally athymic nude mice, *Infect. Immun.,* 2(16), 715, 1977.

44. **Long, G. W. and Dusanic, D. G.,** *Trypanosoma lewisi:* effects of immunosuppression on the serological reactivities of exoantigens and cellular antigens of bloodstream parasites, *Exp. Parasitol.,* 44, 56, 1978.

45. **Dusanic, D. G.,** Precipitin responses of infected mice to exoantigens and cellular antigens of *Trypanosoma musculi, Int. J. Parasitol.,* 8, 297, 1978.

46. **D'Alesandro, P. A.,** *Trypanosoma lewisi:* production of exoantigens during infection in the rat, *Exp. Parasitol.,* 32, 149, 1972.

47. **D'Alesandro, P. A.,** *In vitro* studies of ablastin, the reproduction-inhibiting antibody to *Trypanosoma lewisi, J. Protozool.,* 9, 351, 1962.

48. **Fuson, E. W., Jones, A. W., and Murray, F. A.,** A culture and biochemical assay system for *Trypanosoma lewisi, Exp. Parasitol.,* 40, 225, 1976.

49. **Ferrante, A., Drew, P. A., and Jenkin, C. R.,** A method for the assay of ablastin in the serum of rats infected with *Trypanosoma lewisi, Aust. J. Exp. Biol. Med. Sci.,* 56, 741, 1978.

50. **Ferrante, A., Jenkin, C. R., and Reade, P. C.,** Changes in the activity of the reticulo-endothelial system of rats during an infection with *Trypanosoma lewisi, Aust. J. Exp. Biol. Med. Sci.,* 56, 47, 1978.

51. **Ferrante, A. and Jenkin, C. R.,** The role of the macrophage in immunity to *Trypanosoma lewisi* infection in the rat, *Cell. Immunol.,* 42, 327, 1979.

52. **Dusanic, D. G.,** Homologous and heterologous ablastin effects on *Trypanosoma duttoni (T. musculi)* grown at 37°C, *J. Protozool.,* 21, 422, 1974.

53. **Chang, S. and Dusanic, D. G.,** *In vitro* phagocytosis of *Trypanosoma musculi* by mouse macrophage, *Chin. J. Microbiol.,* 9, 73, 1976.

54. **Dougherty, J., Robson, A. S., and Tyrrel, S. A.,** *Trypanosoma lewisi: in vitro* growth in mammalian cell culture media, *Exp. Parasitol.,* 31, 225, 1972.

55. **El-On, J. and Greenblatt, C. L.,** *Trypanosoma lewisi, Trypanosoma acomys,* and *Trypanosoma cruzi:* a method for their cultivation with mammalian tissue, *Exp. Parasitol.,* 41, 31, 1977.

56. **Viens, P., Lajeunesse, M. C., Richards, R., and Targett, G. A. T.,** *Trypanosoma musculi: in vitro* cultivation of blood forms in cell culture media, *Int. J. Parasitol.,* 7, 109, 1977.

57. **Albright, J. W. and Albright, J. F.,** Growth of *Trypanosoma musculi* in culture of murine spleen cells and analysis of the requirement for supportive spleen cells, *Infect. Immun.,* 22, 343, 1978.

58. **Clayton, C. E.,** A culture system for *in vitro* studies of immunity to *Trypanosoma (herpetosoma) musculi, Trans. R. Soc. Trop. Med. Hyg.,* 74, 125, 1980.

59. **Albright, J. W. and Albright, J. F.,** *In vitro* growth of *Trypanosoma musculi* in cell-free medium conditioned by rodent macrophages and mercapto-ethanol, *Int. J. Parasitol.,* 10, 137, 1980.

60. **Anderson, W. A. and Ellis, R. A.,** Ultrastructure of *Trypanosoma lewisi:* flagellum, microtubules and the kinetoplast, *J. Protozool.,* 12, 483, 1965.

61. **Wilson, V. C., Ellis, D., and Upton, C. P.,** Preliminary observations on the fine structure of the trypomastigote form of *Trypanosoma (herpetosoma) musculi* in the blood stream phase, *Trans. R. Soc. Trop. Med. Hyg.,* 65, 17, 1971.

62. **Watson, S. and Lee, C. M.,** Ultrastructure of *Trypanosoma duttoni, Z. Parasitenkd.,* 46, 133, 1975.

63. **Dwyer, D. M.,** Cell surface saccharides of *Trypanosoma lewisi.* I. Polycation-induced cell agglutination and fine-structure cytochemistry, *J. Cell. Sci.,* 19, 621, 1975.

64. **Dwyer, D. M.,** Cell surface saccharides of *Trypanosoma lewisi.* II. Lectin-mediated agglutination and fine-structure cytochemical detection of lectin-binding site, *J. Cell. Sci.,* 22, 1, 1976.

65. **Dwyer, D. M.,** Immunologic and fine structure evidence of avidly bound host serum proteins in the surface coat of a blood stream trypanosomes, *Proc. Natl. Acad. Sci. U.S.A.,* 73, 1222, 1976.

66. **Giannini, M. S. and D'Alesandro, P. A.,** Unusual antibody-induced modulation of surface antigens in the cell coat of a bloodstream trypanosome, *Science,* 201, 916, 1978.

67. **Giannini, S. H. and D'Alesandro, P. A.,** *Trypanosoma lewisi:* accumulation of antigen-specific host IgG as a component of the surface coat during the course of infection in the rat, *Exp. Parasitol.,* 47, 342, 1979.

68. **Cherian, P. V. and Dusanic, D. G.,** *Trypanosoma lewisi:* immunoelectron microscopic studies on the surface antigens of bloodstream forms, *Exp. Parasitol.,* 43, 128, 1977.

69. **Cherian, P. V. and Dusanic, D. G.,** *Trypanosoma lewisi:* ultrastructural observations of surface antigen movement induced by antibody, *Exp. Parasitol.,* 44, 14, 1978.

70. **Cross, G. A. M.,** Identification, purification, and properties of clone-specific glycoprotein antigens constituting the surface coat of *Trypanosoma brucei, Parasitology,* 71, 393, 1975.

71. **Cross, G. A. M.,** Antigenic variation in trypanosomes, *Am. J. Trop. Med. Hyg.,* 26, 240, 1977.

72. **Borst, P. and Cross, G. A. M.,** Molecular basis for trypanosome antigenic variation, *Cell,* 29, 291, 1982.

73. **Cross, G. A. M.,** New technologies for parasitology, in *Parasites: Their World and Ours,* Mettrick, D. F. and Desser, S. S., Eds., Elsevier, Amsterdam, 1982, 3.

74. **Doyle, J. J., Behim, R., Mauel, J., and Rowe, D. S.,** Antibody induced movement of protozoan surface membrane antigens, *Ann. N.Y. Acad. Sci.* 254, 315, 1974.

75. **Barry, J. D.,** Capping of variable antigen on *Trypanosoma brucei,* and its immunological and biological significance, *J. Cell. Sci.,* 37, 287, 1979.

76. **Dwyer, D. M. and D'Alesandro, P. A.,** Isolation and characterization of pellicular membranes from *Trypanosoma lewisi* bloodstream forms, *J. Parasitol.,* 66, 377, 1980.

77. **Dwyer, D. M. and D'Alesandro, P. A.,** The cell surface of *Trypanosoma musculi* bloodstream forms. I. Fine structure and cytochemistry, *J. Protozool.*, 23, 75, 1976.
78. **Dwyer, D. M. and D'Alesandro, P. A.,** The cell surface of *Trypanosoma musculi* bloodstream forms. II. Lectin and immunologic studies, *J. Protozool.*, 23, 262, 1976.
79. **Watson, L. P. and Lee, C. M.,** *Trypanosoma musculi:* absence of ^{51}Cr binding to bloodstream trypomastigotes, *Z. Parasitenkd.*, 59, 299, 1979.
80. **D'Alesandro, P. A. and Clarkson, A. B.,** *Trypanosoma lewisi:* avidity and absorbability of ablastin, the rat antibody inhibiting parasite reproduction, *Exp. Parasitol.*, 50, 384, 1980.
81. **Davis, C. E., Robbins, R. S., Weller, R. D., and Brande, A. I.,** Thrombocytopenia in experimental trypanosomiasis, *J. Clin. Invest.*, 53, 1359, 1974.
82. **Hirokawa, K., Eishi, Y., Albright, J. W., and Albright, J. F.,** Histopathological and immunocytochemical studies of *Trypanosoma musculi* infection of mice, *Infect. Immun.*, 34, 1008, 1981.
83. **Thoongsuwan, S. and Cox, H. W.,** Anemia, splenomegaly, and glomerulonephritis associated with autoantibody in *Trypanosoma lewisi* infections, *J. Parasitol.*, 64, 669, 1978.
84. **Cox, H. W.,** Roles for immunoconglutinin in diseases from hemoprotozoan infections, in *Parasites: Their World and Ours,* Mettrick, D. F. and Desser, S. S., Eds., Elsevier, Amsterdam, 1982, 242.
85. **Simaren, J. O.,** Ultrastructural demonstration and glomerular cytopathology associated with *Trypanosoma lewisi,* in *Proc. 3rd Int. Congr. Parasitology, Munich,* Facta Publication, Vienna, 1974, 1580.
86. **Greenblatt, C. L.,** *Trypanosoma lewisi:* electron microscopy of the infected spleen, *Exp. Parasitol.*, 38, 342, 1973.
87. **Albright, J. F., Albright, J. W., and Dusanic, D. G.,** Trypanosome-induced splenomegaly and suppression of mouse spleen cell responses to antigen and mitogens, *J. Reticuloendothel. Soc.*, 21, 21, 1977.
88. **Pouliot, P.,** Etude des Mécanismes de la Réponse Immunologique au Cours de L'infection de la Souris par *Trypanosoma musculi,* Ph.D. thesis, Université de Montréal, 1978.
89. **Simaren, J. O.,** Ultrastructure of *Trypanosoma lewisi* localization and alteration in rat livers, *Ann. Parasitol. Hum. Comp.*, 48, 735, 1973.
90. **Lee, C. M. and Barnabas, E.,** *Trypanosoma lewisi:* ultrastructural changes in rat liver, *Z. Parasitenkd.*, 44, 93, 1974.
91. **Taliaferro, W. H.,** A reaction product in infections with *Trypanosoma lewisi* which inhibits the reproduction of trypanosomes, *J. Exp. Med.*, 39, 1, 1924.
92. **Chandler, A. C.,** Some considerations relative to the nature of immunity in *Trypanosoma lewisi* infections, *J. Parasitol.*, 44, 129, 1958.
93. **Ormerod, W. E.,** Initial stages of infection with *Trypanosoma lewisi:* control of parasitemia by the host, in *Immunity to Protozoa,* Vol. 1, Garnham, P. C. C., Pierce, A. E., and Roitt, I., Eds., Blackwell Scientific, Oxford, 1963.
94. **Sanchez, G.,** Physiological and antigenic changes in *Trypanosoma lewisi* mediated by epinephrine, *Comp. Gen. Pharmacol.*, 4, 327, 1973.
95. **D'Alesandro, P. A.,** Ablastin: the phenomenon, *Exp. Parasitol.*, 38, 303, 1975.
96. **D'Alesandro, P. A.,** Electrophoretic and ultracentrifugal studies of antibodies to *Trypanosoma lewisi, J. Infect. Dis.*, 105, 76, 1959.
97. **D'Alesandro, P. A.,** Immunological and biochemical studies of ablastin, the reproduction inhibiting antibody to *Trypanosoma lewisi, Ann. N.Y. Acad. Sci.*, 129, 834, 1966.
98. **Dusanic, D. G.,** Immunosuppression and ablastin, *Exp. Parasitol.*, 38, 322, 1975.
99. **Hsu, S. R. and Dusanic, D. G.,** *Trypanosoma lewisi:* antibody classes which mediate precipitation, agglutination and the inhibition of reproduction, *Exp. Parasitol.*, 53, 45, 1982.
100. **Patton, C. L.,** Inhibition of reproduction in *Trypanosoma lewisi* by ouabain, *Nature (London), New Biol.*, 237, 253, 1972.
101. **Patton, C. L.,** Ouabain and antibody inhibition of active transport and reproduction in the blood protozoan *Trypanosoma lewisi, Fed. Proc., Fed. Am. Soc. Exp.*, 29, 812, 1970.
102. **Patton, C. L.,** The ablastin phenomenon: inhibition of membrane function, *Exp. Parasitol.*, 38, 357, 1975.
103. **Bawden, M. P. and Stauber, L. A.,** *Trypanosoma lewisi:* characteristics of an antigen which induces ablastic antibody, *Exp. Parasitol.*, 36, 397, 1974.
104. **Schraw, W. P. and Vaughan, G. L.,** *Trypanosoma lewisi:* alterations in membrane function in the rat, *Exp. Parasitol.*, 48, 15, 1979.
105. **Ferrante, A. and Jenkin, C. R.,** Surface immunoglobulins, a possible mechanism for the persistence of *Trypanosoma lewisi* in the circulation of rats, *Aust. J. Exp. Biol. Med. Sci.*, 55, 275, 1977.
106. **Ormerod, W. E.,** Ablastin in *Trypanosoma lewisi* and related phenomena in other species of trypanosomes, *Exp. Parasitol.*, 38, 338, 1975.
107. **Greenblatt, C. L. and Tyroler, E.,** *Trypanosoma lewisi: in vitro* behavior of rat spleen cells, *Exp. Parasitol.*, 30, 363, 1971.
108. **Brenier, S. and Viens, P.,** *Trypanosoma musculi:* transfer of immunity from mother mice to litter, *Can. J. Microbiol.*, 26, 1090, 1980.

109. **Brooks, B. O. and Reed, N. D.**, Adsorption of ablastic activity from mouse serum by using a *Trypanosoma musculi* population rich in dividing forms, *Infect. Immun.*, 27, 94, 1980.

110. **Brooks, B. O. and Reed, N. D.**, The effect of trypan blue on the early control of *Trypanosoma musculi* parasitaemia in mice, *J. Reticuloendothel. Soc.*, 25, 325, 1979.

111. **Brooks, B. O., Wassom, D. L., and Cypess, R. H.**, Kinetics of immunoglobulin M and G responses of nude and normal mice to *Trypanosoma musculi, Infect. Immun.*, 36, 667, 1982.

112. **D'Alesandro, P. A.**, The relation of agglutinins to antigenic variations of *Trypanosoma lewisi, J. Protozool.*, 23, 256, 1976.

113. **Clarkson, A. B. and Mellow, G. H.**, Rheumatoid factor-like immunoglobulin M protects previously uninfected rat pups and dams from *Trypanosoma lewisi, Science*, 214, 186, 1981.

114. **Bisen, H. and Tallan, I.**, *Tetrahymena pyriformis* recovers from antibody immobilization by producing univalent antibody fragment, *Nature (London)*, 270, 514, 1977.

115. **Krettli, A. U.**, Complement activation by parasites, in *Parasites: Their World and Ours*, Mettrick, D. F. and Desser, S. S., Eds., Elsevier, Amsterdam, 1982, 37.

116. **Jarvinen, J. A. and Dalmasso, A. P.**, Complement in experimental *Trypanosoma lewisi* infections of rats, *Infect. Immun.*, 14, 894, 1976.

117. **Nielsen, K. and Sheppard, J.**, Activation of complement by trypanosomes, *Experientia*, 33, 769, 1977.

118. **Nielsen, K., Sheppard, J., Tizard, I., and Holmes, W.**, Complement activating factor(s) of *Trypanosoma lewisi:* some physiochemical characteristics of the active components, *Can. J. Comp. Med.*, 42, 74, 1976.

119. **Nielsen, K., Sheppard, J., Tizard, I., and Holmes, W.**, *Trypanosoma lewisi:* characterization of complement-activating components, *Exp. Parasitol.*, 43, 153, 1977.

120. **Nielsen, K., Sheppard, J., Tizard, I., and Holmes, W.**, Direct activation of complement by trypanosomes, *J. Parasitol.*, 64, 544, 1978.

121. **Nielsen, K., Sheppard, J., Holmes, W., and Tizard, I.**, Increased susceptibility of *Trypanosoma lewisi* infected, or decomplemented rats to *Salmonella typhimurium, Experientia*, 34, 118, 1978.

122. **Dusanic, D. G.**, *Trypanosoma musculi* infections in complement-deficient mice, *Exp. Parasitol.*, 2(37), 205, 1975.

123. **Jarvinen, J. A. and Dalmasso, A. P.**, *Trypanosoma musculi* infections in normocomplementemic, C5-deficient and C3-depleted mice, *Infect. Immun.*, 16, 557, 1977.

124. **Jarvinen, J. A. and Dalmasso, A. P.**, *Trypanosoma musculi:* immunologic features of the anemia in infected mice, *Exp. Parasitol.*, 43, 203, 1977a.

125. **Viens, P., Dubois, R., and Kongshavn, P.**, Platelet activity in immune lysis of *Trypanosoma musculi, Int. J. Parasitol.*, in press.

126. **Koj, A.**, Acute phase reactants. Their synthesis, turnover and biological significance, in *Structure and Function of Plasma Proteins*, Allison, A. C., Ed., Plenum Press, London, 1974, 73.

127. **Patton, C. L.**, *Trypanosoma lewisi:* influence of sera and peritoneal exudate cells, *Exp. Parasitol.*, 31, 370, 1972.

128. **Ferrante, A. and Jenkin, C. R.**, Evidence implicating the mononuclear phagocytic system of the rat in immunity to infections with *Trypanosoma lewisi, J. Exp. Biol. Med. Sci.*, 56, 201, 1978.

129. **Bourbonniere, L., Wong, T. C. S., and Tanner, C. E.**, The effect of carrageenan on infection with *Trypanosoma lewisi, Mol. Biochem. Parasitol.*, 5 (Suppl.), 30, 1982.

130. **Bierman, J., MacInnis, A. J., and Lobstein, O. E.**, Effects of lysozyme on *Trypanosoma lewisi, Ann. Clin. Lab. Sci.*, 9, 381, 1979.

131. **Greenblatt, C. L., Spira, D. T., and Tyroler, E.**, *Trypanosoma lewisi:* immune spleen cell transfer in rats, *Exp. Parasitol.*, 32, 131, 1972.

132. **St. Charles, M. H. C., Frank, D., and Tanner, C. E.**, The depressed response of spleen cells from rats infected by *Trypanosoma lewisi* in producing a secondary response *in vitro* to sheep erythrocytes and the ability of soluble products of the trypanosome to induce this depression, *Immunology*, 43, 441, 1981.

133. **Albright, J. W. and Albright, J. F.**, Trypanosome-mediated suppression of murine humoral immunity independent of typical suppressor cells, *J. Immunol.*, 124, 2481, 1980.

134. **Albright, J. M. and Albright, J. F.**, Inhibition of murine humoral immune responses by substances derived from trypanosomes, *J. Immunol.*, 126, 300, 1981.

135. **Albright, J. W., Albright, J. F., and Dusanic, D. G.**, Mechanisms of trypanosome-mediated suppression of humoral immunity in mice, *Proc. Natl. Acad. Sci. U.S.A.*, 75, 3923, 1978.

136. **Albright, J. F., Deitchman, J. W., Hassell, S. A., and Ozato, K.**, Differential antibody production by adherent and non-adherent spleen cells transferred to irradiated and cyclophosphamide-treated recipient mice, *J. Reticuloendothel. Soc.*, 17, 195, 1975.

137. **Targett, G. A. T. and Viens, P.**, The immunological response of CBA mice to *Trypanosoma musculi:* elimination of the parasite from the blood, *Int. J. Parasitol.*, 5, 231, 1975.

138. **Pouliot, P., Viens, P., and Targett, G. A. T.**, T lymphocytes and the transfer of immunity to *Trypanosoma musculi* in mice, *Clin. Exp. Immunol.*, 27, 507, 1977.

139. **Jayawardena, A. N., Waksman, B. H., and Eardley, P. D.,** Activation of distinct helper and suppressor T cells in experimental trypanosomiasis, *J. Immunol.,* 121, 622, 1978.

140. **Vicendeau, P., Caristan, A., and Pautrizel, R.,** Macrophage function during *Trypanosoma musculi* infection in mice, *Infect. Immun.,* 34, 378, 1981.

141. **Viens, P., Pouliot, P., and Targett, G. A. T.,** Cell-mediated immunity during the infection of CBA mice with *Trypanosoma musculi, Can. J. Microbiol.,* 20, 105, 1974.

142. **Pouliot, P., Viens, P., and Targett, G. A. T.,** Lymphocyte transformation and mouse cell-mediated immune response (CMI) to *Trypanosoma musculi* infection, *IRCS Med. Sci.,* 2, 1567, 1974.

143. **Tocantins, L. M.,** The mammalian blood platelet in health and disease, *Medicine,* 17, 155, 1933.

144. **Rieckenberg, H.,** Eine neve Immunitatsreaktion bei experimenteller trypanosomen-infektion: die Blutplat tchenprope, *Z. Immunitatsforsch.,* 26, 53, 1917.

145. **Albright, J. W. and Albright, J. F.,** Basis of the specificity of rodent trypanosomes for their natural hosts, *Infect. Immun.,* 33, 355, 1981.

146. **Hazlett, C. A. and Tizard, I.,** The immunosuppression and mitogenic effects of *Trypanosoma musculi, Clin. Exp. Immunol.,* 33, 225, 1978.

147. **Esuruoso, G. O. E.,** The demonstration *in vitro* of the mitogenic effects of trypanosoma antigen on the spleen cells of normal, athymic and cyclophosphamide treated mice, *Clin. Exp. Immunol.,* 23, 314, 1976.

148. **Hudson, K. M., Byner, C., Freeman, J., and Terry, R. J.,** Immunodepression, high IgM levels, and evasion of the immune response in murine trypanosomiasis, *Nature (London),* 264, 256, 1976.

149. **Goodwin, L. G., Green, D. G., Guy, M. W., and Voller, A.,** Immunosuppression during trypanosomiasis, *Br. J. Exp. Pathol.,* 53, 40, 1972.

150. **Eardley, D. D. and Jayawardena, A. N.,** Suppressor cells in mice infected with *Trypanosoma brucei, J. Immunol.,* 119, 1029, 1977.

151. **Clayton, C. E., Selkirk, M. E., Corsini, C. A., Ogilvie, B. M., and Askonas, B. A.,** Murine trypanosomiasis: cellular proliferation and functional depletion in the blood, peritoneum, and spleen related to changes in bone marrow stem cells, *Infect. Immun.,* 28, 824, 1979.

152. **Clayton, C. E., Sacks, D. L., Ogilvie, B. M., and Askonas, B. A.,** Membrane fractions of trypanosomes mimic the immunosuppressive and mitogenic effects of living parasites on the host, *Parasite Immunol.,* 1, 241, 1979.

153. **Askonas, B. A., Corsini, A. C., Clayton, C. E., and Ogilvie, B. M.,** Functional depletion of T- and B-memory cells and other lymphoid cell subpopulations during trypanosomiasis, *Immunology,* 36, 313, 1979.

154. **Allt, G., Evans, E. M. E., Evans, D. H. C., and Targett, G. A. T.,** Effect of infection with trypanosomes on the development of experimental allergic neuritis in rabbits, *Nature (London),* 233, 197, 1971.

155. **Tarzaali, A., Viens, P., and Quevillon, M.,** Inhibition of the immune response to whooping-cough and tetanus vaccines by malaria infection and the effect of pertusis adjuvant, *Am. J. Trop. Med. Hyg.,* 26, 520, 1977.

156. **Wakelin, D.,** Genetic control of susceptibility and resistance to parasitic infection, *Adv. Parasitol.,* 16, 219, 1978.

157. **Bradley, D. J.,** Genetic control of resistance to protozoal infections, in *Genetic Control of Natural Resistance to Infection and Malignancy,* Skamene, E., Kongshavn, P., and Landry, M., Eds., Academic Press, New York, 1980, 9.

158. **Morrison, W. I. and Murray, M.,** *Trypanosoma congolense:* inheritance of susceptibility to infection in inbred strains of mice, *Exp. Parasitol.,* 48, 364, 1979.

159. **Greenblatt, H. C., Rosenstreich, D. L., and Diggs, C. L.,** Genetic control of natural resistance to *Trypanosoma rhodesiense* in mice, in *Genetic Control of Natural Resistance to Infection and Malignancy,* Skamene, E., Kongshavn, P., and Landy, M., Eds., Academic Press, New York, 1980, 89.

160. **Mellow, G. H. and Clarkson, A. B., Jr.,** *Trypanosoma lewisi:* enhanced resistance in dams lactating rats and their suckling pups, *Exp. Parasitol.,* 53, 217, 1982.

161. **Shaw, G. L.,** *Trypanosoma lewisi:* termination of pregnancy in the infected rats, *Exp. Parasitol.,* 33, 46, 1973.

162. **Krampitz, H. E.,** Experimental study on prenatal infection with *Trypanosoma duttoni* (Sicilian strain) in mice and its immunological aspects, in Proc. 1st Int. Congr. Parasitology, Tamburini, Milan, 1966, 312.

163. **Krampitz, H. E.,** Multiplication foudroyante et formation en rosaces chez *Trypanosoma (herpetosoma) duttoni* Thiroux 1905 dans le sang placentaire de souris blanches, *Acta Trop.,* 26, 361, 1969.

164. **Krampitz, H. E.,** Weiteres zur Vermehrungsaktivität und der besonderen Form multipler Teilungen bei Trypanosomen der Untergattung *Herpetosoma* Doflein 1901 un Plazentarblut des Spezifischen wirtes, *Z. Parasitenkd.,* 34, 296, 1970.

165. **Dubois, R. and Viens, P.,** Influence of pregnancy on mouse immunity to *Trypanosoma musculi, Trans. R. Soc. Trop. Med. Hyg.,* 77(2), 274, 1982.

166. **Viens, P., Roger, M., and Dubois, R.,** unpublished results, 1982.

167. **Meerovitch, E. and Ackerman, S. J.**, Trypanosomiasis in rats with trichinosis, *Trans. R. Soc. Trop. Med. Hyg.*, 68, 417, 1974.
168. **Cox, F. G.**, Enhanced *Trypanosoma musculi* infection in mice with concomitant malaria, *Nature (London)*, 258, 148, 1975.
169. **Bungener, W.**, Verlauf von *Trypanosoma musculi*-infektionen in mit *Plasmodium berghei* infizerten Mansen, *Tropenmed. Parasitol.*, 26, 285, 1975.
170. **Albright, J. W. and Albright, J. F.**, The decline in immunological resistance of aging mice to *Trypanosoma musculi*, *Mol. Biochem. Parasitol.*, 5 (Suppl.), 31, 1982.
171. **Greenblatt, C. L. and Yoffey, J. M.**, *Trypanosoma lewisi:* immunohaematopoetic interrelationships of the infection in normal, hypoxic and rebound animals, *Exp. Parasitol.*, 38, 105, 1975.
172. **Sheppe, W. A. and Adams, J. R.**, The pathogeny of *Trypanosoma duttoni* in hosts under stress conditions, *J. Parasitol.*, 43, 55, 1957.
173. **Jackson, L. A. and Farmer, J. N.**, Effects of host fighting behaviour on the course of infection of *Trypanosoma duttoni* in mice, *Ecology*, 51, 672, 1970.
174. **Sen, D. K., Lyle, J. L., Purohit, V. D., and Lincicome, D. R.**, *Trypanosoma musculi* infections in two mouse strains exposed to various environmental temperatures, *J. Parasitol.*, 67, 744, 1981.
175. **Tizard, I. R. and Ringleberg, C. P.**, The effect of bacterial adjuvants on *Trypanosoma lewisi* infections in rats, *Folia Parasitol. (Prague)*, 22, 323, 1975.
176. **Magluilo, P.**, unpublished data, 1982.
177. **Bloom, B. R.**, Games parasites play: how parasites evade immune surveillance, *Nature (London)*, 279, 21, 1979.
178. **Drew, P. A. and Jenkin, C. R.**, Properties of ablastin — a factor in the serums of rats infected with *Trypanosoma lewisi* which inhibits the parasites' division, *Aust. J. Exp. Biol. Med. Sci.*, 60, 329, 1982.
179. **Olivier, M. and Viens, P.**, unpublished results, 1983.
180. **Joseph, M., Auriault, C., Capron, A., Vorng, H., and Viens, P.**, A new function for platelets: IgE-dependent killing of schistosomes, *Nature (London)*, 303, 810, 1983.
181. **Albright, J. W., Kun-Yen, H., and Albright, J. F.**, Natural killer activity in mice infected with *Trypanosoma musculi*, *Infect. Immun.*, 40, 869, 1983.

225

225

INDEX

A

P

Packed red blood cell volume (PCV), 105
Pancytopenia, 37
Panstrogylus, 146
Parainfluenza 3 virus, 119
Parasite
  antibody response to, 83—84
  differentiation, 115—116
  nonantibody-mediated destruction of, 136
Parasite-associated products, 91
Parasite-induced physiological changes, 2—4
Parasitemia, 84, 105, 115, 167, 215
Parasitosis, 152, 171
  intracardiac neuron, 171
  myofiber, 152
Parasympathetic ganglia, 153
Parasympathetic innervation, 174—175
Parasympathetic myenteric plexus, 154
Parasympathetic neurons, 153
Passive immunization, 216
Pathogenesis, autocoids and, see Autocoids
Pathological consequences of autocoid release, 57—58
Pathology
  Chagas' disease, see Chagas' disease
  nonpathogenic trypanosomes of rodents, 207—208
Pathophysiology, African trypanosomiasis, 1—11
  host changes, 4—6
  parasite-induced changes, 2—4
Penicillamine, 52
Periarteriolar lymphatic sheaths, 79
Peripheral blood leukocytes (PBC), 110
Peritoneal cavity, 210
Peritoneal exudate cells, 88
Peritoneal macrophages, 134, 211
Peroxidase, 190
Petechial hemorrhages, 25, 105
PHA, 84
Phagocytosis, 86, 109, 134, 212
Phenethanolamine-N-methyltransferase. 55
Phenylketonuria (PKU), 4
Phenylpyruvate, 4
Phorbol myristate acetate, 87
Phosphatidylcholine, 69
Phospholipase(s) of trypanosomes, 67—74
  metabolic role, 71—73
  properties, 68—69
Phospholipase-A, 17, 73
Phospholipase A$_1$, 3, 68—71
Phospholipase A$_2$, properties of, 68—69
Physiological changes, 2—8
"Pitos", 147
Pituitary gland, 6
Placenta, 166
Plasma cells, 111
Plasma histamine, 53
Plasma iron turnover, 35, 37
Plasmapheresis, 34

Plasma sialic acid, 17
Plasma volume, 18
  increased, 15, 28
Plasmin, 6, 24, 47
Plasminogen, 22, 24, 47, 56
  activation, 58
Plasminogen activator, 87
Plasmodia, 79, 89
Plasmodium
  berghei, 48, 89
  knowlesi, 46, 48
  yoelli, 90, 212, 215
Plateau phase, 205, 209
Platelet(s), 20, 24—31, 54, 212—213
  abnormal distribution of, 28
  abnormal hemostasis and, 24—26
  aggregation, 29, 30, 55
  function, 30—33
  5-HT release from, 55
  increased destruction of, 26—30
  life span, 26, 28, 29
  production, failure, 28, 30
Platelet count, 22
Platelet storage pool, 31
Pleomorphic populations, 115
Pleomorphic (slender) stumpy strains, 83
Pneumococcal polysaccharide (SIII), 81
Polyclonal activation, 91, 118, 213
  B cell, 60, 80—82, 136, 192
Polyclonal synthesis of antibodies, 59
Polyinosinic:polycytidilic acid (poly I:C), 90
Poor growth, 104—105
Porcine pancreatic phospholipase A, 69
Prednisolone, 153, 159
Pregnancy, role of, 214—215
Prekallikrein, 51
Premunition, 187
"Pro-blastin", 214
Progressive congestive cardiomyopathy, 153
Proliferative glomerulonephritis, 57, 136
Properdin, 137, 189
Prostaglandin(s) (PG), 47, 87
  synthesis, 31
Protamine sulfate test, 23
Protective antibodies, 188
Protective immunity, 106—114
Proteolysis, 3
Prothrombin time (PT), 22
Pseudocyst, 149, 154
  of amastigotes, 160, 165
  cytoplasmic, 169
Purified protein derivative (PPD), 84
  DTH skin reaction to, 117
Pyrogenic substance, 2

R

Radioactive labels, 18
Rats, pregnant, 214
Reaction product, 208